Manual of

SURGERY

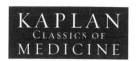

KAPLAN
CLASSICS OF
MEDICINE

Manual of

SURGERY

BY

ALEXIS THOMSON, F.R.C.S.ED.

PROFESSOR OF SURGERY, UNIVERSITY OF EDINBURGH

SURGEON, EDINBURGH ROYAL INFIRMARY

AND

ALEXANDER MILES, F.R.C.S.ED.

SURGEON, EDINBURGH ROYAL INFIRMARY

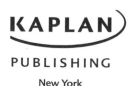

KAPLAN

PUBLISHING

New York

Foreword by Dr. Carlos Pestana © 2008

Published by Kaplan Publishing, a division of Kaplan, Inc.
1 Liberty Plaza, 24th Floor
New York, NY 10006

Printed in the United States of America

August 2008
10 9 8 7 6 5 4 3 2 1

ISBN-13: 978-1-4277-9799-5

Kaplan Publishing books are available at special quantity discounts to use for sales promotions, employee premiums, or educational purposes. Please email our Special Sales Department to order or for more information at kaplanpublishing@kaplan.com, or write to Kaplan Publishing, 1 Liberty Plaza, 24th Floor, New York, NY 10006.

CONTENTS

FOREWORD

Surgery was first developed for the treatment of trauma. It was part and parcel of warfare. Surgery offered the cruel alternative of sacrificing limb to save life. From there, the practice eventually evolved as an option for the management of some diseases.

Although some forms of surgical therapy have existed for thousands of years, operations on civilian patients were actually rare until the middle of the nineteenth century—1846, to be precise, when anesthesia was introduced. Prior to that time, it took a great deal of courage for patients to submit to the knife. Speed was the greatest skill that surgeons could offer. Procedures were completed in mere minutes, sometimes a few seconds. Nitrous oxide, ether, and chloroform changed all that. Remarkably, during an era when news traveled at the speed of a galloping horse or sailing ship, the use of these agents became universal in only a matter of months.

But freedom from pain was not sufficient for surgery to flourish. Longer operations led to infection, ushering the era of "laudable pus" and death by septicemia. Surgery remained of limited use under those circumstances. It took almost fifty years for the cause of infection to be determined and for surgeons to accept Louis Pasteur's germ theory and the pioneering antiseptic discoveries of Joseph Lister. Once that happened, virtually all the major operations that we perform today were invented and successfully introduced in the first decade of the twentieth century. It was during that exciting time, in 1904, that the first edition of *The Manual of Surgery* by Alexander Miles and Alexis Thomson appeared. The book was fittingly published in Edinburgh, where Lister spent much of his distinguished career.

Kaplan Publishing has brought back to life this fascinating glimpse of surgical practice in the pre-antibiotic era, when operations for the complications of tuberculosis or syphilis were far more common than operations for cancer.

Yet, much of the pathology that is described and illustrated remains recognizable today, albeit portrayed at much more advanced stages of the disease. That is what makes the book so entertaining. Obviously one wouldn't use *The Manual of Surgery* as a current reference, but to contrast what we know today with what was known in 1921, when this sixth edition of the book was published, puts our profession in perspective. We have indeed come a long way.

But let's not get too proud of our surgical practice in the first decade of the twenty-first century. When our textbooks are reprinted a hundred years from now, their pages will look as quaint and dated as those that you now hold in your hands. We are no better than Miles and Thomson. We simply build upon what they built. *The Manual of Surgery* is not only fascinating to read, but it also represents the foundations of what we do today.

Interestingly enough, as the process of medical discovery is repeated every century, surgery itself will eventually come full circle to where it began. The operations that we perform today will gradually disappear as we develop better means to prevent diseases or treat them medically. The surgical option will become a thing of the past. But trauma will never go away. Neither will warfare; humans have a nasty tendency to resolve their differences with violence. Thus, surgeons will always be needed to take care of the injured. Like Miles and Thompson, surgeons of the future will surely continue to write books. Oh, what would I give to read one of them!

Carlos Pestana, M.D., Ph.D.
March, 2008

PREFACE TO SIXTH EDITION

Much has happened since this Manual was last revised, and many surgical lessons have been learned in the hard school of war. Some may yet have to be unlearned, and others have but little bearing on the problems presented to the civilian surgeon. Save in its broadest principles, the surgery of warfare is a thing apart from the general surgery of civil life, and the exhaustive literature now available on every aspect of it makes it unnecessary that it should receive detailed consideration in a manual for students. In preparing this new edition, therefore, we have endeavoured to incorporate only such additions to our knowledge and resources as our experience leads us to believe will prove of permanent value in civil practice.

For the rest, the text has been revised, condensed, and in places rearranged; a number of old illustrations have been discarded, and a greater number of new ones added. Descriptions of operative procedures have been omitted from the *Manual,* as they are to be found in the companion volume on *Operative Surgery,* the third edition of which appeared some months ago.

We have retained the Basle anatomical nomenclature, as extended experience has confirmed our preference for it. For the convenience of readers who still employ the old terms, these are given in brackets after the new.

This edition of the *Manual* appears in three volumes; the first being devoted to General Surgery, the other two to Regional Surgery. This arrangement has enabled us to deal in a more consecutive manner than hitherto with the surgery of the Extremities, including Fractures and Dislocations.

PREFACE

We have once more to express our thanks to colleagues in the Edinburgh School and to other friends for aiding us in providing new illustrations, and for other valuable help, as well as to our publishers for their generosity in the matter of illustrations.

EDINBURGH,

March, 1921

REPAIR

INTRODUCTION

To prolong human life and to alleviate suffering are the ultimate objects of scientific medicine. The two great branches of the healing art—Medicine and Surgery—are so intimately related that it is impossible to draw a hard-and-fast line between them, but for convenience Surgery may be defined as "the art of treating lesions and malformations of the human body by manual operations, mediate and immediate." To apply his art intelligently and successfully, it is essential that the surgeon should be conversant not only with the normal anatomy and physiology of the body and with the various pathological conditions to which it is liable, but also with the nature of the process by which repair of injured or diseased tissues is effected. Without this knowledge he is unable to recognise such deviations from the normal as result from mal-development, injury, or disease, or rationally to direct his efforts towards the correction or removal of these.

PROCESS OF REPAIR

The process of repair in living tissue depends upon an inherent power possessed by vital cells of reacting to the irritation caused by injury or disease. The cells of the damaged tissues, under the influence of this irritation, undergo certain proliferative changes, which are designed to restore the normal structure and configuration of the part. The process by which this restoration is effected is essentially the same in all tissues, but the extent to which different tissues can carry the recuperative process varies. Simple structures, such as skin, cartilage, bone, periosteum, and tendon, for example, have a high power of regeneration, and in them the reparative process may result in almost perfect restitution to the normal. More complex structures, on the other hand, such as secreting glands, muscle, and the tissues of the central nervous system, are but imperfectly restored, simple cicatricial connective tissue taking the place of what has been lost or destroyed. Any given tissue can be replaced only by tissue of a similar kind, and in a damaged part each element takes its share in the reparative process by producing new material which approximates more or less closely to the normal according to the recuperative capacity of the particular tissue. The normal process of repair may be interfered with by various extraneous agencies, the most important of which are infection by disease-producing micro-organisms, the presence of foreign substances, undue movement of the affected part, and improper applications and dressings. The effect of these agencies is to delay repair or to prevent the individual tissues carrying the process to the furthest degree of which they are capable.

In the management of wounds and other diseased conditions the main object of the surgeon is to promote the natural reparative process by preventing or eliminating any factor by which it may be disturbed.

Healing by Primary Union.—The most favourable conditions for the progress of the reparative process are to be found in a clean-cut wound of the integument, which is uncomplicated by loss of tissue, by the presence of foreign substances, or by infection with disease-producing micro-organisms, and its edges are in contact. Such a wound in virtue of the absence of infection is said to be *aseptic*, and under these conditions healing takes place by what is called "primary union"—the "healing by first intention" of the older writers.

Granulation Tissue.—The essential and invariable medium of repair in all structures is an elementary form of new tissue known as *granulation tissue*, which is produced in the damaged area in response to the irritation caused by injury or disease. The vital reaction induced by such irritation results in dilatation of the vessels of the part, emigration of leucocytes, transudation of lymph, and certain proliferative changes in the fixed tissue cells. These changes are common to the processes of inflammation and repair; no hard-and-fast line can be drawn between these processes, and the two may go on together. It is, however, only when the proliferative changes have come to predominate that the reparative process is effectively established by the production of healthy granulation tissue.

Formation of Granulation Tissue.—When a wound is made in the integument under aseptic conditions, the passage of the knife through the tissues is immediately followed by an oozing of blood, which soon coagulates on the cut surfaces. In each of the divided vessels a clot forms, and extends as far as the nearest collateral branch; and on the surface of the wound there is a microscopic layer of bruised and devitalised tissue. If the wound is closed, the narrow space between its edges is occupied by blood-clot, which consists of red and white corpuscles mixed with a quantity of fibrin, and this forms a temporary uniting medium between the divided surfaces. During the first twelve hours, the minute vessels in the vicinity of the wound dilate, and from them lymph exudes and leucocytes migrate into the tissues. In from twenty-four to thirty-six hours, the capillaries of the part adjacent to the wound begin to throw out minute buds and fine processes, which bridge the gap and form a firmer, but still temporary, connection between the two sides. Each bud begins in the wall of the capillary as a small accumulation of granular protoplasm, which gradually elongates into a filament containing a nucleus. This filament either joins with a neighbouring capillary or with a similar filament, and in time these become hollow and are filled with blood from the vessels that gave them origin. In this way a series of young *capillary loops* is formed.

The spaces between these loops are filled by cells of various kinds, the most important being the *fibroblasts*, which are destined to form cicatricial fibrous tissue. These fibroblasts are large irregular nucleated cells derived mainly from the proliferation of the fixed connective-tissue cells of the part, and to a less extent from the lymphocytes and other mononuclear cells which have migrated from the vessels. Among the fibroblasts, larger multi-nucleated cells—*giant cells*—are sometimes found, particularly when resistant substances, such as silk ligatures or fragments of bone, are embedded in the tissues, and their function seems to be to soften such substances preliminary to their being removed by the phagocytes. Numerous *polymorpho-nuclear leucocytes*, which have wandered from the vessels, are also present in the spaces. These act as phagocytes, their function being to remove the red corpuscles and fibrin of the original clot, and this performed, they either pass back into the circulation in virtue of their amoeboid movement, or are themselves eaten up by the growing fibroblasts. Beyond this phagocytic action, they do not appear to play any direct part in the reparative process. These young capillary loops, with their supporting cells and fluids, constitute granulation tissue, which is usually fully formed in from three to five days, after which it begins to be replaced by cicatricial or scar tissue.

Formation of Cicatricial Tissue.—The transformation of this temporary granulation tissue into scar tissue is effected by the fibroblasts, which become elongated and spindle-shaped, and produce in and around them a fine fibrillated material which gradually increases in quantity till it replaces the cell protoplasm. In this way white fibrous tissue is formed, the cells of which are arranged in parallel lines and eventually become grouped in bundles, constituting fully formed white fibrous tissue. In its growth it gradually obliterates the capillaries, until at the end of two, three, or four weeks both vessels and cells have almost entirely disappeared, and the original wound is occupied by cicatricial tissue. In course of time this tissue becomes consolidated, and the cicatrix undergoes a certain amount of contraction—*cicatricial contraction.*

Healing of Epidermis.—While these changes are taking place in the deeper parts of the wound, the surface is being covered over by *epidermis* growing in from the margins. Within twelve hours the cells of the rete Malpighii close to the cut edge begin to sprout on to the surface of the wound, and by their proliferation gradually cover the granulations with a thin pink pellicle. As the epithelium increases in thickness it assumes a bluish hue and eventually the cells become cornified and the epithelium assumes a greyish-white colour.

Clinical Aspects.—So long as the process of repair is not complicated by infection with micro-organisms, there is no interference with the general health of the patient. The temperature remains normal; the circulatory, gastro-intestinal, nervous, and other functions are undisturbed; locally, the part is cool, of natural colour and free from pain.

Modifications of the Process of Repair.—The process of repair by primary union, above described, is to be looked upon as the type of all reparative processes, such modifications as are met with depending merely upon incidental differences in the conditions present, such as loss of tissue, infection by micro-organisms, etc.

Repair after Loss or Destruction of Tissue.—When the edges of a wound cannot be approximated either because tissue has been lost, for example in excising a tumour or because a drainage tube or gauze packing has been necessary, a greater amount of granulation tissue is required to fill the gap, but the process is essentially the same as in the ideal method of repair.

The raw surface is first covered by a layer of coagulated blood and fibrin. An extensive new formation of capillary loops and fibroblasts takes place towards the free surface, and goes on until the gap is filled by a fine velvet-like mass of granulation tissue. This granulation tissue is gradually replaced by young cicatricial tissue, and the surface is covered by the ingrowth of epithelium from the edges.

This modification of the reparative process can be best studied clinically in a recent wound which has been packed with gauze. When the plug is introduced, the walls of the cavity consist of raw tissue with numerous oozing blood vessels. On removing the packing on the fifth or sixth day, the surface is found to be covered with minute, red, papillary granulations, which are beginning to fill up the cavity. At the edges the epithelium has proliferated and is covering over the newly formed granulation tissue. As lymph and leucocytes escape from the exposed surface there is a certain amount of serous or sero-purulent discharge. On examining the wound at intervals of a few days, it is found that the granulation tissue gradually increases in amount till the gap is completely filled up, and that coincidently the epithelium spreads in and covers over its surface. In course of time the epithelium thickens, and as the granulation tissue is slowly replaced by young cicatricial tissue, which has a peculiar tendency to contract and so to obliterate the blood vessels in it, the scar that is left becomes smooth, pale, and depressed. This method of healing is sometimes spoken of as "healing by granulation"—although, as we have seen, it is by granulation that all repair takes place.

Healing by Union of two Granulating Surfaces.—In gaping wounds union is sometimes obtained by bringing the two surfaces into apposition after each has become covered with healthy granulations. The exudate on the surfaces causes them to adhere, capillary loops pass from one to the other, and their final fusion takes place by the further development of granulation and cicatricial tissue.

Reunion of Parts entirely Separated from the Body.—Small portions of tissue, such as the end of a finger, the tip of the nose or a portion of the external ear, accidentally separated from the body, if accurately replaced and fixed in position, occasionally adhere by primary union.

In the course of operations also, portions of skin, fascia, or bone, or even a complete joint may be transplanted, and unite by primary union.

Healing under a Scab.—When a small superficial wound is exposed to the air, the blood and serum exuded on its surface may dry and form a hard crust or *scab*, which serves to protect the surface from external irritation in the same way as would a dry pad of sterilised gauze. Under this scab the formation of granulation tissue, its transformation into cicatricial tissue, and the growth of epithelium on the surface, go on until in the course of time the crust separates, leaving a scar.

Healing by Blood-clot.—In subcutaneous wounds, for example tenotomy, in amputation wounds, and in wounds made in excising tumours or in operating upon bones, the space left between the divided tissues becomes filled with blood-clot, which acts as a temporary scaffolding in which granulation tissue is built up. Capillary loops grow into the coagulum, and migrated leucocytes from the adjacent blood vessels destroy the red corpuscles, and are in turn disposed of by the developing fibroblasts, which by their growth and proliferation fill up the gap with young connective tissue. It will be evident that this process only differs from healing by primary union in the *amount* of blood-clot that is present.

Presence of a Foreign Body.—When an aseptic foreign body is present in the tissues, *e.g.* a piece of unabsorbable chromicised catgut, the healing process may be modified. After primary union has taken place the scar may broaden, become raised above the surface, and assume a bluish-brown colour; the epidermis gradually thins and gives way, revealing the softened portion of catgut, which can be pulled out in pieces, after which the wound rapidly heals and resumes a normal appearance.

REPAIR IN INDIVIDUAL TISSUES

Skin and Connective Tissue.—The mode of regeneration of these tissues under aseptic conditions has already been described as the type of ideal repair. In highly vascular parts, such as the face, the reparative process goes on with great rapidity, and even extensive wounds may be firmly united in from three to five days. Where the anastomosis is less free the process is more prolonged. The more highly organised elements of the skin, such as the hair follicles, the sweat and sebaceous glands, are imperfectly reproduced; hence the scar remains smooth, dry, and hairless.

Epithelium.—Epithelium is only reproduced from pre-existing epithelium, and, as a rule, from one of a similar type, although metaplastic transformation of cells of one kind of epithelium into another kind can take place. Thus a granulating surface may be covered entirely by the ingrowing of the cutaneous epithelium from the margins; or islets, originating in surviving cells of sebaceous glands or sweat glands, or of hair follicles, may spring up in the centre of the raw area. Such islets may also be due to the accidental transference of loose epithelial cells from the edges. Even the fluid from a blister, in virtue of the isolated cells of the rete Malpighii which it contains, is capable of starting epithelial growth on a granulating surface. Hairs and nails may be completely regenerated if a sufficient amount of the hair follicles or of the nail matrix has escaped destruction. The epithelium of a mucous membrane is regenerated in the same way as that on a cutaneous surface.

Epithelial cells have the power of living for some time after being separated from their normal surroundings, and of growing again when once more placed in favourable circumstances. On this fact the practice of skin grafting is based (p. 11).

Cartilage.—When an articular cartilage is divided by incision or by being implicated in a fracture involving the articular end of a bone, it is repaired by ordinary cicatricial fibrous tissue derived from the proliferating cells of the perichondrium. Cartilage being a non-vascular tissue, the reparative process goes on slowly, and it may be many weeks before it is complete.

It is possible for a metaplastic transformation of connective-tissue cells into cartilage cells to take place, the characteristic hyaline matrix being secreted by the new cells. This is sometimes observed as an intermediary stage in the healing of fractures, especially in young bones. It may also take place in the regeneration of lost portions of cartilage, provided the new tissue is so situated as to constitute part of a joint and to be subjected to pressure by an opposing cartilaginous surface. This is illustrated by what takes place after excision of joints where it is desired to restore the function of the articulation. By carrying out movements between the constituent parts, the fibrous tissue covering the ends of the bones becomes moulded into shape, its cells take on the characters of cartilage cells, and, forming a matrix, so develop a new cartilage.

Conversely, it is observed that when articular cartilage is no longer subjected to pressure by an opposing cartilage, it tends to be transformed into fibrous tissue, as may be seen in deformities attended with displacement of articular surfaces, such as hallux valgus and club-foot.

After fractures of costal cartilage or of the cartilages of the larynx the cicatricial tissue may be ultimately replaced by bone.

Tendons.—When a tendon is divided, for example by subcutaneous tenotomy, the end nearer the muscle fibres is drawn away from the other, leaving a gap which is speedily filled by blood-clot. In the course of a few days this clot becomes permeated by granulation tissue, the fibroblasts of which are derived from the sheath of the tendon, the surrounding connective tissue, and probably also from the divided ends of the tendon itself. These fibroblasts ultimately develop into typical tendon cells, and the fibres which they form constitute the new tendon fibres. Under aseptic conditions repair is complete in from two to three weeks. In the course of the reparative process the tendon and its sheath may become adherent, which leads to impaired movement and stiffness. If the ends of an accidentally divided tendon are at once brought into accurate apposition and secured by sutures, they unite directly with a minimum amount of scar tissue, and function is perfectly restored.

Muscle.—Unstriped muscle does not seem to be capable of being regenerated to any but a moderate degree. If the ends of a divided striped muscle are at once brought into apposition by stitches, primary union takes place with a minimum of intervening fibrous tissue. The nuclei of the muscle fibres in close proximity to this young cicatricial tissue proliferate, and a few new muscle fibres may be developed, but any gross loss of muscular tissue is replaced by a fibrous cicatrix. It would appear that portions of muscle transplanted from animals to fill up gaps in human muscle are similarly replaced by fibrous tissue. When a muscle is paralysed from loss of its nerve supply and undergoes complete degeneration, it is not capable of being regenerated, even should the integrity of the nerve be restored, and so its function is permanently lost.

Secretory Glands.—The regeneration of secretory glands is usually incomplete, cicatricial tissue taking the place of the glandular substance which has been destroyed. In wounds of the liver, for example, the gap is filled by fibrous tissue, but towards the periphery of the wound the liver cells proliferate and a certain amount of regeneration takes place. In the kidney also, repair mainly takes place by cicatricial tissue, and although a few collecting tubules may be reformed, no regeneration of secreting tissue takes place. After the operation of decapsulation of the kidney a new capsule is formed, and during the process young blood vessels permeate the superficial parts of the kidney and temporarily increase its blood supply, but in the consolidation of the new fibrous tissue these vessels are ultimately obliterated. This does not prove that the operation is useless, as the temporary improvement of the circulation in the kidney may serve to tide the patient over a critical period of renal insufficiency.

Stomach and Intestine.—Provided the peritoneal surfaces are accurately apposed, wounds of the stomach and intestine heal with great rapidity. Within a few hours the peritoneal surfaces are glued together by a thin layer of fibrin and leucocytes, which is speedily organised and replaced by fibrous tissue. Fibrous tissue takes the place of the muscular elements, which are not regenerated. The mucous lining is restored by ingrowth from the margins, and there is evidence that some of the secreting glands may be reproduced.

Hollow viscera, like the oesophagus and urinary bladder, in so far as they are not covered by peritoneum, heal less rapidly.

Nerve Tissues.—There is no trustworthy evidence that regeneration of the tissues of the brain or spinal cord in man ever takes place. Any loss of substance is replaced by cicatricial tissue.

The repair of *Bone*, *Blood Vessels*, and *Peripheral Nerves* is more conveniently considered in the chapters dealing with these structures.

Rate of Healing.—While the rate at which wounds heal is remarkably constant there are certain factors that influence it in one direction or the other. Healing is more rapid when the edges are in contact, when there is a minimum amount of blood-clot between them, when the patient is in normal health and the vitality of the tissues has not been impaired. Wounds heal slightly more quickly in the young than in the old, although the difference is so small that it can only be demonstrated by the most careful observations.

Certain tissues take longer to heal than others: for example, a fracture of one of the larger long bones takes about six weeks to unite, and divided nerve trunks take much longer—about a year.

Wounds of certain parts of the body heal more quickly than others: those of the scalp, face, and neck, for example, heal more quickly than those over the buttock or sacrum, probably because of their greater vascularity.

The extent of the wound influences the rate of healing; it is only natural that a long and deep wound should take longer to heal than a short and superficial one, because there is so much more work to be done in the conversion of blood-clot into granulation tissue, and this again into scar tissue that will be strong enough to stand the strain on the edges of the wound.

THE TRANSPLANTATION OR GRAFTING OF TISSUES

Conditions are not infrequently met with in which healing is promoted and restoration of function made possible by the transference of a portion of tissue from one part of the body to another; the tissue transferred is known as the *graft* or the *transplant*. The simplest example of grafting is the transplantation of skin.

In order that the graft may survive and have a favourable chance of "taking," as it is called, the transplanted tissue must retain its vitality until it has formed an organic connection with the tissue in which it is placed, so that it may derive the necessary nourishment from its new bed. When these conditions are fulfilled the tissues of the graft continue to proliferate, producing new tissue elements to replace those that are lost and making it possible for the graft to become incorporated with the tissue with which it is in contact.

Dead tissue, on the other hand, can do neither of these things; it is only capable of acting as a model, or, at the most, as a scaffolding for such mobile tissue elements as may be derived from, the parent tissue with which the graft is in contact: a portion of sterilised marine sponge, for example, may be observed to become permeated with granulation tissue when it is embedded in the tissues.

A successful graft of living tissue is not only capable of regeneration, but it acquires a system of lymph and blood vessels, so that in time it bleeds when cut into, and is permeated by new nerve fibres spreading in from the periphery towards the centre.

It is instructive to associate the period of survival of the different tissues of the body after death, with their capacity of being used for grafting purposes; the higher tissues such as those of the central nervous system and highly specialised glandular tissues like those of the kidney lose their vitality quickly after death and are therefore useless for grafting; connective tissues, on the other hand, such as fat, cartilage, and bone retain their vitality for several hours after death, so that when they are transplanted, they readily "take" and do all that is required of them: the same is true of the skin and its appendages.

Sources of Grafts.—It is convenient to differentiate between *autoplastic* grafts, that is those derived from the same individual; *homoplastic* grafts, derived from another animal of the same species; and *heteroplastic* grafts, derived from an animal of another species. Other conditions being equal, the prospects of success are greatest with autoplastic grafts, and these are therefore preferred whenever possible.

There are certain details making for success that merit attention: the graft must not be roughly handled or allowed to dry, or be subjected to chemical irritation; it must be brought into accurate contact with the new soil, no blood-clot intervening between the two, no movement of the one upon the other should be possible and all infection must be excluded; it will be observed that these are exactly the same conditions that permit of the primary healing of wounds, with which of course the healing of grafts is exactly comparable.

Preservation of Tissues for Grafting.—It was at one time believed that tissues might be taken from the operating theatre and kept in cold storage until they were required. It is now agreed that tissues which have been separated from the body for some time inevitably lose their vitality, become incapable of regeneration, and are therefore unsuited for grafting purposes. If it is intended to preserve a portion of tissue for future grafting, it should be embedded in the subcutaneous tissue of the abdominal wall until it is wanted; this has been carried out with portions of costal cartilage and of bone.

INDIVIDUAL TISSUES AS GRAFTS

The Blood lends itself in an ideal manner to transplantation, or, as it has long been called, *transfusion*. Being always a homoplastic transfer, the new blood is not always tolerated by the old, in which case biochemical changes occur, resulting in hæmolysis, which corresponds to the disintegration of other unsuccessful homoplastic grafts. (See article on Transfusion, *Op. Surg.*, p. 37.)

The Skin.—The skin was the first tissue to be used for grafting purposes, and it is still employed with greater frequency than any other, as lesions causing defects of skin are extremely common and without the aid of grafts are tedious in healing.

Skin grafts may be applied to a raw surface or to one that is covered with granulations.

Skin grafting of raw surfaces is commonly indicated after operations for malignant disease in which considerable areas of skin must be sacrificed, and after accidents, such as avulsion of the scalp by machinery.

Skin grafting of granulating surfaces is chiefly employed to promote healing in the large defects of skin caused by severe burns; the grafting is carried out when the surface is covered by a uniform layer of healthy granulations and before the inevitable contraction of scar tissue makes itself manifest. Before applying the grafts it is usual to scrape away the granulations until the young fibrous tissue underneath is exposed, but, if the granulations are healthy and can be rendered aseptic, the grafts may be placed on them directly.

If it is decided to scrape away the granulations, the oozing must be arrested by pressure with a pad of gauze, a sheet of dental rubber or green protective is placed next the raw surface to prevent the gauze adhering and starting the bleeding afresh when it is removed.

Methods of Skin-Grafting.—Two methods are employed: one in which the epidermis is mainly or exclusively employed—epidermis or epithelial grafting; the other, in which the graft consists of the whole thickness of the true skin—cutis-grafting.

Epidermis or Epithelial Grafting.—The method introduced by the late Professor Thiersch of Leipsic is that almost universally practised. It consists in transplanting strips of epidermis shaved from the surface of the skin, the razor passing through the tips of the papillæ, which appear as tiny red points yielding a moderate ooze of blood.

The strips are obtained from the front and lateral aspects of the thigh or upper arm, the skin in those regions being pliable and comparatively free from hairs.

They are cut with a sharp hollow-ground razor or with Thiersch's grafting knife, the blade of which is rinsed in alcohol and kept moistened with warm saline solution. The cutting is made easier if the skin is well stretched and kept flat and perfectly steady, the operator's left hand exerting traction on the skin behind, the hands of the assistant on the skin in front, one above and the other below the seat of operation. To ensure uniform strips being cut, the razor is kept parallel with the surface and used with a short, rapid, sawing movement, so that, with a little practice, grafts six or eight inches long by one or two inches broad can readily be cut. The patient is given a general anæsthetic, or regional anæsthesia is obtained by injections of a solution of one per cent. novocain into the line of the lateral and middle cutaneous nerves; the disinfection of the skin is carried out on the usual lines, any chemical agent being finally got rid of, however, by means of alcohol followed by saline solution.

The strips of epidermis wrinkle up on the knife and are directly transferred to the surface, for which they should be made to form a complete carpet, slightly overlapping the edges of the area and of one another; some blunt instrument is used to straighten out the strips, which are then subjected to firm pressure with a pad of gauze to express blood and air-bells and to ensure accurate contact, for this must be as close as that between a postage stamp and the paper to which it is affixed.

As a dressing for the grafted area and of that also from which the grafts have been taken, gauze soaked in *liquid paraffin*—the patent variety known as *ambrine* is excellent—appears to be the best; the gauze should be moistened every other day or so with fresh paraffin, so that, at the end of a week, when the grafts should have united, the gauze can be removed without risk of detaching them. *Dental wax* is another useful type of dressing; as is also *picric acid* solution. Over the gauze, there is applied a thick layer of cotton wool, and the whole dressing is kept in place by a firmly applied bandage, and in the case of the limbs some form of splint should be added to prevent movement.

A dressing may be dispensed with altogether, the grafts being protected by a wire cage such as is used after vaccination, but they tend to dry up and come to resemble a scab.

When the grafts have healed, it is well to protect them from injury and to prevent them drying up and cracking by the liberal application of lanoline or vaseline.

The new skin is at first insensitive and is fixed to the underlying connective tissue or bone, but in course of time (from six weeks onwards) sensation returns and the formation of elastic tissue beneath renders the skin pliant and movable so that it can be pinched up between the finger and thumb. *Reverdin's* method consists in planting out pieces of skin not bigger than a pin-head over a granulating surface. It is seldom employed.

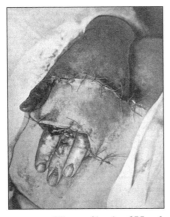

FIG. I. Ulcer of back of Hand covered by flap of skin raised from anterior abdominal wall. The lateral edges of the flap are divided after the graft has adhered.

Grafts of the Cutis Vera.—Grafts consisting of the entire thickness of the true skin were specially advocated by Wolff and are often associated with his name. They should be cut oval or spindle-shaped, to facilitate the approximation of the edges of the resulting wound. The graft should be cut to the exact size of the surface it is to cover; Gillies believes that tension of the graft favours its taking. These grafts may be placed either on a fresh raw surface or on healthy granulations. It is sometimes an advantage to stitch them in position, especially on the face. The dressing and the after-treatment are the same as in epidermis grafting.

There is a degree of uncertainty about the graft retaining its vitality long enough to permit of its deriving the necessary nourishment from its new surroundings; in a certain number of cases the flap dies and is thrown off as a slough—moist or dry according to the presence or absence of septic infection.

The technique for cutis-grafting must be without a flaw, and the asepsis absolute; there must not only be a complete absence of movement, but there must be no traction on the flap that will endanger its blood supply.

Owing to the uncertainty in the results of cutis-grafting the *two-stage* or *indirect method* has been introduced, and its almost uniform success has led to its sphere of application being widely extended. The flap is raised as in the direct method but is left attached at one of its margins for a period ranging from 14 to 21 days until its blood supply from its new bed is assured; the detachment is then made complete. The blood supply of the proposed flap may influence its selection and the way in which it is fashioned; for example, a flap cut from the side of the head to fill a defect in the cheek, having in its margin of attachment or pedicle the superficial temporal artery, is more likely to take than a flap cut with its base above.

Another modification is to raise the flap but leave it connected at both ends like the piers of a bridge; this method is well suited to defects of skin on the dorsum of the fingers, hand and forearm, the bridge of skin is raised from the abdominal wall and the hand is passed beneath it and securely fixed in position; after an interval of 14 to 21 days, when the flap is assured of its blood supply, the piers of the bridge are divided (Fig. 1). With undermining it is usually easy to bring the edges of the gap in the abdominal wall together, even in children; the skin flap on the dorsum of the hand appears rather thick and prominent—almost like the pad of a boxing-glove—for some time, but the restoration of function in the capacity to flex the fingers is gratifying in the extreme.

The indirect element of this method of skin-grafting may be carried still further by transferring the flap of skin first to one part of the body and then, after it has taken, transferring it to a third part. Gillies has especially developed this method in the remedying of deformities of the face caused by gunshot wounds and by petrol burns in air-men. A rectangular flap of skin is marked out in the neck and chest, the lateral margins of the flap are raised sufficiently to enable them to be brought together so as to form a tube of skin: after the circulation has been restored, the lower end of the tube is detached and is brought up to the lip or cheek, or eyelid, where it is wanted; when this end has derived its new blood supply, the other end is detached from the neck and brought up to where it is wanted. In this way, skin from the chest may be brought up to form a new forehead and eyelids.

Grafts of *mucous membrane* are used to cover defects in the lip, cheek, and conjunctiva. The technique is similar to that employed in skin-grafting; the sources of mucous membrane are limited and the element of septic infection cannot always be excluded.

Fat.—Adipose tissue has a low vitality, but it is easily retained and it readily lends itself to transplantation. Portions of fat are often obtainable at operations—from the omentum, for example, otherwise the subcutaneous fat of the buttock is the most accessible; it may be employed to fill up cavities of all kinds in order to obtain more rapid and sounder healing and also to remedy deformity, as in filling up a depression in the cheek or forehead. It is ultimately converted into ordinary connective tissue *pari passu* with the absorption of the fat.

The *fascia lata of the thigh* is widely and successfully used as a graft to fill defects in the dura mater, and interposed between the bones of a joint—if the articular cartilage has been destroyed—to prevent the occurrence of ankylosis.

The *peritoneum* of hydrocele and hernial sacs and of the omentum readily lends itself to transplantation.

Cartilage and bone, next to skin, are the tissues most frequently employed for grafting purposes; their sphere of action is so extensive and includes so much of technical detail in their employment, that they will be considered later with the surgery of the bones and joints and with the methods of re-forming the nose.

Tendons and blood vessels readily lend themselves to transplantation and will also be referred to later.

Muscle and nerve, on the other hand, do not retain their vitality when severed from their surroundings and do not functionate as grafts except for their connective-tissue elements, which it goes without saying are more readily obtainable from other sources.

Portions of the *ovary* and of the *thyreoid* have been successfully transplanted into the subcutaneous cellular tissue of the abdominal wall by Tuffier and others. In these new surroundings, the ovary or thyreoid is vascularised and has been shown to functionate, but there is not sufficient regeneration of the essential tissue elements to "carry on"; the secreting tissue is gradually replaced by connective tissue and the special function comes to an end. Even such temporary function may, however, tide a patient over a difficult period.

CONDITIONS WHICH INTERFERE WITH REPAIR

SURGICAL BACTERIOLOGY

Want of Rest ◆ *Irritation*
Unhealthy Tissues ◆ *Pathogenic Bacteria*
Surgical Bacteriology ◆ *General Characters of Bacteria*
Classification of Bacteria ◆ *Conditions of Bacterial Life*
Pathogenic Powers of Bacteria
Results of Bacterial Growth
Death of Bacteria ◆ *Immunity*
Antitoxic Sera ◆ *Identification of Bacteria*
Pyogenic Bacteria

In the management of wounds and other surgical conditions it is necessary to eliminate various extraneous influences which tend to delay or arrest the natural process of repair.

Of these, one of the most important is undue movement of the affected part. "The first and great requisite for the restoration of injured parts is *rest*," said John Hunter; and physiological and mechanical rest as the chief of natural therapeutic agents was the theme of John Hilton's classical work—*Rest and Pain*. In this connection it must be understood that "rest" implies more than the mere state of physical repose: all physiological as well as mechanical function must be prevented as far as is possible. For instance, the constituent bones of a joint affected with tuberculosis must be controlled by splints or other appliances so that no movement can take place between them, and the limb may not be used for any purpose; physiological rest may be secured to an inflamed colon by making an artificial anus in the cæcum; the activity of a diseased kidney may be diminished by regulating the quantity and quality of the fluids taken by the patient.

Another source of interference with repair in wounds is *irritation*, either by mechanical agents such as rough, unsuitable dressings, bandages, or ill-fitting splints; or by chemical agents in the form of strong lotions or other applications.

An *unhealthy or devitalised condition of the patient's tissues* also hinders the reparative process. Bruised or lacerated skin heals less kindly than skin cut with a smooth, sharp instrument; and persistent venous congestion of a part, such as occurs, for example, in the leg when the veins are varicose, by preventing the access of healthy blood, tends to delay the healing of open wounds. The existence of grave constitutional disease, such as Bright's disease, diabetes, syphilis, scurvy, or alcoholism, also impedes healing.

Infection by disease-producing micro-organisms or *pathogenic bacteria* is, however, the most potent factor in disturbing the natural process of repair in wounds.

SURGICAL BACTERIOLOGY

The influence of micro-organisms in the causation of disease, and the rôle played by them in interfering with the natural process of repair, are so important that the science of applied bacteriology has now come to dominate every department of surgery, and it is from the standpoint of bacteriology that nearly all surgical questions have to be considered.

The term *sepsis* as now used in clinical surgery no longer retains its original meaning as synonymous with "putrefaction," but is employed to denote all conditions in which bacterial infection has taken place, and more particularly those in which pyogenic bacteria are present. In the same way the term *aseptic* conveys the idea of freedom from all forms of bacteria, putrefactive or otherwise; and the term *antiseptic* is used to denote a power of counteracting bacteria and their products.

General Characters of Bacteria.—A *bacterium* consists of a finely granular mass of protoplasm, enclosed in a thin gelatinous envelope. Many forms are motile—some in virtue of fine thread-like flagella, and others through contractility of the protoplasm. The great majority multiply by simple fission, each parent cell giving rise to two daughter cells, and this process goes on with extraordinary rapidity. Other varieties, particularly bacilli, are propagated by the formation of *spores*. A spore is a minute mass of protoplasm surrounded by a dense, tough membrane, developed in the interior of the parent cell. Spores are remarkable for their tenacity of life, and for the resistance they offer to the action of heat and chemical germicides.

Bacteria are most conveniently classified according to their shape. Thus we recognise (1) those that are globular—*cocci*; (2) those that resemble a rod—*bacilli*; (3) the spiral or wavy forms—*spirilla*.

Cocci or *micrococci* are minute round bodies, averaging about 1 μ in diameter. The great majority are non-motile. They multiply by fission; and when they divide in such a way that the resulting cells remain in pairs, are called *diplococci*, of which the bacteria of gonorrhoea and pneumonia are examples (Fig. 5). When they divide irregularly, and form grape-like bunches, they are known as *staphylococci*, and to this variety the commonest pyogenic or pus-forming organisms belong (Fig. 2). When division takes place only in one axis, so that long chains are formed, the term *streptococcus* is applied (Fig. 3). Streptococci are met with in erysipelas and various other inflammatory and suppurative processes of a spreading character.

Bacilli are rod-shaped bacteria, usually at least twice as long as they are broad (Fig. 4). Some multiply by fission, others by sporulation. Some forms are motile, others are non-motile. Tuberculosis, tetanus, anthrax, and many other surgical diseases are due to different forms of bacilli.

Spirilla are long, slender, thread-like cells, more or less spiral or wavy. Some move by a screw-like contraction of the protoplasm, some by flagellæ. The spirochæte associated with syphilis (Fig. 36) is the most important member of this group.

Conditions of Bacterial Life.—Bacteria require for their growth and development a suitable food-supply in the form of proteins, carbohydrates, and salts of calcium and potassium which they break up into simpler elements. An alkaline medium favours bacterial growth; and moisture is a necessary condition; spores, however, can survive the want of water for much longer periods than fully developed bacteria. The necessity for oxygen varies in different species. Those that require oxygen are known as *aërobic bacilli* or *aërobes*; those that cannot live in the presence of oxygen are spoken of as *anaërobes*.

The great majority of bacteria, however, while they prefer to have oxygen, are able to live without it, and are called *facultative anaërobes*.

The most suitable temperature for bacterial life is from 95° to 102° F., roughly that of the human body. Extreme or prolonged cold paralyses but does not kill micro-organisms. Few, however, survive being raised to a temperature of 134½° F. Boiling for ten to twenty minutes will kill all bacteria, and the great majority of spores. Steam applied in an autoclave under a pressure of two atmospheres destroys even the most resistant spores in a few minutes. Direct sunlight, electric light, or even diffuse daylight, is inimical to the growth of bacteria, as are also Röntgen rays and radium emanations.

Pathogenic Properties of Bacteria.—We are now only concerned with pathogenic bacteria—that is, bacteria capable of producing disease in the human subject. This capacity depends upon two sets of factors—(1) certain features peculiar to the invading bacteria, and (2) others peculiar to the host. Many bacteria have only the power of living upon dead matter, and are known as *saprophytes*. Such as do nourish in living tissue are, by distinction, known as *parasites*. The power a given parasitic micro-organism has of multiplying in the body and giving rise to disease is spoken of as its *virulence*, and this varies not only with different species, but in the same species at different times and under varying circumstances. The actual number of organisms introduced is also an important factor in determining their pathogenic power. Healthy tissues can resist the invasion of a certain number of bacteria of a given species, but when that number is exceeded, the organisms get the upper hand and disease results. When the organisms gain access directly to the blood-stream, as a rule they produce their effects more certainly and with greater intensity than when they are introduced into the tissues.

Further, the virulence of an organism is modified by the condition of the patient into whose tissues it is introduced. So long as a person is in good health, the tissues are able to resist the attacks of moderate numbers of most bacteria. Any lowering of the vitality of the individual, however, either locally or generally, at once renders him more susceptible to infection. Thus bruised or torn tissue is much more liable to infection with pus-producing organisms than tissues clean-cut with a knife; also, after certain diseases, the liability to infection by the organisms of diphtheria, pneumonia, or erysipelas is much increased. Even such slight depression of vitality as results from bodily fatigue, or exposure to cold and damp, may be sufficient to turn the scale in the battle between the tissues and the bacteria. Age is an important factor in regard to the action of certain bacteria. Young subjects are attacked by diphtheria, tuberculosis, acute osteomyelitis, and some other diseases with greater frequency and severity than those of more advanced years.

In different races, localities, environment, and seasons, the pathogenic powers of certain organisms, such as those of erysipelas, diphtheria, and acute osteomyelitis, vary considerably.

There is evidence that a *mixed infection*—that is, the introduction of more than one species of organism, for example, the tubercle bacillus and a pyogenic staphylococcus—increases the severity of the resulting disease. If one of the varieties gain the ascendancy, the poisons produced by the others so devitalise the tissue cells, and diminish their power of resistance, that the virulence of the most active organisms is increased. On the other hand, there is reason to believe that the products of certain organisms antagonise one another—for example, an attack of erysipelas may effect the cure of a patch of tuberculous lupus.

Lastly, in patients suffering from chronic wasting diseases, bacteria may invade the internal organs by the blood-stream in enormous numbers and with great rapidity, during the period of extreme debility which shortly precedes death. The discovery of such collections of organisms on post-mortem examination may lead to erroneous conclusions being drawn as to the cause of death.

Results of Bacterial Growth.—Some organisms, such as those of tetanus and erysipelas, and certain of the pyogenic bacteria, show little tendency to pass far beyond the point at which they gain an entrance to the body. Others, on the contrary—for example, the tubercle bacillus and the organism of acute osteomyelitis—although frequently remaining localised at the seat of inoculation, tend to pass to distant parts, lodging in the capillaries of joints, bones, kidney, or lungs, and there producing their deleterious effects.

In the human subject, multiplication in the blood-stream does not occur to any great extent. In some general acute pyogenic infections, such as osteomyelitis, cellulitis, etc., pure cultures of staphylococci or of streptococci may be obtained from the blood. In pneumococcal and typhoid infections, also, the organisms may be found in the blood.

It is by the vital changes they bring about in the parts where they settle that micro-organisms disturb the health of the patient. In deriving nourishment from the complex organic compounds in which they nourish, the organisms evolve, probably by means of a ferment, certain chemical products of unknown composition, but probably colloidal in nature, and known as *toxins*. When these poisons are absorbed into the general circulation they give rise to certain groups of symptoms—such as rise of temperature, associated circulatory and respiratory derangements, interference with the gastro-intestinal functions and also with those of the nervous system—which go to make up the condition known as blood-poisoning, toxæmia, or *bacterial intoxication*. In addition to this, certain bacteria produce toxins that give rise to definite and distinct groups of symptoms—such as the convulsions of tetanus, or the paralyses that follow diphtheria.

Death of Bacteria.—Under certain circumstances, it would appear that the accumulation of the toxic products of bacterial action tends to interfere with the continued life and growth of the organisms themselves, and in this way the natural cure of certain diseases is brought about. Outside the body, bacteria may be killed by starvation, by want of moisture, by being subjected to high temperature, or by the action of certain chemical agents of which carbolic acid, the perchloride and biniodide of mercury, and various chlorine preparations are the most powerful.

Immunity.—Some persons are insusceptible to infection by certain diseases, from which they are said to enjoy a *natural immunity*. In many acute diseases one attack protects the patient, for a time at least, from a second attack—*acquired immunity*.

Phagocytosis.—In the production of immunity the leucocytes and certain other cells play an important part in virtue of the power they possess of ingesting bacteria and of destroying them by a process of intra-cellular digestion. To this process Metchnikoff gave the name of *phagocytosis*, and he recognised two forms of *phagocytes*: (1) the *microphages*, which are the polymorpho-nuclear leucocytes of the blood; and (2) the *macrophages*, which include the larger hyaline leucocytes, endothelial cells, and connective-tissue corpuscles.

During the process of phagocytosis, the polymorpho-nuclear leucocytes in the circulating blood increase greatly in numbers (*leucocytosis*), as well as in their phagocytic action, and in the course of destroying the bacteria they produce certain ferments which enter the blood serum. These are known as *opsonins* or *alexins*, and they act on the bacteria by a process comparable to narcotisation, and render them an easy prey for the phagocytes.

Artificial or Passive Immunity.—A form of immunity can be induced by the introduction of protective substances obtained from an animal which has been actively immunised. The process by which passive immunity is acquired depends upon the fact that as a result of the reaction between the specific virus of a particular disease (the *antigen*) and the tissues of the animal attacked, certain substances—*antibodies*—are produced, which when transferred to the body of a susceptible animal protect it against that disease. The most important of these antibodies are the *antitoxins*. From the study of the processes by which immunity is secured against the effects of bacterial action the serum and vaccine methods of treating certain infective diseases have been evolved. The *serum treatment* is designed to furnish the patient with a sufficiency of antibodies to neutralise the infection. The anti-diphtheritic and the anti-tetanic act by neutralising the specific toxins of the disease— *antitoxic serums*; the anti-streptcoccic and the serum for anthrax act upon the bacteria—*anti-bacterial serums*.

A *polyvalent* serum, that is, one derived from an animal which has been immunised by numerous strains of the organism derived from various sources, is much more efficacious than when a single strain has been used.

Clinical Use of Serums.—Every precaution must be taken to prevent organismal contamination of the serum or of the apparatus by means of which it is injected. Syringes are so made that they can be sterilised by boiling. The best situations for injection are under the skin of the abdomen, the thorax, or the buttock, and the skin should be purified at the seat of puncture. If the bulk of the full dose is large, it should be divided and injected into different parts of the body, not more than 20 c.c. being injected at one place. The serum may be introduced directly into a vein, or into the spinal canal, *e.g.* anti-tetanic serum. The immunity produced by injections of antitoxic sera lasts only for a comparatively short time, seldom longer than a few weeks.

"Serum Disease" and Anaphylaxis.—It is to be borne in mind that some patients exhibit a supersensitiveness with regard to protective sera, an injection being followed in a few days by the appearance of an urticarial or erythematous rash, pain and swelling of the joints, and a variable degree of fever. These

symptoms, to which the name *serum disease* is applied, usually disappear in the course of a few days.

The term *anaphylaxis* is applied to an allied condition of supersensitiveness which appears to be induced by the injection of certain substances, including toxins and sera, that are capable of acting as antigens. When a second injection is given after an interval of some days, if anaphylaxis has been established by the first dose, the patient suddenly manifests toxic symptoms of the nature of profound shock which may even prove fatal. The conditions which render a person liable to develop anaphylaxis and the mechanism by which it is established are as yet imperfectly understood.

Vaccine Treatment.—The vaccine treatment elaborated by A. E. Wright consists in injecting, while the disease is still active, specially prepared dead cultures of the causative organisms, and is based on the fact that these "vaccines" render the bacteria in the tissues less able to resist the attacks of the phagocytes. The method is most successful when the vaccine is prepared from organisms isolated from the patient himself, *autogenous vaccine*, but when this is impracticable, or takes a considerable time, laboratory-prepared polyvalent *stock vaccines* may be used.

Clinical Use of Vaccines.—Vaccines should not be given while a patient is in a negative phase, as a certain amount of the opsonin in the blood is used up in neutralising the substances injected, and this may reduce the opsonic index to such an extent that the vaccines themselves become dangerous. As a rule, the propriety of using a vaccine can be determined from the general condition of the patient. The initial dose should always be a small one, particularly if the disease is acute, and the subsequent dosage will be regulated by the effect produced. If marked constitutional disturbance with rise of temperature follows the use of a vaccine, it indicates a negative phase, and calls for a diminution in the next dose. If, on the other hand, the local as well as the general condition of the patient improves after the injection, it indicates a positive phase, and the original dose may be repeated or even increased. Vaccines are best introduced subcutaneously, a part being selected which is not liable to pressure, as there is sometimes considerable local reaction. Repeated doses may be necessary at intervals of a few days.

The vaccine treatment has been successfully employed in various tuberculous lesions, in pyogenic infections such as acne, boils, sycosis, streptococcal, pneumococcal, and gonococcal conditions, in infections of the accessory air sinuses, and in other diseases caused by bacteria.

PYOGENIC BACTERIA

From the point of view of the surgeon the most important varieties of micro-organisms are those that cause inflammation and suppuration—the *pyogenic bacteria*. This group includes a great many species, and these are so widely distributed that they are to be met with under all conditions of everyday life.

The nature of the inflammatory and suppurative processes will be considered in detail later; suffice it here to say that they are brought about by the action of one or other of the organisms that we have now to consider.

It is found that the *staphylococci*, which cluster into groups, tend to produce localised lesions; while the chain-forms—*streptococci*—give rise to diffuse, spreading conditions. Many varieties of pyogenic bacteria have now been differentiated, the best known being the staphylococcus aureus, the streptococcus, and the bacillus coli communis.

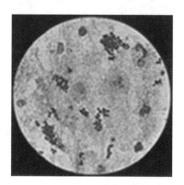

FIG. 2. Staphylococcus aureus in Pus from case of Osteomyelitis. × 1000 diam. Gram's stain.

Staphylococcus Aureus.—This is the commonest organism found in localised inflammatory and suppurative conditions. It varies greatly in its virulence, and is found in such widely different conditions as skin pustules, boils, carbuncles, and some acute inflammations of bone. As seen by the microscope it occurs in grape-like clusters, fission of the individual cells taking place irregularly (Fig. 2). When grown in artificial media, the colonies assume an orange-yellow colour—hence the name *aureus*. It is of high vitality and resists more prolonged exposure to high temperatures than most non-sporing bacteria. It is capable of lying latent in the tissues for long periods, for example, in the marrow of long bones, and of again becoming active and causing a fresh outbreak of suppuration. This organism is widely distributed: it is found on the skin, in the mouth, and in other situations in the body, and as it is present in the dust of the air and on all objects upon which dust has settled, it is a continual source of infection unless means are taken to exclude it from wounds.

The *staphylococcus albus* is much less common than the aureus, but has the same properties and characters, save that its growth on artificial media assumes a white colour. It is the common cause of stitch abscesses, the skin being its normal habitat.

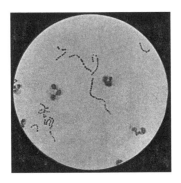

FIG. 3. Streptococci in Pus from an acute abscess in subcutaneous tissue. × 1000 diam. Gram's stain.

Streptococcus Pyogenes.—This organism also varies greatly in its virulence; in some instances—for example in erysipelas—it causes a sharp attack of acute spreading inflammation, which soon subsides without showing any tendency to end in suppuration; under other conditions it gives rise to a generalised infection which rapidly proves fatal. The streptococcus has less capacity of liquefying the tissues than the staphylococcus, so that pus formation takes place more slowly. At the same time its products are very potent in destroying the tissues in their vicinity, and so interfering with the exudation of leucocytes which would otherwise exercise their protective influence. Streptococci invade the lymph spaces, and are associated with acute spreading conditions such as phlegmonous or erysipelatous inflammations and suppurations, lymphangitis and suppuration in lymph glands, and inflammation of serous and synovial membranes, also with a form of pneumonia which is prone to follow on severe operations in the mouth and throat. Streptococci are also concerned in the production of spreading gangrene and pyæmia.

Division takes place in one axis, so that chains of varying length are formed (Fig. 3). It is less easily cultivated by artificial media than the staphylococcus; it forms a whitish growth.

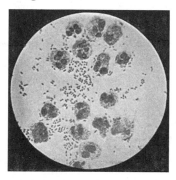

FIG. 4. Bacillus coli communis in Urine, from a case of Cystitis. × 1000 diam. Leishman's stain.

Bacillus Coli Communis.—This organism, which is a normal inhabitant of the intestinal tract, shows a great tendency to invade any organ or tissue whose vitality is lowered. It is causatively associated with such conditions as peritonitis and peritoneal suppuration resulting from strangulated hernia, appendicitis, or perforation in any part of the alimentary canal. In cystitis, pyelitis, abscess of the kidney, suppuration in the bile-ducts or liver, and in many other abdominal conditions, it plays a most important part. The discharge from wounds infected by this organism has usually a foetid, or even a fæcal odour, and often contains gases resulting from putrefaction.

It is a small rod-shaped organism with short flagellæ, which render it motile (Fig. 4). It closely resembles the typhoid bacillus, but is distinguished from it by its behaviour in artificial culture media.

Pneumo-bacteria.—Two forms of organism associated with pneumonia—*Fraenkel's pneumococcus* (one of the diplococci) (Fig. 5) and *Friedländer's pneumo-bacillus* (a short rod-shaped form)—are frequently met with in inflammations of the serous and synovial membranes, in suppuration in the liver, and in various other inflammatory and suppurative conditions.

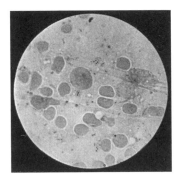

FIG. 5. Fraenkel's Pneumococci in Pus from Empyema following Pneumonia. × 100 diam. Stained with Muir's capsule stain.

Bacillus Typhosus.—This organism has been found in pure culture in suppurative conditions of bone, of cellular tissue, and of internal organs, especially during convalescence from typhoid fever. Like the staphylococcus, it is capable of lying latent in the tissues for long periods.

Other Pyogenic Bacteria.—It is not necessary to do more than name some of the other organisms that are known to be pyogenic, such as the bacillus pyocyaneus, which is found in green and blue pus, the micrococcus tetragenus, the gonococcus, actinomyces, the glanders bacillus, and the tubercle bacillus. Most of these will receive further mention in connection with the diseases to which they give rise.

Leucocytosis.—Most bacterial diseases, as well as certain other pathological conditions, are associated with an increase in the number of leucocytes in the blood throughout the circulatory system. This condition of the blood, which is known as *leucocytosis*, is believed to be due to an excessive output and rapid formation of leucocytes by the bone marrow, and it probably has as its object the arrest and destruction of the invading organisms or toxins. To increase the resisting power of the system to pathogenic organisms, an artificial leucocytosis may be induced by subcutaneous injection of a solution of nucleinate of soda (16 minims of a 5 per cent. solution).

The *normal* number of leucocytes per cubic millimetre varies in different individuals, and in the same individual under different conditions, from 5000 to 10,000: 7500 is a normal average, and anything above 12,000 is considered abnormal. When leucocytosis is present, the number may range from 12,000 to 30,000 or even higher; 40,000 is looked upon as a high degree of leucocytosis. According to Ehrlich, the following may be taken as the standard proportion of the various forms of leucocytes in normal blood: polynuclear neutrophile leucocytes, 70 to 72 per cent.; lymphocytes, 22 to 25 per cent.; eosinophile cells, 2 to 4 per cent.; large mononuclear and transitional leucocytes, 2 to 4 per cent.; mast-cells, 0.5 to 2 per cent.

In estimating the clinical importance of a leucocytosis, it is not sufficient merely to count the aggregate number of leucocytes present. A differential count must be made to determine which variety of cells is in excess. In the majority of surgical affections it is chiefly the granular polymorpho-nuclear neutrophile leucocytes that are in excess (*ordinary leucocytosis*). In some cases, and particularly in parasitic diseases such as trichiniasis and hydatid disease, the eosinophile leucocytes also show a proportionate increase (*eosinophilia*). The term *lymphocytosis* is applied when there is an increase in the number of circulating lymphocytes, as occurs, for example, in lymphatic leucæmia, and in certain cases of syphilis.

Leucocytosis is met with in nearly all acute infective diseases, and in acute pyogenic inflammatory affections, particularly in those attended with suppuration. In exceptionally acute septic conditions the extreme virulence of the toxins may prevent the leucocytes reacting, and leucocytosis may be absent. The absence of leucocytosis in a disease in which it is usually present is therefore to be looked upon as a grave omen, particularly when the general symptoms are severe. In some cases of malignant disease the number of leucocytes is increased to 15,000 or 20,000. A few hours after a severe hæmorrhage also there is usually a leucocytosis of from 15,000 to 30,000, which lasts for three or four days (Lyon). In cases of hæmorrhage the leucocytosis is increased by infusion of fluids into the circulation. After all operations there is at least a transient leucocytosis (*post-operative leucocytosis*) (F. I. Dawson).

The leucocytosis begins soon after the infection manifests itself—for example, by shivering, rigor, or rise of temperature. The number of leucocytes rises somewhat rapidly, increases while the condition is progressing, and remains high during the febrile period, but there is no constant correspondence between the number of leucocytes and the height of the temperature. The arrest of the inflammation and its resolution are accompanied by a fall in the number of leucocytes, while the occurrence of suppuration is attended with a further increase in their number.

In interpreting the "blood count," it is to be kept in mind that a *physiological leucocytosis* occurs within three or four hours of taking a meal, especially one rich in proteins, from 1500 to 2000 being added to the normal number. In this *digestion leucocytosis* the increase is chiefly in the polynuclear neutrophile leucocytes. Immediately before and after delivery, particularly in primiparæ, there is usually a moderate degree of leucocytosis. If the labour is normal and the puerperium uncomplicated, the number of leucocytes regains the normal in about a week. Lactation has no appreciable effect on the number of leucocytes. In new-born infants the leucocyte count is abnormally high, ranging from 15,000 to 20,000. In children under one year of age, the normal average is from 10,000 to 20,000.

Absence of Leucocytosis—Leucopenia.—In certain infective diseases the number of leucocytes in the circulating blood is abnormally low—3000 or 4000—and this condition is known as *leucopenia*. It occurs in typhoid fever, especially in the later stages of the disease, in tuberculous lesions unaccompanied by suppuration, in malaria, and in most cases of uncomplicated influenza. The occurrence of leucocytosis in any of these conditions is to be looked upon as an indication that a mixed infection has taken place, and that some suppurative process is present.

The absence of leucocytosis in some cases of virulent septic poisoning has already been referred to.

It will be evident that too much reliance must not be placed upon a single observation, particularly in emergency cases. Whenever possible, a series of observations should be made, the blood being examined about four hours after meals, and about the same hour each day.

The clinical significance of the blood count in individual diseases will be further referred to.

The Iodine or Glycogen Reaction.—The leucocyte count may be supplemented by staining films of the blood with a watery solution of iodine and potassium iodide. In all advancing purulent conditions, in septic poisonings, in pneumonia, and in cancerous growths associated with ulceration, a certain number of the polynuclear leucocytes are stained a brown or reddish-brown colour, due to the action of the iodine on some substance in the cells of the nature of glycogen. This reaction is absent in serous effusions, in unmixed tuberculous infections, in uncomplicated typhoid fever, and in the early stages of cancerous growths.

INFLAMMATION

Definition
Nature of Inflammation from Surgical Point of View
Sequence of Changes in Bacterial Inflammation
Clinical Aspects of Inflammation
General Principles of Treatment ◆ *Chronic Inflammation.*

Inflammation may be defined as the series of vital changes that occurs in the tissues in response to irritation. These changes represent the reaction of the tissue elements to the irritant, and constitute the attempt made by nature to arrest or to limit its injurious effects, and to repair the damage done by it.

The phenomena which characterise the inflammatory reaction can be induced by any form of irritation—such, for example, as mechanical injury, the application of heat or of chemical substances, or the action of pathogenic bacteria and their toxins—and they are essentially similar in kind whatever the irritant may be. The extent to which the process may go, however, and its effects on the part implicated and on the system as a whole, vary with different irritants and with the intensity and duration of their action. A mechanical, a thermal, or a chemical irritant, acting alone, induces a degree of reaction directly proportionate to its physical properties, and so long as it does not completely destroy the vitality of the part involved, the changes in the tissues are chiefly directed towards repairing the damage done to the part, and the inflammatory reaction is not only compatible with the occurrence of ideal repair, but may be looked upon as an integral step in the reparative process.

The irritation caused by infection with bacteria, on the other hand, is cumulative, as the organisms not only multiply in the tissues, but in addition produce chemical poisons (toxins) which aggravate the irritative effects. The resulting reaction is correspondingly progressive, and has as its primary object the expulsion of the irritant and the limitation of its action. If the natural protective effort is successful, the resulting tissue changes subserve the process of repair, but if the bacteria gain the upper hand in the struggle, the inflammatory reaction becomes more intense, certain of the tissue elements succumb, and the process for the time being is a destructive one. During the stage of bacterial inflammation, reparative processes are in abeyance, and it is only after the inflammation has been allayed, either by natural means or by the aid of the surgeon, that repair takes place.

In applying the antiseptic principle to the treatment of wounds, our main object is to exclude or to eliminate the bacterial factor, and so to prevent the inflammatory reaction going beyond the stage in which it is protective, and just in proportion as we succeed in attaining this object, do we favour the occurrence of ideal repair.

Sequence of Changes in Bacterial Inflammation.—As the form of inflammation with which we are most concerned is that due to the action of bacteria, in describing the process by which the protective influence of the inflammatory reaction is brought into play, we shall assume the presence of a bacterial irritant.

The introduction of a colony of micro-organisms is quickly followed by an accumulation of wandering cells, and proliferation of connective-tissue cells in the tissues at the site of infection. The various cells are attracted to the bacteria by a peculiar chemical or biological power known as *chemotaxis*, which seems to result from variations in the surface tension of different varieties of cells, probably caused by some substance produced by the micro-organisms. Changes in the blood vessels then ensue, the arteries becoming dilated and the rate of the current in them being for a time increased—*active hyperæmia*. Soon, however, the rate of the blood flow becomes slower than normal, and in course of time the current may cease (*stasis*), and the blood in the vessels may even coagulate (*thrombosis*). Coincidently with these changes in the vessels, the leucocytes in the blood of the inflamed part rapidly increase in number, and they become viscous and adhere to the vessel wall, where they may accumulate in large numbers. In course of time the leucocytes pass through the vessel wall—*emigration of leucocytes*—and move towards the seat of infection, giving rise to a marked degree of *local leucocytosis*. Through the openings by which the leucocytes have escaped from the vessels, red corpuscles may be passively extruded—*diapedesis of red corpuscles*. These processes are accompanied by changes in the endothelium of the vessel walls, which result in an increased formation of lymph, which transudes into the meshes of the connective tissue giving rise to an *inflammatory oedema*, or, if the inflammation is on a free surface, forming an *inflammatory exudate*. The quantity and characters of this exudate vary in different parts of the body, and according to the nature, virulence, and location of the organisms causing the inflammation. Thus it may be *serous*, as in some forms of synovitis; *sero-fibrinous*, as in certain varieties of peritonitis, the fibrin tending to limit the spread of the inflammation by forming adhesions; *croupous*, when it coagulates on a free surface and forms a false membrane, as in diphtheria; *hæmorrhagic* when mixed with blood; or *purulent*, when suppuration has occurred. The protective effects of the inflammatory reaction depend for the most part upon the transudation of lymph and the emigration of leucocytes. The lymph contains the opsonins which act on the bacteria and render them less able to resist the attack of the phagocytes, as well as the various protective antibodies which neutralise the toxins. The polymorph leucocytes are the principal agents in the process of phagocytosis (p. 22), and together with the other forms of phagocytes they ingest and destroy the bacteria.

If the attempt to repel the invading organisms is successful, the irritant effects are overcome, the inflammation is arrested, and *resolution* is said to take place.

Certain of the vascular and cellular changes are now utilised to restore the condition to the normal, and *repair* ensues after the manner already described. In certain situations, notably in tendon sheaths, in the cavities of joints, and in the interior of serous cavities, for example the pleura and peritoneum, the restoration to the normal is not perfect, adhesions forming between the opposing surfaces.

If, however, the reaction induced by the infection is insufficient to check the growth and spread of the organisms, or to inhibit their toxin production, local necrosis of tissue may take place, either in the form of suppuration or of gangrene, or the toxins absorbed into the circulation may produce blood-poisoning, which may even prove fatal.

Clinical Aspects of Inflammation.—It must clearly be understood that inflammation is not to be looked upon as a disease in itself, but rather as an evidence of some infective process going on in the tissues in which it occurs, and of an effort on the part of these tissues to overcome the invading organisms and their products. The chief danger to the patient lies, not in the reactive changes that constitute the inflammatory process, but in the fact that he is liable to be poisoned by the toxins of the bacteria at work in the inflamed area.

Since the days of Celsus (first century A.D.), heat, redness, swelling, and pain have been recognised as cardinal signs of inflammation, and to these may be added, interference with function in the inflamed part, and general constitutional disturbance. Variations in these signs and symptoms depend upon the acuteness of the condition, the nature of the causative organism and of the tissue attacked, the situation of the part in relation to the surface, and other factors.

The *heat* of the inflamed part is to be attributed to the increased quantity of blood present in it, and the more superficial the affected area the more readily is the local increase of temperature detected by the hand. This clinical point is best tested by placing the palm of the hand and fingers for a few seconds alternately over an uninflamed and an inflamed area, otherwise under similar conditions as to coverings and exposure. In this way even slight differences may be recognised.

Redness, similarly, is due to the increased afflux of blood to the inflamed part. The shade of colour varies with the stage of the inflammation, being lighter and brighter in the early, hyperæmic stages, and darker and duskier when the blood flow is slowed or when stasis has occurred and the oxygenation of the blood is defective. In the thrombotic stage the part may assume a purplish hue.

The *swelling* is partly due to the increased amount of blood in the affected part and to the accumulation of leucocytes and proliferated tissue cells, but chiefly to the exudate in the connective tissue—*inflammatory oedema*. The more open the structure of the tissue of the part, the greater is the amount of swelling—witness the marked degree of oedema that occurs in such parts as the scrotum or the eyelids.

Pain is a symptom seldom absent in inflammation. *Tenderness*—that is, pain elicited on pressure—is one of the most valuable diagnostic signs we possess, and is often present before pain is experienced by the patient. That the area of tenderness corresponds to the area of inflammation is almost an axiom of surgery. Pain and tenderness are due to the irritation of nerve filaments of the part, rendered all the more sensitive by the abnormal conditions of their blood supply. In inflammatory conditions of internal organs, for example the abdominal viscera, the pain is frequently referred to other parts, usually to an area supplied by branches from the same segment of the cord as that supplying the inflamed part.

For purposes of diagnosis, attention should be paid to the terms in which the patient describes his pain. For example, the pain caused by an inflammation of the skin is usually described as of a *burning* or *itching* character; that of inflammation in dense tissues like periosteum or bone, or in encapsuled organs, as *dull*, *boring*, or *aching*. When inflammation is passing on to suppuration the pain assumes a *throbbing* character, and as the pus reaches the surface, or "points," as it is called, sharp, *darting*, or *lancinating* pains are experienced. Inflammation involving a nerve-trunk may cause a *boring* or a *tingling* pain; while the implication of a serous membrane such as the pleura or peritoneum gives rise to a pain of a sharp, *stabbing* character.

Interference with the function of the inflamed part is always present to a greater or less extent.

Constitutional Disturbances.—Under the term constitutional disturbances are included the presence of fever or elevation of temperature; certain changes in the pulse rate and the respiration; gastro-intestinal and urinary disturbances; and derangements of the central nervous system. These are all due to the absorption of toxins into the general circulation.

Temperature.—A marked rise of temperature is one of the most constant and important concomitants of acute inflammatory conditions, and the temperature chart forms a fairly reliable index of the state of the patient. The toxins interfere with the nerve-centres in the medulla that regulate the balance between the production and the loss of body heat.

Clinically the temperature is estimated by means of a self-registering thermometer placed, for from one to five minutes, in close contact with the skin in the axilla, or in the mouth. Sometimes the thermometer is inserted into the rectum, where, however, the temperature is normally ¾° F. higher than in the axilla.

In health the temperature of the body is maintained at a mean of about 98.4° F. (37° C.) by the heat-regulating mechanism. It varies from hour to hour even in health, reaching its maximum between four and eight in the evening, when it may rise to 99° F., and is at its lowest between four and six in the morning, when it may be about 97° F.

The temperature is more easily disturbed in children than in adults, and may become markedly elevated (104° or 105° F.) from comparatively slight causes; in the aged it is less liable to change, so that a rise to 103° or 104° F. is to be looked upon as indicating a high state of fever.

A sudden rise of temperature is usually associated with a feeling of chilliness down the back and in the limbs, which may be so marked that the patient shivers violently, while the skin becomes cold, pale, and shrivelled— *cutis anserina*. This is a nervous reaction due to a want of correspondence between the internal and the surface temperature of the body, and is known clinically as a *rigor*. When the temperature rises gradually the chill is usually slight and may be unobserved. Even during the cold stage, however, the internal temperature is already raised, and by the time the chill has passed off its maximum has been reached.

The *pulse* is always increased in frequency, and usually varies directly with the height of the temperature. *Respiration* is more active during the progress of an inflammation; and bronchial catarrh is common apart from any antecedent respiratory disease.

Gastro-intestinal disturbances take the form of loss of appetite, vomiting, diminished secretion of the alimentary juices, and weakening of the peristalsis of the bowel, leading to thirst, dry, furred tongue, and constipation. Diarrhoea is sometimes present. The *urine* is usually scanty, of high specific gravity, rich in nitrogenous substances, especially urea and uric acid, and in calcium salts, while sodium chloride is deficient. Albumin and hyaline casts may be present in cases of severe inflammation with high temperature. The significance of general *leucocytosis* has already been referred to.

General Principles of Treatment.—The capacity of the inflammatory reaction for dealing with bacterial infections being limited, it often becomes necessary for the surgeon to aid the natural defensive processes, as well as to counteract the local and general effects of the reaction, and to relieve symptoms.

The ideal means of helping the tissues is by removing the focus of infection, and when this can be done, as for example in a carbuncle or an anthrax pustule, the infected area may be completely excised. When the focus is not sufficiently limited to admit of this, the infected tissue may be scraped away with the sharp spoon, or destroyed by caustics or by the actual cautery. If this is inadvisable, the organisms may be attacked by strong antiseptics, such as pure carbolic acid.

Moist dressings favour the removal of bacteria by promoting the escape of the inflammatory exudate, in which they are washed out.

Artificial Hyperæmia.—When such direct means as the above are impracticable, much can be done to aid the tissues in their struggle by improving the condition of the circulation in the inflamed area, so as to ensure that a plentiful supply of fresh arterial blood reaches it. The beneficial effects of *hot fomentations and poultices* depend on their causing a dilatation of the vessels, and so inducing a hyperæmia in the affected area. It has been shown experimentally that repeated, short applications of moist heat (not exceeding 106° F.) are more efficacious than continuous application. It is now believed that the so-called *counter-irritants*—mustard, iodine, cantharides, actual cautery—act in the same way; and the method of treating erysipelas by applying a strong solution of iodine around the affected area is based on the same principle.

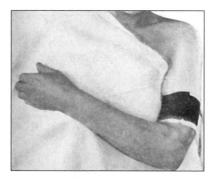

FIG. 6. Passive Hyperæmia of Hand and Forearm induced by Bier's Bandage.

While these and similar methods have long been employed in the treatment of inflammatory conditions, it is only within comparatively recent years that their mode of action has been properly understood, and to August Bier belongs the credit of having put the treatment of inflammation on a scientific and rational basis. Recognising the "beneficent intention" of the inflammatory reaction, and the protective action of the leucocytosis which accompanies the hyperæmic stages of the process, Bier was led to study the effects of increasing the hyperæmia by artificial means. As a result of his observations, he has formulated a method of treatment which consists in inducing an artificial hyperæmia in the inflamed area, either by obstructing the venous return from the part (*passive hyperæmia*), or by stimulating the arterial flow through it (*active hyperæmia*).

Bier's Constricting Bandage.—To induce a *passive hyperæmia* in a limb, an elastic bandage is applied some distance above the inflamed area sufficiently tightly to obstruct the venous return from the distal parts without arresting in any way the inflow of arterial blood (Fig. 6). If the constricting band is correctly applied, the parts beyond become swollen and oedematous, and assume a bluish-red hue, but they retain their normal temperature, the pulse is unchanged, and there is no pain. If the part becomes blue, cold, or painful, or if any existing pain is increased, the band has been applied too tightly. The hyperæmia is kept up from twenty to twenty-two hours out of the twenty-four, and in the intervals the limb is elevated to get rid of the oedema and to empty it of impure blood, and so make room for a fresh supply of healthy blood when the bandage is re-applied. As the inflammation subsides, the period during which the band is kept on each day is diminished; but the treatment should be continued for some days after all signs of inflammation have subsided.

This method of treating acute inflammatory conditions necessitates close supervision until the correct degree of tightness of the band has been determined.

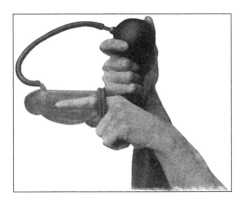

FIG. 7. Passive Hyperæmia of Finger induced by Klapp's Suction Bell.

Klapp's Suction Bells.—In inflammatory conditions to which the constricting band cannot be applied, as for example an acute mastitis, a bubo in the groin, or a boil on the neck, the affected area may be rendered hyperæmic by an appropriately shaped glass bell applied over it and exhausted by means of a suction-pump, the rarefaction of the air in the bell determining a flow of blood into the tissues enclosed within it (Figs. 7 and 8). The edge of the bell is smeared with vaseline, and the suction applied for from five to ten minutes at a time, with a corresponding interval between the applications. Each sitting lasts for from half an hour to an hour, and the treatment may be carried out once or twice a day according to circumstances. This apparatus acts in the same way as the old-fashioned *dry cup*, and is more convenient and equally efficacious.

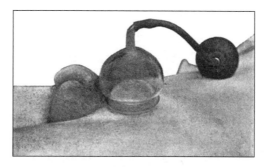

FIG. 8. Passive Hyperæmia induced by Klapp's Suction Bell for Inflammation of Inguinal Gland.

Active hyperæmia is induced by the local application of heat, particularly by means of hot air. It has not proved so useful in acute inflammation as passive hyperæmia, but is of great value in hastening the absorption of inflammatory products and in overcoming adhesions and stiffness in tendons and joints.

General Treatment.—The patient should be kept at rest, preferably in bed, to diminish the general tissue waste; and the diet should be restricted to fluids, such as milk, beef-tea, meat juices or gruel, and these may be rendered more easily assimilable by artificial digestion if necessary. To counteract the general effect of toxins absorbed into the circulation, specific antitoxic sera are employed in certain forms of infection, such as diphtheria, streptococcal septicæmia, and tetanus. In other forms of infection, vaccines are employed to increase the opsonic power of the blood. When such means are not available, the circulating toxins may to some extent be diluted by giving plenty of bland fluids by the mouth or normal salt solution by the rectum.

The elimination of the toxins is promoted by securing free action of the emunctories. A saline purge, such as half an ounce of sulphate of magnesium in a small quantity of water, ensures a free evacuation of the bowels. The kidneys are flushed by such diluent drinks as equal parts of milk and lime water, or milk with a dram of liquor calcis saccharatus added to each tumblerful. Barley-water and "Imperial drink," which consists of a dram and a half of cream of tartar added to a pint of boiling water and sweetened with sugar after cooling, are also useful and non-irritating diuretics. The skin may be stimulated by Dover's powder (10 grains) or liquor ammoniæ acetatis in three-dram doses every four hours.

Various drugs administered internally, such as quinine, salol, salicylate of iron, and others, have a reputation, more or less deserved, as internal antiseptics.

Weakness of the heart, as indicated by the condition of the pulse, is treated by the use of such drugs as digitalis, strophanthus, or strychnin, according to circumstances.

Gastro-intestinal disturbances are met by ordinary medical means. Vomiting, for example, can sometimes be checked by effervescing drinks, such as citrate of caffein, or by dilute hydrocyanic acid and bismuth. In severe cases, and especially when the vomited matter resembles coffee-grounds from admixture with altered blood—the so-called post-operative hæmatemesis—the best means of arresting the vomiting is by washing out the stomach. Thirst is relieved by rectal injections of saline solution. The introduction of saline solution into the veins or by the rectum is also useful in diluting and hastening the elimination of circulating toxins.

In surgical inflammations, as a rule, nothing is gained by lowering the temperature, unless at the same time the cause is removed. When severe or prolonged pyrexia becomes a source of danger, the use of hot or cold sponging, or even the cold bath, is preferable to the administration of drugs.

Relief of Symptoms.—For the relief of *pain*, rest is essential. The inflamed part should be placed in a splint or other appliance which will prevent movement, and steps must be taken to reduce its functional activity as far as possible. Locally, warm and moist dressings, such as a poultice or fomentation, may be used. To make a fomentation, a piece of flannel or lint is wrung out of very hot water or antiseptic lotion and applied under a sheet of mackintosh. Fomentations should be renewed as often as they cool. An ordinary india-rubber bag filled with hot water and fixed over the fomentation, by retaining the heat, obviates the necessity of frequently changing the application. The addition of a few drops of laudanum sprinkled on the flannel has a soothing effect. Lead and opium lotion is a useful, soothing application employed as a fomentation. We prefer the application of lint soaked in a 10 per cent. aqueous or glycerine solution of ichthyol, or smeared with ichthyol ointment (1 in 3). Belladonna and glycerine, equal parts, may be used.

Dry cold obtained by means of icebags, or by Leiter's lead tubes through which a continuous stream of ice-cold water is kept flowing, is sometimes soothing to the patient, but when the vessels in the inflamed part are greatly congested its use is attended with considerable risk, as it not only contracts the arterioles supplying the part, but also diminishes the outflow of venous blood, and so may determine gangrene of tissues already devitalised.

A milder form of employing cold is by means of evaporating lotions: a thin piece of lint or gauze is applied over the inflamed part and kept constantly moist with the lotion, the dressing being left freely exposed to allow of continuous evaporation. A useful evaporating lotion is made up as follows: take of chloride of ammonium, half an ounce; rectified spirit, one ounce; and water, seven ounces.

The administration of opiates may be necessary for the relief of pain.

The accumulation of an excessive amount of inflammatory exudate may endanger the vitality of the tissues by pressing on the blood vessels to such an extent as to cause stasis, and by concentrating the local action of the toxins. Under such conditions the tension should be relieved and the exudate with its contained toxins removed by making an incision into the inflamed tissues, and applying a suction bell. When the exudate has collected in a synovial cavity, such as a joint or bursa, it may be withdrawn by means of a trocar and cannula. There are other methods of withdrawing blood and exudate from an inflamed area, for example by leeches or wet-cupping, but they are seldom employed now.

Before applying leeches the part must be thoroughly cleansed, and if the leech is slow to bite, may be smeared with cream. The leech is retained in position under an inverted wine-glass or wide test-tube till it takes hold. After it has sucked its fill it usually drops off, having withdrawn a dram or a dram and a half of blood. If it be desirable to withdraw more blood, hot fomentations should be applied to the bite. As it is sometimes necessary to employ considerable pressure to stop the bleeding, leeches should, if possible, be applied over a bone which will furnish the necessary resistance. The use of styptics may be called for.

Wet-cupping has almost entirely been superseded by the use of Klapp's suction bells.

General blood-letting consists in opening a superficial vein (venesection) and allowing from eight to ten ounces of blood to flow from it. It is seldom used in the treatment of surgical forms of inflammation.

Counter-irritants.—In deep-seated inflammations, counter-irritants are sometimes employed in the form of mustard leaves or blisters, according to the degree of irritation required. A mustard leaf or plaster should not be left on longer than ten or fifteen minutes, unless it is desired to produce a blister. Blistering may be produced by a *cantharides plaster*, or by painting with *liquor epispasticus*. The plaster should be left on from eight to ten hours, and if it has failed to raise a blister, a hot fomentation should be applied to the part. *Liquor epispasticus*, alone or mixed with equal parts of collodion, is painted on the part with a brush. Several paintings are often required before a blister is raised. The preliminary removal of the natural grease from the skin favours the action of these applications.

The treatment of inflammation in special tissues and organs will be considered in the sections devoted to regional surgery.

Chronic Inflammation.—A variety of types of chronic and subacute inflammation are met with which, owing to ignorance of their causations, cannot at present be satisfactorily classified.

The best defined group is that of the *granulomata*, which includes such important diseases as tuberculosis and syphilis, and in which different types of chronic inflammation are caused by infection with a specific organism, all having the common character, however, that abundant granulation tissue is formed in which cellular changes are more in evidence than changes in the blood vessels, and in which the subsequent degeneration and necrosis of the granulation tissue results in the breaking down and destruction of the tissue in which it is formed. Another group is that in which chronic inflammation is due to mild or attenuated forms of pyogenic infection affecting especially the lymph glands and the bone marrow. In the glands of the groin, for example, associated with various forms of irritation about the external genitals, different types of *chronic lymphadenitis* are met with; they do not frankly suppurate as do the acute types, but are attended with a hyperplasia of the tissue elements which results in enlargement of the affected glands of a persistent, and sometimes of a relapsing character. Similar varieties of *osteomyelitis* are met with that do not, like the acute forms, go on to suppuration or to death of bone, but result in thickening of the bone affected, both on the surface and in the interior, resulting in obliteration of the medullary canal.

A third group of chronic inflammations are those that begin as an acute pyogenic inflammation, which, instead of resolving completely, persists in a chronic form. It does so apparently because there is some factor aiding the organisms and handicapping the tissues, such as the presence of a foreign body, a piece of glass or metal, or a piece of dead bone; in these circumstances the inflammation persists in a chronic form, attended with the formation of fibrous tissue, and, in the case of bone, with the formation of new bone in excess. It will be evident that in this group, chronic inflammation and repair are practically interchangeable terms.

There are other groups of chronic inflammation, the origin of which continues to be the subject of controversy. Reference is here made to the chronic inflammations of the synovial membrane of joints, of tendon sheaths and of bursæ—*chronic synovitis, teno-synovitis* and *bursitis*; of the fibrous tissues of joints—chronic forms of *arthritis*; of the blood vessels—chronic forms of *endarteritis* and of *phlebitis* and of the peripheral nerves—*neuritis*. Also in the breast and in the prostate, with the waning of sexual life there may occur a formation of fibrous tissue—chronic *interstitial mastitis, chronic prostatitis*, having analogies with the chronic interstitial inflammations of internal organs like the kidney—*chronic interstitial nephritis*; and in the breast and prostate, as in the kidney, the formation of fibrous tissue leads to changes in the secreting epithelium resulting in the formation of cysts.

Lastly, there are still other types of chronic inflammation attended with the formation of fibrous tissue on such a liberal scale as to suggest analogies with new growths. The best known of these are the systematic forms of fibromatosis met with in the central nervous system and in the peripheral nerves—*neuro-fibromatosis*; in the submucous coat of the stomach—*gastric fibromatosis*; and in the colon—*intestinal fibromatosis*.

These conditions will be described with the tissues and organs in which they occur.

In the *treatment of chronic inflammations*, pending further knowledge as to their causation, and beyond such obvious indications as to help the tissues by removing a foreign body or a piece of dead bone, there are employed— empirically—a number of procedures such as the induction of hyperæmia, exposure to the X-rays, and the employment of blisters, cauteries, and setons. Vaccines may be had recourse to in those of bacterial origin.

· IV ·

SUPPURATION

Suppuration, or the formation of pus, is one of the results of the action of bacteria on the tissues. The invading organism is usually one of the staphylococci, less frequently a streptococcus, and still less frequently one of the other bacteria capable of producing pus, such as the bacillus coli communis, the gonococcus, the pneumococcus, or the typhoid bacillus.

So long as the tissues are in a healthy condition they are able to withstand the attacks of moderate numbers of pyogenic bacteria of ordinary virulence, but when devitalised by disease, by injury, or by inflammation due to the action of other pathogenic organisms, suppuration ensues.

It would appear, for example, that pyogenic organisms can pass through the healthy urinary tract without doing any damage, but if the pelvis of the kidney, the ureter, or the bladder is the seat of stone, they give rise to suppuration. Similarly, a calculus in one of the salivary ducts frequently results in an abscess forming in the floor of the mouth. When the lumen of a tubular organ, such as the appendix or the Fallopian tube is blocked also, the action of pyogenic organisms is favoured and suppuration ensues.

Pus.—The fluid resulting from the process of suppuration is known as *pus*. In its typical form it is a yellowish creamy substance, of alkaline reaction,

45

with a specific gravity of about 1030, and it has a peculiar mawkish odour. If allowed to stand in a test-tube it does not coagulate, but separates into two layers: the upper, transparent, straw-coloured fluid, the *liquor puris* or pus serum, closely resembling blood serum in its composition, but containing less protein and more cholestrol; it also contains leucin, tyrosin, and certain albumoses which prevent coagulation.

The layer at the bottom of the tube consists for the most part of polymorph leucocytes, and proliferated connective tissue and endothelial cells (*pus corpuscles*). Other forms of leucocytes may be present, especially in long-standing suppurations; and there are usually some red corpuscles, dead bacteria, fat cells and shreds of tissue, cholestrol crystals, and other detritus in the deposit.

If a film of fresh pus is examined under the microscope, the pus cells are seen to have a well-defined rounded outline, and to contain a finely granular protoplasm and a multi-partite nucleus; if still warm, the cells may exhibit amoeboid movement. In stained films the nuclei take the stain well. In older pus cells the outline is irregular, the protoplasm coarsely granular, and the nuclei disintegrated, no longer taking the stain.

Variations from Typical Pus.—Pus from old-standing sinuses is often watery in consistence (ichorous), with few cells. Where the granulations are vascular and bleed easily, it becomes sanious from admixture with red corpuscles; while, if a blood-clot be broken down and the debris mixed with the pus, it contains granules of blood pigment and is said to be "grumous." The *odour* of pus varies with the different bacteria producing it. Pus due to ordinary pyogenic cocci has a mawkish odour; when putrefactive organisms are present it has a putrid odour; when it forms in the vicinity of the intestinal canal it usually contains the bacillus coli communis and has a fæcal odour.

The *colour* of pus also varies: when due to one or other of the varieties of the bacillus pyocyaneus, it is usually of a blue or green colour; when mixed with bile derivatives or altered blood pigment, it may be of a bright orange colour. In wounds inflicted with rough iron implements from which rust is deposited, the pus often presents the same colour.

The pus may form and collect within a circumscribed area, constituting a localised *abscess*; or it may infiltrate the tissues over a wide area—*diffuse suppuration*.

ACUTE CIRCUMSCRIBED ABSCESS

Any tissue of the body may be the seat of an acute abscess, and there are many routes by which the bacteria may gain access to the affected area. For example: an abscess in the integument or subcutaneous cellular tissue usually results from infection by organisms which have entered through a wound or abrasion of the surface, or along the ducts of the skin; an abscess in the breast from organisms which have passed along the milk ducts opening on the nipple, or along the lymphatics which accompany these. An abscess in a lymph gland is usually due to infection passing by way of the lymph channels from the area of skin or mucous membrane drained by them. Abscesses in internal organs, such as the kidney, liver, or brain, usually result from organisms carried in the blood-stream from some focus of infection elsewhere in the body.

A knowledge of the possible avenues of infection is of clinical importance, as it may enable the source of a given abscess to be traced and dealt with. In suppuration in the Fallopian tube (pyosalpynx), for example, the fact that the most common origin of the infection is in the genital passage, leads to examination for vaginal discharge; and if none is present, the abscess is probably due to infection carried in the blood-stream from some primary focus about the mouth, such as a gumboil or an infective sore throat.

The exact location of an abscess also may furnish a key to its source; in axillary abscess, for example, if the suppuration is in the lymph glands the infection has come through the afferent lymphatics; if in the cellular tissue, it has spread from the neck or chest wall; if in the hair follicles, it is a local infection through the skin.

Formation of an Abscess.—When pyogenic bacteria are introduced into the tissue there ensues an inflammatory reaction, which is characterised by dilatation of the blood vessels, exudation of large numbers of leucocytes, and proliferation of connective-tissue cells. These wandering cells soon accumulate round the focus of infection, and form a protective barrier which tends to prevent the spread of the organisms and to restrict their field of action. Within the area thus circumscribed the struggle between the bacteria and the phagocytes takes place, and in the process toxins are formed by the organisms, a certain number of the leucocytes succumb, and, becoming degenerated, set free certain proteolytic enzymes or ferments. The toxins cause coagulation-necrosis of the tissue cells with which they come in contact, the

47

ferments liquefy the exudate and other albuminous substances, and in this way *pus* is formed.

If the bacteria gain the upper hand, this process of liquefaction which is characteristic of suppuration, extends into the surrounding tissues, the protective barrier of leucocytes is broken down, and the suppurative process spreads. A fresh accession of leucocytes, however, forms a new barrier, and eventually the spread is arrested, and the collection of pus so hemmed in constitutes an *abscess*.

Owing to the swelling and condensation of the parts around, the pus thus formed is under considerable pressure, and this causes it to burrow along the lines of least resistance. In the case of a subcutaneous abscess the pus usually works its way towards the surface, and "points," as it is called. Where it approaches the surface the skin becomes soft and thin, and eventually sloughs, allowing the pus to escape.

An abscess forming in the deeper planes is prevented from pointing directly to the surface by the firm fasciæ and other fibrous structures. The pus therefore tends to burrow along the line of the blood vessels and in the connective-tissue septa, till it either finds a weak spot or causes a portion of fascia to undergo necrosis and so reaches the surface. Accordingly, many abscess cavities resulting from deep-seated suppuration are of irregular shape, with pouches and loculi in various directions—an arrangement which interferes with their successful treatment by incision and drainage.

The relief of tension which follows the bursting of an abscess, the removal of irritation by the escape of pus, and the casting off of bacteria and toxins, allow the tissues once more to assert themselves, and a process of repair sets in. The walls of the abscess fall in; granulation tissue grows into the space and gradually fills it; and later this is replaced by cicatricial tissue. As a result of the subsequent contraction of the cicatricial tissue, the scar is usually depressed below the level of the surrounding skin surface.

If an abscess is prevented from healing—for example, by the presence of a foreign body or a piece of necrosed bone—a sinus results, and from it pus escapes until the foreign body is removed.

Clinical Features of an Acute Circumscribed Abscess.—In the initial stages the usual symptoms of inflammation are present. Increased elevation of temperature, with or without a rigor, progressive leucocytosis, and sweating, mark the transition between inflammation and suppuration. An increasing leucocytosis is evidence that a suppurative process is spreading.

The local symptoms vary with the seat of the abscess. When it is situated superficially—for example, in the breast tissue—the affected area is hot, the redness of inflammation gives place to a dusky purple colour, with a pale, sometimes yellow, spot where the pus is near the surface. The swelling increases in size, the firm brawny centre becomes soft, projects as a cone beyond the level of the rest of the swollen area, and is usually surrounded by a zone of induration.

By gently palpating with the finger-tips over the softened area, a fluid wave may be detected—*fluctuation*—and when present this is a certain indication of the existence of fluid in the swelling. Its recognition, however, is by no means easy, and various fallacies are to be guarded against in applying this test clinically. When, for example, the walls of the abscess are thick and rigid, or when its contents are under excessive tension, the fluid wave cannot be elicited. On the other hand, a sensation closely resembling fluctuation may often be recognised in oedematous tissues, in certain soft, solid tumours such as fatty tumours or vascular sarcomata, in aneurysm, and in a muscle when it is palpated in its transverse axis.

When pus has formed in deeper parts, and before it has reached the surface, oedema of the overlying skin is frequently present, and the skin pits on pressure.

With the formation of pus the continuous burning or boring pain of inflammation assumes a throbbing character, with occasional sharp, lancinating twinges. Should doubt remain as to the presence of pus, recourse may be had to the use of an exploring needle.

Differential Diagnosis of Acute Abscess.—A practical difficulty which frequently arises is to decide whether or not pus has actually formed. It may be accepted as a working rule in practice that when an acute inflammation has lasted for four or five days without showing signs of abatement, suppuration has almost certainly occurred. In deep-seated suppuration, marked oedema of the skin and the occurrence of rigors and sweating may be taken to indicate the formation of pus.

There are cases on record where rapidly growing sarcomatous and angiomatous tumours, aneurysms, and the bruises that occur in hæmophylics, have been mistaken for acute abscesses and incised, with disastrous results.

Treatment of Acute Abscesses.—The dictum of John Bell, "Where there is pus, let it out," summarises the treatment of abscess. The extent and situ-

49

ation of the incision and the means taken to drain the cavity, however, vary with the nature, site, and relations of the abscess. In a superficial abscess, for example a bubo, or an abscess in the breast or face where a disfiguring scar is undesirable, a small puncture should be made where the pus threatens to point, and a Klapp's suction bell be applied as already described (p. 39). A drain is not necessary, and in the intervals between the applications of the bell the part is covered with a moist antiseptic dressing.

In abscesses deeply placed, as for example under the gluteal or pectoral muscles, one or more incisions should be made, and the cavity drained by glass or rubber tubes or by strips of rubber tissue.

The wound should be dressed the next day, and the tube shortened, in the case of a rubber tube, by cutting off a portion of its outer end. On the second day or later, according to circumstances, the tube is removed, and after this the dressing need not be repeated oftener than every second or third day.

Where pus has formed in relation to important structures—as, for example, in the deeper planes of the neck—*Hilton's method* of opening the abscess may be employed. An incision is made through the skin and fascia, a grooved director is gently pushed through the deeper tissues till pus escapes along its groove, and then the track is widened by passing in a pair of dressing forceps and expanding the blades. A tube, or strip of rubber tissue, is introduced, and the subsequent treatment carried out as in other abscesses. When the drain lies in proximity to a large blood vessel, care must be taken not to leave it in position long enough to cause ulceration of the vessel wall by pressure.

In some abscesses, such as those in the vicinity of the anus, the cavity should be laid freely open in its whole extent, stuffed with iodoform or bismuth gauze, and treated by the open method.

It is seldom advisable to wash out an abscess cavity, and squeezing out the pus is also to be avoided, lest the protective zone be broken down and the infection be diffused into the surrounding tissues.

The importance of taking precautions against further infection in opening an abscess can scarcely be exaggerated, and the rapidity with which healing occurs when the access of fresh bacteria is prevented is in marked contrast to what occurs when such precautions are neglected and further infection is allowed to take place.

Acute Suppuration in a Wound.—If in the course of an operation infection of the wound has occurred, a marked inflammatory reaction soon manifests itself, and the same changes as occur in the formation of an acute abscess take place, modified, however, by the fact that the pus can more readily reach the surface. In from twenty-four to forty-eight hours the patient is conscious of a sensation of chilliness, or may even have a rigor. At the same time he feels generally out of sorts, with impaired appetite, headache, and it may be looseness of the bowels. His temperature rises to 100° or 101° F., and the pulse quickens to 100 or 110.

On exposing the wound it is found that the parts for some distance around are red, glazed, and oedematous. The discoloration and swelling are most intense in the immediate vicinity of the wound, the edges of which are everted and moist. Any stitches that may have been introduced are tight, and the deep ones may be cutting into the tissues. There is heat, and a constant burning or throbbing pain, which is increased by pressure. If the stitches be cut, pus escapes, the wound gapes, and its surfaces are found to be inflamed and covered with pus.

The open method is the only safe means of treating such wounds. The infected surface may be sponged over with pure carbolic acid, the excess of which is washed off with absolute alcohol, and the wound either drained by tubes or packed with iodoform gauze. The practice of scraping such surfaces with the sharp spoon, squeezing or even of washing them out with antiseptic lotions, is attended with the risk of further diffusing the organisms in the tissue, and is only to be employed under exceptional circumstances. Continuous irrigation of infected wounds or their immersion in antiseptic baths is sometimes useful. The free opening up of the wound is almost immediately followed by a fall in the temperature. The surrounding inflammation subsides, the discharge of pus lessens, and healing takes place by the formation of granulation tissue—the so-called "healing by second intention."

Wound infection may take place from *catgut* which has not been efficiently prepared. The local and general reactions may be slight, and, as a rule, do not appear for seven or eight days after the operation, and, it may be, not till after the skin edges have united. The suppuration is strictly localised to the part of the wound where catgut was employed for stitches or ligatures, and shows little tendency to spread. The infected part, however, is often long of healing. The irritation in these cases is probably due to toxins in the catgut and not to bacteria.

When suppuration occurs in connection with buried sutures of unabsorbable materials, such as silk, silkworm gut, or silver wire, it is apt to persist till the foreign material is cast off or removed.

Suppuration may occur in the track of a skin stitch, producing a *stitch abscess*. The infection may arise from the material used, especially catgut or silk, or, more frequently perhaps, from the growth of staphylococcus albus from the skin of the patient when this has been imperfectly disinfected. The formation of pus under these conditions may not be attended with any of the usual signs of suppuration, and beyond some induration around the wound and a slight tenderness on pressure there may be nothing to suggest the presence of an abscess.

Acute Suppuration of a Mucous Membrane.—When pyogenic organisms gain access to a mucous membrane, such as that of the bladder, urethra, or middle ear, the usual phenomena of acute inflammation and suppuration ensue, followed by the discharge of pus on the free surface. It would appear that the most marked changes take place in the submucous tissue, causing the covering epithelium in places to die and leave small superficial ulcers, for example in gonorrhoeal urethritis, the cicatricial contraction of the scar subsequently leading to the formation of stricture. When mucous glands are present in the membrane, the pus is mixed with mucus—*muco-pus*.

DIFFUSE CELLULITIS AND DIFFUSE SUPPURATION

Cellulitis is an acute affection resulting from the introduction of some organism—commonly the *streptococcus pyogenes*—into the cellular connective tissue of the integument, intermuscular septa, tendon sheaths, or other structures. Infection always takes place through a breach of the surface, although this may be superficial and insignificant, such as a pin-prick, a scratch, or a crack under a nail, and the wound may have been healed for some time before the inflammation becomes manifest. The cellulitis, also, may develop at some distance from the seat of inoculation, the organisms having travelled by the lymphatics.

The virulence of the organisms, the loose, open nature of the tissues in which they develop, and the free lymphatic circulation by means of which they are spread, account for the diffuse nature of the process. Sometimes numbers of cocci are carried for a considerable distance from the primary area before they are arrested in the lymphatics, and thus several patches of inflammation may appear with healthy areas between.

The pus infiltrates the meshes of the cellular tissue, there is sloughing of considerable portions of tissue of low vitality, such as fat, fascia, or tendon, and if the process continues for some time several collections of pus may form.

Clinical Features.—The reaction in cases of diffuse cellulitis is severe, and is usually ushered in by a distinct chill or even a rigor, while the temperature rises to 103°, 104°, or 105° F. The pulse is proportionately increased in frequency, and is small, feeble, and often irregular. The face is flushed, the tongue dry and brown, and the patient may become delirious, especially during the night. Leucocytosis is present in cases of moderate severity; but in severe cases the virulence of the toxins prevents reaction taking place, and leucocytosis is absent.

The local manifestations vary with the relation of the seat of the inflammation to the surface. When the superficial cellular tissue is involved, the skin assumes a dark bluish-red colour, is swollen, oedematous, and the seat of burning pain. To the touch it is firm, hot, and tender. When the primary focus is in the deeper tissues, the constitutional disturbance is aggravated, while the local signs are delayed, and only become prominent when pus forms and approaches the surface. It is not uncommon for blebs containing dark serous fluid to form on the skin. The infection frequently spreads along the line of the main lymph vessels of the part (*septic lymphangitis*) and may reach the lymph glands (*septic lymphadenitis*).

With the formation of pus the skin becomes soft and boggy at several points, and eventually breaks, giving exit to a quantity of thick grumous discharge. Sometimes several small collections under the skin fuse, and an abscess is formed in which fluctuation can be detected. Occasionally gases are evolved in the tissues, giving rise to emphysema. It is common for portions of fascia, ligaments, or tendons to slough, and this may often be recognised clinically by a peculiar crunching or grating sensation transmitted to the fingers on making firm pressure on the part.

If it is not let out by incision, the pus, travelling along the lines of least resistance, tends to point at several places on the surface, or to open into joints or other cavities.

Prognosis.—The occurrence of *septicæmia* is the most serious risk, and it is in cases of diffuse suppurative cellulitis that this form of blood-poisoning assumes its most aggravated forms. The toxins of the streptococci are exceedingly virulent, and induce local death of tissue so rapidly that the protective emigration of leucocytes fails to take place. In some cases the passage of masses of free cocci in the lymphatics, or of infective emboli in the blood vessels, leads to the formation of *pyogenic abscesses* in vital organs, such as the brain, lungs, liver, kidneys, or other viscera. *Hæmorrhage* from erosion of arterial or venous trunks may take place and endanger life.

Treatment.—The treatment of diffuse cellulitis depends to a large extent on the situation and extent of the affected area, and on the stage of the process.

In the limbs, for example, where the application of a constricting band is practicable, Bier's method of inducing passive hyperæmia yields excellent results. If pus is formed, one or more small incisions are made and a light moist dressing placed over the wounds to absorb the discharge, but no drain is inserted. The whole of the inflamed area should be covered with gauze wrung out of a 1 in 10 solution of ichthyol in glycerine. The dressing is changed as often as necessary, and in the intervals when the band is off, gentle active and passive movements should be carried out to prevent the formation of adhesions. After incisions have been made, we have found the *immersion* of the limb, for a few hours at a time, in a water-bath containing warm boracic lotion or eusol a useful adjuvant to the passive hyperæmia.

Continuous irrigation of the part by a slow, steady stream of lotion, at the body temperature, such as eusol, or Dakin's solution, or boracic acid, or frequent washing with peroxide of hydrogen, has been found of value.

A suitably arranged splint adds to the comfort of the patient; and the limb should be placed in the attitude which, in the event of stiffness resulting, will least interfere with its usefulness. The elbow, for example, should be flexed to a little less than a right angle; at the wrist, the hand should be dorsiflexed and the fingers flexed slightly towards the palm.

Massage, passive movement, hot and cold douching, and other measures, may be necessary to get rid of the chronic ocdema, adhesions of tendons, and stiffness of joints which sometimes remain.

In situations where a constricting band cannot be applied, for example, on the trunk or the neck, Klapp's suction bells may be used, small incisions being made to admit of the escape of pus.

If these measures fail or are impracticable, it may be necessary to make one or more free incisions, and to insert drainage-tubes, portions of rubber dam, or iodoform worsted.

The general treatment of toxæmia must be carried out, and in cases due to infection by streptococci, anti-streptococcic serum may be used.

In a few cases, amputation well above the seat of disease, by removing the source of toxin production, offers the only means of saving the patient.

WHITLOW

The clinical term whitlow is applied to an acute infection, usually followed by suppuration, commonly met with in the fingers, less frequently in the toes. The point of infection is often trivial—a pin-prick, a puncture caused by a splinter of wood, a scratch, or even an imperceptible lesion of the skin.

Several varieties of whitlow are recognised, but while it is convenient to describe them separately, it is to be clearly understood that clinically they merge one into another, and it is not always possible to determine in which connective-tissue plane a given infection has originated.

Initial Stage.—Attention is usually first attracted to the condition by a sensation of tightness in the finger and tenderness when the part is squeezed or knocked against anything. In the course of a few hours the part becomes red and swollen; there is continuous pain, which soon assumes a throbbing character, particularly when the hand is dependent, and may be so severe as to prevent sleep, and the patient may feel generally out of sorts.

If a constricting band is applied at this stage, the infection can usually be checked and the occurrence of suppuration prevented. If this fails, or if the condition is allowed to go untreated, the inflammatory reaction increases and terminates in suppuration, giving rise to one or other of the forms of whitlow to be described.

The Purulent Blister.—In the most superficial variety, pus forms between the rete Malpighii and the stratum corneum of the skin, the latter being raised as a blister in which fluctuation can be detected (Fig. 9, a). This is commonly met with in the palm of the hand of labouring men who have recently resumed work after a spell of idleness. When the blister forms near the tip of the finger, the pus burrows under the nail—which corresponds to the stratum corneum—raising it from its bed.

There is some local heat and discoloration, and considerable pain and tenderness, but little or no constitutional disturbance. Superficial lymphangitis may extend a short distance up the forearm. By clipping away the raised epidermis, and if necessary the nail, the pus is allowed to escape, and healing speedily takes place.

Whitlow at the Nail Fold.—This variety, which is met with among those who handle septic material, occurs in the sulcus between the nail and the skin, and is due to the introduction of infective matter at the root of the nail (Fig. 9, b). A small focus of suppuration forms under the nail, with swelling and redness of the nail fold, causing intense pain and discomfort, interfering with sleep, and producing a constitutional reaction out of all proportion to the local lesion.

To allow the pus to escape, it is necessary, under local anæsthesia, to cut away the nail fold as well as the portion of nail in the infected area, or, it may be, to remove the nail entirely. If only a small opening is made in the nail it is apt to be blocked by granulations.

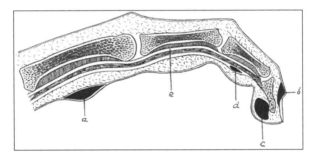

FIG. 9. Diagram of various forms of Whitlow.
a = Purulent blister.
b = Suppuration at nail fold.
c = Subcutaneous whitlow.
d = Whitlow in sheath of flexor tendon (e).

Subcutaneous Whitlow.—In this variety the infection manifests itself as a cellulitis of the pulp of the finger (Fig. 9, c), which sometimes spreads towards the palm of the hand. The finger becomes red, swollen, and tense; there is severe throbbing pain, which is usually worst at night and prevents sleep, and the part is extremely tender on pressure. When the palm is invaded there may be marked oedema of the back of the hand, the dense integument of the palm preventing the swelling from appearing on the front. The pus may be under such tension that fluctuation cannot be detected. The patient is usually able to flex the finger to a certain extent without increasing the pain—a point which indicates that the tendon sheaths have not been invaded. The suppurative process may, however, spread to the tendon sheaths, or even to the bone. Sometimes the excessive tension and virulent toxins induce actual gangrene of the distal part, or even of the whole finger. There is considerable constitutional disturbance, the temperature often reaching 101° or 102° F.

The treatment consists in applying a constriction band and making an incision over the centre of the most tender area, care being taken to avoid opening the tendon sheath lest the infection be conveyed to it. Moist dressings should be employed while the suppuration lasts. Carbolic fomentations, however, are to be avoided on account of the risk of inducing gangrene.

Whitlow of the Tendon Sheaths.—In this form the main incidence of the infection is on the sheaths of the flexor tendons, but it is not always possible to determine whether it started there or spread thither from the subcutaneous cellular tissue (Fig. 9, d). In some cases both connective tissue planes are involved. The affected finger becomes red, painful, and swollen, the swelling spreading to the dorsum. The involvement of the tendon sheath is usually indicated by the patient being unable to flex the finger, and by the pain being increased when he attempts to do so. On account of the anatomical arrangement of the tendon sheaths, the process may spread into the forearm—directly in the case of the thumb and little finger, and after invading the palm in the case of the other fingers—and there give rise to a diffuse cellulitis which may result in sloughing of fasciæ and tendons. When the infection spreads into the common flexor sheath under the transverse carpal (anterior annular) ligament, it is not uncommon for the intercarpal and wrist joints to become implicated. Impaired movement of tendons and joints is, therefore, a common sequel to this variety of whitlow.

The *treatment* consists in inducing passive hyperæmia by Bier's method, and, if this is done early, suppuration may be avoided. If pus forms, small incisions are made, under local anæsthesia, to relieve the tension in the sheath and to diminish the risk of the tendons sloughing. No form of drain should be inserted. In the fingers the incisions should be made in the middle line, and in the palm they should be made over the metacarpal bones to avoid the digital vessels and nerves. If pus has spread under the transverse carpal ligament, the incision must be made above the wrist. Passive movements and massage must be commenced as early as possible and be perseveringly employed to diminish the formation of adhesions and resulting stiffness.

Subperiosteal Whitlow.—This form is usually an extension of the subcutaneous or of the thecal variety, but in some cases the inflammation begins in the periosteum—usually of the terminal phalanx. It may lead to necrosis of a portion or even of the entire phalanx. This is usually recognised by the persistence of suppuration long after the acute symptoms have passed off, and by feeling bare bone with the probe. In such cases one or more of the joints are usually implicated also, and lateral mobility and grating may be elicited. Recovery does not take place until the dead bone is removed, and the usefulness of the finger is often seriously impaired by fibrous or bony ankylosis of the interphalangeal joints. This may render amputation advisable when a stiff finger is likely to interfere with the patient's occupation.

SUPPURATIVE CELLULITIS IN DIFFERENT SITUATIONS

Cellulitis of the forearm is usually a sequel to one of the deeper varieties of whitlow.

In the *region of the elbow-joint*, cellulitis is common around the olecranon. It may originate as an inflammation of the olecranon bursa, or may invade the bursa secondarily. In exceptional cases the elbow-joint is also involved.

Cellulitis of the *axilla* may originate in suppuration in the lymph glands, following an infected wound of the hand, or it may spread from a septic wound on the chest wall or in the neck. In some cases it is impossible to discover the primary seat of infection. A firm, brawny swelling forms in the armpit and extends on to the chest wall. It is attended with great pain, which is increased on moving the arm, and there is marked constitutional disturbance. When suppuration occurs, its spread is limited by the attachments of the axillary fascia, and the pus tends to burrow on to the chest wall beneath the pectoral muscles, and upwards towards the shoulder-joint, which may become infected. When the pus forms in the axillary space, the treatment consists in making free incisions, which should be placed on the thoracic side of the axilla to avoid the axillary vessels and nerves. If the pus spreads on to the chest wall, the abscess should be opened below the clavicle by Hilton's method, and a counter opening may be made in the axilla.

Cellulitis of the *sole of the foot* may follow whitlow of the toes.

In the *region of the ankle* cellulitis is not common; but *around the knee* it frequently occurs in relation to the prepatellar bursa and to the popliteal lymph glands, and may endanger the knee-joint. It is also met with in the *groin* following on inflammation and suppuration of the inguinal glands, and cases are recorded in which the sloughing process has implicated the femoral vessels and led to secondary hæmorrhage.

Cellulitis of the scalp, orbit, neck, pelvis, and perineum will be considered with the diseases of these regions.

CHRONIC SUPPURATION

While it is true that a chronic pyogenic abscess is sometimes met with—for example, in the breast and in the marrow of long bones—in the great majority of instances the formation of a chronic or cold abscess is the result of the action of the tubercle bacillus. It is therefore more convenient to study this form of suppuration with tuberculosis (p. 139).

SINUS AND FISTULA

Sinus.—A sinus is a track leading from a focus of suppuration to a cutaneous or mucous surface. It usually represents the path by which the discharge escapes from an abscess cavity that has been prevented from closing completely, either from mechanical causes or from the persistent formation of discharge which must find an exit. A sinus is lined by granulation tissue, and when it is of long standing the opening may be dragged below the level of the surrounding skin by contraction of the scar tissue around it. As a sinus will persist until the obstacle to closure of the original abscess is removed, it is necessary that this should be sought for. It may be a foreign body, such as a piece of dead bone, an infected ligature, or a bullet, acting mechanically or by keeping up discharge, and if the body is removed the sinus usually heals. The presence of a foreign body is often suggested by a mass of redundant granulations at the mouth of the sinus. If a sinus passes through a muscle, the repeated contractions tend to prevent healing until the muscle is kept at rest by a splint, or put out of action by division of its fibres. The sinuses associated with empyema are prevented from healing by the rigidity of the chest wall, and will only close after an operation which admits of the cavity being obliterated. In any case it is necessary to disinfect the track, and, it may be, to remove the unhealthy granulations lining it, by means of the sharp spoon, or to excise it bodily. To encourage healing from the bottom the cavity should be packed with bismuth or iodoform gauze. The healing of long and tortuous sinuses is often hastened by the injection of Beck's bismuth paste (p. 145). If disfigurement is likely to follow from cicatricial contraction—for example, in a sinus over the lower jaw associated with a carious tooth—the sinus should be excised and the raw surfaces approximated with stitches.

The *tuberculous sinus* is described under Tuberculosis.

A **fistula** is an abnormal canal passing from a mucous surface to the skin or to another mucous surface. Fistulæ resulting from suppuration usually occur near the natural openings of mucous canals—for example, on the cheek, as a salivary fistula; beside the inner angle of the eye, as a lacrymal fistula; near the ear, as a mastoid fistula; or close to the anus, as a fistula-in-ano. Intestinal fistulæ are sometimes met with in the abdominal wall after strangulated hernia, operations for appendicitis, tuberculous peritonitis, and other conditions. In the perineum, fistulæ frequently complicate stricture of the urethra.

Fistulæ also occur between the bladder and vagina (*vesico-vaginal fistula*), or between the bladder and the rectum (*recto-vesical fistula*).

The *treatment* of these various forms of fistula will be described in the sections dealing with the regions in which they occur.

Congenital fistulæ, such as occur in the neck from imperfect closure of branchial clefts, or in the abdomen from unobliterated foetal ducts such as the urachus or Meckel's diverticulum, will be described in their proper places.

CONSTITUTIONAL MANIFESTATIONS OF PYOGENIC INFECTION

We have here to consider under the terms Sapræmia, Septicæmia, and Pyæmia certain general effects of pyogenic infection, which, although their clinical manifestations may vary, are all associated with the action of the same forms of bacteria. They may occur separately or in combination, or one may follow on and merge into another.

Sapræmia, or septic intoxication, is the name applied to a form of poisoning resulting from the absorption into the blood of the toxic products of pyogenic bacteria. These products, which are of the nature of alkaloids, act immediately on their entrance into the circulation, and produce effects in direct proportion to the amount absorbed. As the toxins are gradually eliminated from the body the symptoms abate, and if no more are introduced they disappear. Sapræmia in these respects, therefore, is comparable to poisoning by any other form of alkaloid, such as strychnin or morphin.

Clinical Features.—The symptoms of sapræmia seldom manifest themselves within twenty-four hours of an operation or injury, because it takes some time for the bacteria to produce a sufficient dose of their poisons. The onset of the condition is marked by a feeling of chilliness, sometimes amounting to a rigor, and a rise of temperature to 102°, 103°, or 104° F., with morning remissions (Fig. 10). The heart's action is markedly depressed, and the pulse is soft and compressible. The appetite is lost, the tongue dry and covered with a thin brownish-red fur, so that it has the appearance of "dried beef." The urine is scanty and loaded with urates. In severe cases diarrhoea and vomiting of dark coffee-ground material are often prominent features. Death is usually impending when the skin becomes cold and clammy, the mucous membranes livid, the pulse feeble and fluttering, the discharges involuntary, and when a low form of muttering delirium is present.

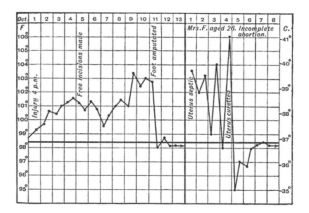

FIG. 10. Charts of Acute sapræmia from (a) case of crushed foot, and (b) case of incomplete abortion.

A local form of septic infection is always present—it may be an abscess, an infected compound fracture, or an infection of the cavity of the uterus, for example, from a retained portion of placenta.

Treatment.—The first indication is the immediate and complete removal of the infected material. The wound must be freely opened, all blood-clot, discharge, or necrosed tissue removed, and the area disinfected by washing with sterilised salt solution, peroxide of hydrogen, or eusol. Stronger lotions are to be avoided as being likely to depress the tissues, and so interfere with protective phagocytosis. On account of its power of neutralising toxins, iodoform is useful in these cases, and is best employed by packing the wound with iodoform gauze, and treating it by the open method, if this is possible.

The general treatment is carried out on the same lines as for other infective conditions.

Chronic sapræmia or Hectic Fever.—Hectic fever differs from acute sapræmia merely in degree. It usually occurs in connection with tuberculous conditions, such as bone or joint disease, psoas abscess, or empyema, which have opened externally, and have thereby become infected with pyogenic organisms. It is gradual in its development, and is of a mild type throughout.

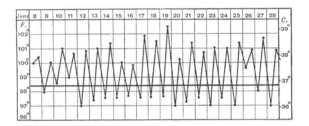

FIG. 11. Chart of Hectic Fever.

The pulse is small, feeble, and compressible, and the temperature rises in the afternoon or evening to 102° or 103° F. (Fig. 11), the cheeks becoming characteristically flushed. In the early morning the temperature falls to normal or below it, and the patient breaks into a profuse perspiration, which leaves him pale, weak, and exhausted. He becomes rapidly and markedly emaciated, even although in some cases the appetite remains good and is even voracious.

The poisons circulating in the blood produce *waxy degeneration* in certain viscera, notably the liver, spleen, kidneys, and intestines. The process begins in the arterial walls, and spreads thence to the connective-tissue structures, causing marked enlargement of the affected organs. Albuminuria, ascites, oedema of the lower limbs, clubbing of the fingers, and diarrhoea are among the most prominent symptoms of this condition.

The *prognosis* in hectic fever depends on the completeness with which the further absorption of toxins can be prevented. In many cases this can only be effected by an operation which provides for free drainage, and, if possible, the removal of infected tissues. The resulting wound is best treated by the open method. Even advanced waxy degeneration does not contra-indicate this line of treatment, as the diseased organs usually recover if the focus from which absorption of toxic material is taking place is completely eradicated.

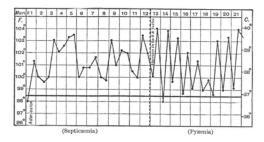

FIG. 12. Chart of case of Septicæmia followed by Pyæmia.

Septicæmia.—This form of blood-poisoning is the result of the action of pyogenic bacteria, which not only produce their toxins at the primary seat of infection, but themselves enter the blood-stream and are carried to other parts, where they settle and produce further effects.

Clinical Features.—There may be an incubation period of some hours between the infection and the first manifestation of acute septicæmia. In such conditions as acute osteomyelitis or acute peritonitis, we see the most typical clinical pictures of this condition. The onset is marked by a chill, or a rigor, which may be repeated, while the temperature rises to 103° or 104° F., although in very severe cases the temperature may remain subnormal throughout, the virulence of the toxins preventing reaction. It is in the general appearance of the patient and in the condition of the pulse that we have our best guides as to the severity of the condition. If the pulse remains firm, full, and regular, and does not exceed 110 or even 120, while the temperature is moderately raised, the outlook is hopeful; but when the pulse becomes small and compressible, and reaches 130 or more, especially if at the same time the temperature is low, a grave prognosis is indicated. The tongue is often dry and coated with a black crust down the centre, while the sides are red. It is a good omen when the tongue becomes moist again. Thirst is most distressing, especially in septicæmia of intestinal origin. Persistent vomiting of dark-brown material is often present, and diarrhoea with blood-stained stools is not uncommon. The urine is small in amount, and contains a large proportion of urates. As the poisons accumulate, the respiration becomes shallow and laboured, the face of a dull ashy grey, the nose pinched, and the skin cold and clammy. Capillary hæmorrhages sometimes take place in the skin or mucous membranes; and in a certain proportion of cases cutaneous eruptions simulating those of scarlet fever or measles appear, and are apt to lead to errors in diagnosis. In other cases there is slight jaundice. The mental state is often one of complete apathy, the patient failing to realise the gravity of his condition; sometimes there is delirium.

The *prognosis* is always grave, and depends on the possibility of completely eradicating the focus of infection, and on the reserve force the patient has to carry him over the period during which he is eliminating the poison already circulating in his blood.

The *treatment* is carried out on the same lines as in sapræmia, but it is less likely to be successful owing to the organisms having entered the circulation. When possible, the primary focus of infection should be dealt with.

Pyæmia is a form of blood-poisoning characterised by the development of secondary foci of suppuration in different parts of the body. Toxins are thus introduced into the blood, not only at the primary seat of infection, but also from each of these metastatic collections. Like septicæmia, this condition is due to pyogenic bacteria, the *streptococcus pyogenes* being the commonest organism found. The primary infection is usually in a wound—for example, a compound fracture—but cases occur in which the point of entrance of the bacteria is not discoverable. The dissemination of the organisms takes place through the medium of infected emboli which form in a thrombosed vein in the vicinity of the original lesion, and, breaking loose, are carried thence in the blood-stream. These emboli lodge in the minute vessels of the lungs, spleen, liver, kidneys, pleura, brain, synovial membranes, or cellular tissue, and the bacteria they contain give rise to secondary foci of suppuration. Secondary abscesses are thus formed in those parts, and these in turn may be the starting-point of new emboli which give rise to fresh areas of pus formation. The organs above named are the commonest situations of pyæmic abscesses, but these may also occur in the bone marrow, the substance of muscles, the heart and pericardium, lymph glands, subcutaneous tissue, or, in fact, in any tissue of the body. Organisms circulating in the blood are prone to lodge on the valves of the heart and give rise to endocarditis.

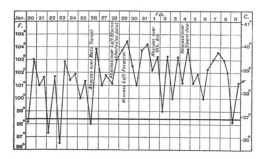

FIG. 13. Chart of Pyæmia following on Acute Osteomyelitis.

Clinical Features.—Before antiseptic surgery was practised, pyæmia was a common complication of wounds. In the present day it is not only infinitely less common, but appears also to be of a less severe type. Its rarity and its mildness may be related as cause and effect, because it was formerly found that pyæmia contracted from a pyæmic patient was more virulent than that from other sources.

In contrast with sapræmia and septicæmia, pyæmia is late of developing, and it seldom begins within a week of the primary infection. The first sign is a feeling of chilliness, or a violent rigor lasting for perhaps half an hour, during which time the temperature rises to 103°, 104°, or 105° F. In the course of an hour it begins to fall again, and the patient breaks into a profuse sweat. The temperature may fall several degrees, but seldom reaches the normal. In a few days there is a second rigor with rise of temperature, and another remission, and such attacks may be repeated at diminishing intervals during the course of the illness (Figs. 12 and 13). The pulse is soft, and tends to remain abnormally rapid even when the temperature falls nearly to normal.

The face is flushed, and wears a drawn, anxious expression, and the eyes are bright. A characteristic sweetish odour, which has been compared to that of new-mown hay, can be detected in the breath and may pervade the patient. The appetite is lost; there may be sickness and vomiting and profuse diarrhoea; and the patient emaciates rapidly. The skin is continuously hot, and has often a peculiar pungent feel. Patches of erythema sometimes appear scattered over the body. The skin may assume a dull sallow or earthy hue, or a bright yellow icteric tint may appear. The conjunctivæ also may be yellow. In the latter stages of the disease the pulse becomes small and fluttering; the tongue becomes dry and brown; sordes collect on the teeth; and a low muttering form of delirium supervenes.

Secondary infection of the parotid gland frequently occurs, and gives rise to a suppurative parotitis. This condition is associated with severe pain, gradually extending from behind the angle of the jaw on to the face. There is also swelling over the gland, and eventually suppuration and sloughing of the gland tissue and overlying skin.

Secondary abscesses in the lymph glands, subcutaneous tissue, or joints are often so insidious and painless in their development that they are only discovered accidentally. When the abscess is evacuated, healing often takes place with remarkable rapidity, and with little impairment of function.

The general symptoms may be simulated by an attack of malaria.

Prognosis.—The prognosis in acute pyæmia is much less hopeless than it once was, a considerable proportion of the patients recovering. In acute cases the disease proves fatal in ten days or a fortnight, death being due to toxæmia. Chronic cases often run a long course, lasting for weeks or even months, and prove fatal from exhaustion and waxy disease following on prolonged suppuration.

Treatment.—In such conditions as compound fractures and severe lacerated wounds, much can be done to avert the conditions which lead to pyæmia, by applying a Bier's constricting bandage as soon as there is evidence of infection having taken place, or even if there is reason to suspect that the wound is not aseptic.

If sepsis is already established, and evidence of general infection is present, the wound should be opened up sufficiently to admit of thorough disinfection and drainage, and the constricting bandage applied to aid the defensive processes going on in the tissues. If these measures fail, amputation of the limb may be the only means of preventing further dissemination of infective material from the primary source of infection.

Attempts have been made to interrupt the channel along which the infective emboli spread, by ligating or resecting the main vein of the affected part, but this is seldom feasible except in the case of the internal jugular vein for infection of the transverse sinus.

Secondary abscesses must be aspirated or opened and drained whenever possible.

The general treatment is conducted on the same lines as on other forms of pyogenic infection.

· V ·

ULCERATION AND ULCERS

The process of *ulceration* may be defined as the molecular or cellular death of tissue taking place on a free surface. It is essentially of the same nature as the process of suppuration, only that the purulent discharge, instead of collecting in a closed cavity and forming an abscess, at once escapes on the surface.

An *ulcer* is an open wound or sore in which there are present certain conditions tending to prevent it undergoing the natural process of repair. Of these, one of the most important is the presence of pathogenic bacteria, which by their action not only prevent healing, but so irritate and destroy the tissues as to lead to an actual increase in the size of the sore. Interference with the nutrition of a part by oedema or chronic venous congestion may impede healing; as may also induration of the surrounding area, by preventing the contraction which is such an important factor in repair. Defective innervation, such as occurs in injuries and diseases of the spinal cord, also plays an important part in delaying repair. In certain constitutional conditions, too—for example, Bright's disease, diabetes, or syphilis—the vitiated state of the tissues is an impediment to repair. Mechanical causes, such as unsuitable dressings or ill-fitting appliances, may also act in the same direction.

Clinical Examination of an Ulcer.—In examining any ulcer, we observe—
(1) Its *base* or *floor*, noting the presence or absence of granulations, their dis-

position, size, colour, vascularity, and whether they are depressed or elevated in relation to the surrounding parts. (2) The *discharge* as to quantity, consistence, colour, composition, and odour. (3) The *edges*, noting particularly whether or not the marginal epithelium is attempting to grow over the surface; also their shape, regularity, thickness, and whether undermined or overlapping, everted or depressed. (4) The *surrounding tissues*, as to whether they are congested, oedematous, inflamed, indurated, or otherwise. (5) Whether or not there is *pain* or tenderness in the raw surface or its surroundings. (6) The *part of the body* on which it occurs, because certain ulcers have special seats of election—for example, the varicose ulcer in the lower third of the leg, the perforating ulcer on the sole of the foot, and so on.

The Healing Sore.—If a portion of skin be excised aseptically, and no attempt made to close the wound, the raw surface left is soon covered over with a layer of coagulated blood and lymph. In the course of a few days this is replaced by the growth of *granulations*, which are of uniform size, of a pinkish-red colour, and moist with a slight serous exudate containing a few dead leucocytes. They grow until they reach the level of the surrounding skin, and so fill the gap with a fine velvety mass of granulation tissue. At the edges, the young epithelium may be seen spreading in over the granulations as a fine bluish-white pellicle, which gradually covers the sore, becoming paler in colour as it thickens, and eventually forming the smooth, non-vascular covering of the cicatrix. There is no pain, and the surrounding parts are healthy.

This may be used as a type with which to compare the ulcers seen at the bedside, so that we may determine how far, and in what particulars, these differ from the type; and that we may in addition recognise the conditions that have to be counteracted before the characters of the typical healing sore are assumed.

For purposes of contrast we may indicate the characters of an open sore in which bacterial infection with pathogenic bacteria has taken place. The layer of coagulated blood and lymph becomes liquefied and is thrown off, and instead of granulations being formed, the tissues exposed on the floor of the ulcer are destroyed by the bacterial toxins, with the formation of minute sloughs and a quantity of pus.

The discharge is profuse, thin, acrid, and offensive, and consists of pus, broken-down blood-clot, and sloughs. The edges are inflamed, irregular, and ragged, showing no sign of growing epithelium—on the contrary, the sore may be actually increasing in area by the breaking-down of the tissues at its margins. The surrounding parts are hot, red, swollen, and oedematous; and there is pain and tenderness both in the sore itself and in the parts around.

Classification of Ulcers.—The nomenclature of ulcers is much involved and gives rise to great confusion, chiefly for the reason that no one basis of classification has been adopted. Thus some ulcers are named according to the causes at work in producing or maintaining them—for example, the traumatic, the septic, and the varicose ulcer; some from the constitutional element present, as the gouty and the diabetic ulcer; and others according to the condition in which they happen to be when seen by the surgeon, such as the weak, the inflamed, and the callous ulcer.

So long as we retain these names it will be impossible to find a single basis for classification; and yet many of the terms are so descriptive and so generally understood that it is undesirable to abolish them. We must therefore remain content with a clinical arrangement of ulcers,—it cannot be called a classification,—considering any given ulcer from two points of view: first its *cause*, and second its *present condition*. This method of studying ulcers has the practical advantage that it furnishes us with the main indications for treatment as well as for diagnosis: the cause must be removed, and the condition so modified as to convert the ulcer into an aseptic healing sore.

A. Arrangement of Ulcers according to their Cause.—Although any given ulcer may be due to a combination of causes, it is convenient to describe the following groups:

Ulcers due to Traumatism.—Traumatism in the form of a *crush* or *bruise* is a frequent cause of ulcer formation, acting either by directly destroying the skin, or by so diminishing its vitality that it is rendered a suitable soil for bacteria. If these gain access, in the course of a few days the damaged area of skin becomes of a greyish colour, blebs form on it, and it undergoes necrosis, leaving an unhealthy raw surface when the slough separates.

Heat and *prolonged exposure to the Röntgen rays* or *to radium emanations* act in a similar way.

The *pressure* of improperly padded splints or other appliances may so far interfere with the circulation of the part pressed upon, that the skin sloughs, leaving an open sore. This is most liable to occur in patients who suffer from some nerve lesion—such as anterior poliomyelitis, or injury of the spinal cord or nerve-trunks. Splint-pressure sores are usually situated over bony prominences, such as the malleoli, the condyles of the femur or humerus, the head of the fibula, the dorsum of the foot, or the base of the fifth metatarsal bone. On removing the splint, the skin of the part pressed upon is found to be of a red or pink colour, with a pale grey patch in the centre, which eventually sloughs and leaves an ulcer. Certain forms of *bed-sore* are also due to prolonged pressure.

Pressure sores are also known to have been produced artificially by malingerers and hysterical subjects.

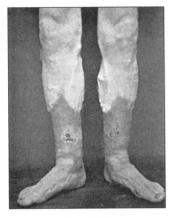

FIG. 14. Leg Ulcers associated with Varicose Veins and Pigmentation of the Skin.

Ulcers due to Imperfect Circulation.—Imperfect circulation is an important causative factor in ulceration, especially when it is the *venous return* that is defective. This is best illustrated in the so-called *leg ulcer*, which occurs most frequently on the front and medial aspect of the lower third of the leg. At this point the anastomosis between the superficial and deep veins of the leg is less free than elsewhere, so that the extra stress thrown upon the surface veins interferes with the nutrition of the skin (Hilton). The importance of imperfect venous return in the causation of such ulcers is evidenced by the fact that as soon as the condition of the circulation is improved by confining the patient to bed and elevating the limb, the ulcer begins to heal, even although all methods of local treatment have hitherto proved ineffectual. In a considerable number of cases, but by no means in all, this form of ulcer is associated with the presence of varicose veins, and in such cases it is spoken of as the *varicose ulcer* (Fig. 14). The presence of varicose veins is frequently associated with a diffuse brownish or bluish pigmentation of the skin of the lower third of the leg, or with an obstinate form of dermatitis (*varicose eczema*), and the scratching or rubbing of the part is liable to cause a breach of the surface and permit of infection which leads to ulceration. Varicose ulcers may also originate from the bursting of a small peri-phlebitic abscess.

Varicose veins in immediate relation to the base of a large chronic ulcer usually become thrombosed, and in time are reduced to fibrous cords, and therefore in such cases hæmorrhage is not a common complication. In smaller and more superficial ulcers, however, the destructive process is liable to implicate the wall of the vessel before the occurrence of thrombosis, and to lead to profuse and it may be dangerous bleeding.

These ulcers are at first small and superficial, but from want of care, from continued standing or walking, or from injudicious treatment, they gradually become larger and deeper. They are not infrequently multiple, and this, together with their depth, may lead to their being mistaken for ulcers due to syphilis. The base of the ulcer is covered with imperfectly formed, soft, oedematous granulations, which give off a thin sero-purulent discharge. The edges are slightly inflamed, and show no evidence of healing. The parts around are usually pigmented and slightly oedematous, and as a rule there is little pain. This variety of ulcer is particularly prone to pass into the condition known as callous.

In *anæmic* patients, especially young girls, ulcers are occasionally met with which have many of the clinical characters of those associated with imperfect venous return. They are slow to heal, and tend to pass into the condition known as weak.

Ulcers due to Interference with Nerve-Supply.—Any interference with the nerve-supply of the superficial tissues predisposes to ulceration. For example, *trophic* ulcers are liable to occur in injuries or diseases of the spinal cord, in cerebral paralysis, in limbs weakened by poliomyelitis, in ascending or peripheral neuritis, or after injuries of nerve-trunks.

The *acute bed-sore* is a rapidly progressing form of ulceration, often amounting to gangrene, of portions of skin exposed to pressure when their trophic nerve-supply has been interfered with.

The *perforating ulcer of the foot* is a peculiar type of sore which occurs in association with the different forms of peripheral neuritis, and with various lesions of the brain and spinal cord, such as general paralysis, locomotor ataxia, or syringo-myelia (Fig. 15). It also occurs in patients suffering from glycosuria, and is usually associated with arterio-sclerosis—local or general. Perforating ulcer is met with most frequently under the head of the metatarsal bone of the great toe. A callosity forms and suppura-

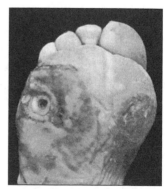

FIG. 15. Perforating Ulcers of Sole of Foot. (From Photograph lent by Sir Montagu Cotterill.)

tion occurs under it, the pus escaping through a small hole in the centre. The process slowly and gradually spreads deeper and deeper, till eventually the bone or joint is reached, and becomes implicated in the destructive process—hence the term "perforating ulcer." The flexor tendons are sometimes destroyed, the toe being dorsiflexed by the unopposed extensors. The depth of the track being so disproportionate to its superficial area, the condition closely simulates a tuberculous sinus, for which it is liable to be mistaken. The raw surface is absolutely insensitive, so that the probe can be freely employed without the patient even being aware of it or suffering the least discomfort—a significant fact in diagnosis. The cavity is filled with effete and decomposing epidermis, which has a most offensive odour. The chronic and intractable character of the ulcer is due to interference with the trophic nerve-supply of the parts, and to the fact that the epithelium of the skin grows in and lines the track leading down to the deepest part of the ulcer and so prevents closure. While they are commonest on the sole of the foot and other parts subjected to pressure, perforating ulcers are met with on the sides and dorsum of the foot and toes, on the hands, and on other parts where no pressure has been exerted.

The *tuberculous ulcer*, so often seen in the neck, in the vicinity of joints, or over the ribs and sternum, usually results from the bursting through the skin of a tuberculous abscess. The base is soft, pale, and covered with feeble granulations and grey shreddy sloughs. The edges are of a dull blue or purple colour, and gradually thin out towards their free margins, and in addition are characteristically undermined, so that a probe can be passed for some distance between the floor of the ulcer and the thinned-out edges. Thin, devitalised tags of skin often stretch from side to side of the ulcer. The outline is irregular; small perforations often occur through the skin, and a thin, watery discharge, containing grey shreds of tuberculous debris, escapes.

Bazin's Disease.—This term is applied to an affection of the skin and subcutaneous tissue which bears certain resemblances to tuberculosis. It is met with almost exclusively between

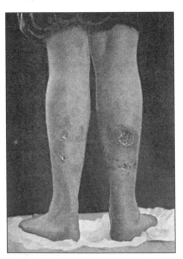

FIG. 16. Bazin's Disease in a girl æt. 16.

the knee and the ankle, and it usually affects both legs. It is commonest in girls of delicate constitution, in whose family history there is evidence of a tuberculous taint. The patient often presents other lesions of a tuberculous character, notably enlarged cervical glands, and phlyctenular ophthalmia. The tubercle bacillus has rarely been found, but we have always observed characteristic epithelioid cells and giant cells in sections made from the edge or floor of the ulcer.

The condition begins by the formation in the skin and subcutaneous tissue of dusky or livid nodules of induration, which soften and ulcerate, forming small open sores with ragged and undermined edges, not unlike those resulting from the breaking down of superficial syphilitic gummata (Fig. 16). Fresh crops of nodules appear in the neighbourhood of the ulcers, and in turn break down. While in the nodular stage the affection is sometimes painful, but with the formation of the ulcer the pain subsides.

The disease runs a chronic course, and may slowly extend over a wide area in spite of the usual methods of treatment. After lasting for some months, or even years, however, it may eventually undergo spontaneous cure. The most satisfactory treatment is to excise the affected tissues and fill the gap with skin-grafts.

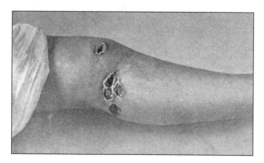

FIG. 17. Syphilitic Ulcers in region of Knee, showing punched-out appearance and raised indurated edges.

The *syphilitic ulcer* is usually formed by the breaking down of a cutaneous or subcutaneous gumma in the tertiary stage of syphilis. When the gummatous tissue is first exposed by the destruction of the skin or mucous membrane covering it, it appears as a tough greyish slough, compared to "wash leather," which slowly separates and leaves a more or less circular, deep, punched-out gap which shows a few feeble unhealthy granulations and small sloughs on its floor. The edges are raised and indurated; and the discharge is thick, glairy, and peculiarly offensive. The parts around the ulcer are congested and of a dark brown colour. There are usually several such ulcers together, and as they tend to heal at one part while they spread at another, the affected area assumes a sinuous or serpiginous outline. Syphilitic ulcers may be met with in any part of the body, but are most frequent in the upper part of the leg (Fig. 17), especially around the knee-joint in women, and over the ribs and sternum. On healing, they usually leave a depressed and adherent cicatrix.

The *scorbutic ulcer* occurs in patients suffering from scurvy, and is characterised by its prominent granulations, which show a marked tendency to bleed, with the formation of clots, which dry and form a spongy crust on the surface.

In *gouty* patients small ulcers which are exceedingly irritable and painful are liable to occur.

Ulcers associated with Malignant Disease.—Cancer and sarcoma when situated in the subcutaneous tissue may destroy the overlying skin so that the substance of the tumour is exposed. The fungating masses thus produced are sometimes spoken of as malignant ulcers, but as they are essentially different in their nature from all other forms of ulcers, and call for totally different treatment, it is best to consider them along with the tumours with which they are associated. Rodent ulcer, which is one form of cancer of the skin, will be discussed with new growths of the skin.

B. **Arrangement of Ulcers according to their Condition.**—Having arrived at an opinion as to the cause of a given ulcer, and placed it in one or other of the preceding groups, the next question to ask is, In what condition do I find this ulcer at the present moment?

Any ulcer is in one of three states—healing, stationary, or spreading; although it is not uncommon to find healing going on at one part while the destructive process is extending at another.

The Healing Condition.—The process of healing in an ulcer has already been studied, and we have learned that it takes place by the formation of granulation tissue, which becomes converted into connective tissue, and is covered over by epithelium growing in from the edges.

Those ulcers which are *stationary*—that is, neither healing nor spreading—may be in one of several conditions.

The Weak Condition.—Any ulcer may get into a weak state from receiving a blood supply which is defective either in quantity or in quality. The granulations are small and smooth, and of a pale yellow or grey colour, the discharge is small in amount, and consists of thin serum and a few pus cells, and as this dries on the edges it forms scabs which interfere with the growth of epithelium.

Should the part become oedematous, either from general causes, such as heart or kidney disease, or from local causes, such as varicose veins, the granulations share in the oedema, and there is an abundant serous discharge.

The excessive use of moist dressings leads to a third variety of weak ulcer—namely, one in which the granulations become large, soft, pale, and flabby, projecting beyond the level of the skin and overlapping the edges, which become pale and sodden. The term "proud flesh" is popularly applied to such redundant granulations.

The Callous Condition.—This condition is usually met with in ulcers on the lower third of the leg, and is often associated withthe presence of varicose veins. It is chiefly met with in hospital practice. The want of healing is mainly due to impeded venous return and to oedema and induration of the surrounding skin and cellular tissues (Fig. 18). The induration results from coagulation and partial organisation of the inflammatory effusion, and prevents the necessary contraction of the sore. The base of a callous ulcer lies at some distance below the level of the swollen, thickened, and white edges, and presents a glazed appearance, such granulations as are present being unhealthy and irregular. The discharge is usually watery, and cakes in the dressing. When from neglect and want of cleanliness the ulcer becomes inflamed,

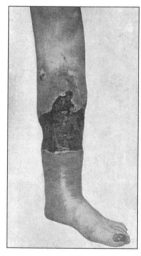

FIG. 18. Callous Ulcer showing thickened edges and indurated swelling of surrounding parts.

there is considerable pain, and the discharge is purulent and often offensive.

The prolonged hyperæmia of the tissues in relation to a callous ulcer of the leg often leads to changes in the underlying bones. The periosteum is abnormally thick and vascular, the superficial layers of the bone become injected and porous, and the bones, as a whole, are thickened. In the macerated bone "the surface is covered with irregular, stalactite-like processes or foliaceous masses, which, to a certain extent, follow the line of attachment of the interosseous membrane and of the intermuscular septa" (Cathcart) (Fig. 19). When the whole thickness of the soft tissues is destroyed by the ulcerative process, the area of bone that comes to form the base of the ulcer projects as a flat, porous node, which in its turn may be eroded. These changes as seen in the macerated specimen are often mistaken for disease originating in the bone.

The *irritable condition* is met with in ulcers which occur, as a rule, just above the external malleolus in women of neurotic temperament. They are small in size and have prominent granulations, and by the aid of a probe points of excessive tenderness may be discovered. These, Hilton believed, correspond to exposed nerve filaments.

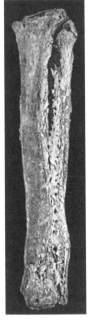

FIG. 19. Tibia and Fibula, showing changes due to chronic ulcer of leg.

Ulcers which are spreading may be met with in one of several conditions.

The Inflamed Condition.—Any ulcer may become acutely inflamed from the access of fresh organisms, aided by mechanical irritation from trauma, ill-fitting splints or bandages, or want of rest, or from chemical irritants, such as strong antiseptics. The best clinical example of an inflamed ulcer is the venereal soft sore. The base of the ulcer becomes red and angry-looking, the granulations disappear, and a copious discharge of thin yellow pus, mixed with blood, escapes. Sloughs of granulation tissue or of connective tissue may form. The edges become red, ragged, and everted, and the ulcer increases in size by spreading into the inflamed and oedematous surrounding tissues. Such ulcers are frequently multiple. Pain is a constant symptom, and is often severe, and there is usually some constitutional disturbance.

The *phagedænic condition* is the result of an ulcer being infected with specially virulent bacteria. It occurs in syphilitic ulcers, and rapidly leads to a widespread destruction of tissue. It is also met with in the throat in some cases of scarlet fever, and may give rise to fatal hæmorrhage by ulcerating into large blood vessels. All the local and constitutional signs of a severe septic infection are present.

Treatment of Ulcers.—An ulcer is not only an immediate cause of suffering to the patient, crippling and incapacitating him for his work, but is a distinct and constant menace to his health: the prolonged discharge reduces his strength; the open sore is a possible source of infection by the organisms of suppuration, erysipelas, or other specific diseases; phlebitis, with formation of septic emboli, leading to pyæmia, is liable to occur; and in old persons it is not uncommon for ulcers of long standing to become the seat of cancer. In addition, the offensive odour of many ulcers renders the patient a source of annoyance and discomfort to others. The primary object of treatment in any ulcer is to bring it into the condition of a healing sore. When this has been effected, nature will do the rest, provided extraneous sources of irritation are excluded.

Steps must be taken to facilitate the venous return from the ulcerated part, and to ensure that a sufficient supply of fresh, healthy blood reaches it. The septic element must be eliminated by disinfecting the ulcer and its surroundings, and any other sources of irritation must be removed.

If the patient's health is below par, good nourishing food, tonics, and general hygienic treatment are indicated.

Management of a Healing Sore.—Perhaps the best dressing for a healing sore is a layer of Lister's perforated oiled-silk protective, which is made to cover the raw surface and the skin for about a quarter of an inch beyond the margins of the sore. Over this three or four thicknesses of sterilised gauze, wrung out of eusol, creolin, or sterilised water, are applied, and covered by a pad of absorbent wool. As far as possible the part should be kept at rest, and the position should be adjusted so as to favour the circulation in the affected area.

The dressing may be renewed at intervals, and care must be taken to avoid any rough handling of the sore. Any discharge that lies on the surface should be removed by a gentle stream of lotion rather than by wiping. The area round the sore should be cleansed before the fresh dressing is applied.

In some cases, healing goes on more rapidly under a dressing of weak boracic ointment (one-quarter the strength of the pharmacopoeial preparation). The growth of epithelium may be stimulated by a 6 to 8 per cent. ointment of scarlet-red.

Dusting powders and poultice dressings are best avoided in the treatment of healing sores.

In extensive ulcers resulting from recent burns, if the granulations are healthy and aseptic, skin-grafts may safely be placed on them directly. If, however, their asepticity cannot be relied upon, it is necessary to scrape away the superficial layer of the granulations, the young fibrous tissue underneath being conserved, as it is sufficiently vascular to nourish the grafts placed on it.

Treatment of Special Varieties of Ulcers.—Before beginning to treat a given ulcer, two questions have to be answered—first, What are the causative conditions present? and second, In what condition do I find the ulcer?—in other words, In what particulars does it differ from a healthy healing sore?

If the cause is a local one, it must be removed; if a constitutional one, means must be taken to counteract it. This done, the condition of the ulcer must be so modified as to bring it into the state of a healing sore, after which it will be managed on the lines already laid down.

Treatment in relation to the Cause of the Ulcer.—*Traumatic Group.*—The *prophylaxis* of these ulcers consists in excluding bacteria, by cleansing crushed or bruised parts, and applying sterilised dressings and properly adjusted splints. If there is reason to fear that the disinfection has not been complete, a Bier's constricting bandage should be applied for some hours each day. These measures will often prevent a grossly injured portion of skin dying, and will ensure asepticity should it do so. In the event of the skin giving way, the same form of dressing should be continued till the slough has separated and a healthy granulating surface is formed. The protective dressing appropriate to a healing sore is then substituted. *Pressure sores* are treated on the same lines.

The treatment of ulcers caused by *burns and scalds* will be described later.

In *ulcers of the leg due to interference with the venous return*, the primary indication is to elevate the limb in order to facilitate the flow of the blood in the veins, and so admit of fresh blood reaching the part. The limb may be placed on pillows, or the foot of the bed raised on blocks, so that the ulcer lies on a higher level than the heart. Should varicose veins be present, the question of operative treatment must be considered.

When an *imperfect nerve supply* is the main factor underlying ulcer formation, prophylaxis is the chief consideration. In patients suffering from spinal injuries or diseases, cerebral paralysis, or affections of the peripheral nerves, all sources of irritation, such as ill-fitting splints, tight bandages, moist applications, and hot bottles, should be avoided. Any part liable to pressure, from the position of the patient or otherwise, must be carefully protected by pads of wool, air-cushions, or water-bags, and must be kept absolutely dry. The skin should be hardened by daily applications of methylated spirit.

Should an ulcer form in spite of these precautions, the mildest antiseptics must be employed for bathing and dressing it, and as far as possible all dressings should be dry.

The *perforating ulcer* of the foot calls for special treatment. To avoid pressure on the sole of the foot, the patient must be confined to bed. As the main local obstacle to healing is the down-growth of epithelium along the sides of the ulcer, this must be removed by the knife or sharp spoon. The base also should be excised, and any bone which may have become involved should be gouged away, so as to leave a healthy and vascular surface. The cavity thus formed is stuffed with bismuth or iodoform gauze and encouraged to heal from the bottom. As the parts are insensitive an anæsthetic is not required. After the ulcer has healed, the patient should wear in his boot a thick felt sole with a hole cut out opposite the situation of the cicatrix. When a joint has been opened into, the difficulty of thoroughly getting rid of all unhealthy and infected granulations is so great that amputation may be advisable, but it is to be remembered that ulceration may recur in the stump if pressure is put upon it. The treatment of any nervous disease or glycosuria which may coexist is, of course, indicated.

Exposure of the plantar nerves by an incision behind the medial malleolus, and subjecting them to forcible stretching, has been employed by Chipault and others in the treatment of perforating ulcers of the foot.

The ulcer that forms in relation to callosities on the sole of the foot is treated by paring away all the thickened skin, after softening it with soda fomentations, removing the unhealthy granulations, and applying stimulating dressings.

Treatment of Ulcers due to Constitutional Causes.—When ulcers are associated with such diseases as tuberculosis, syphilis, diabetes, Bright's disease, scurvy, or gout, these must receive appropriate treatment.

The local treatment of the *tuberculous ulcer* calls for special mention. If the ulcer is of limited extent and situated on an exposed part of the body, the most satisfactory method is complete removal, by means of the knife, scissors, or sharp spoon, of the ulcerated surface and of all the infected area around it, so as to leave a healthy surface from which granulations may spring up. Should the raw surface left be likely to result in an unsightly scar or in cicatricial contraction, skin-grafting should be employed.

For extensive ulcers on the limbs, the chest wall, or on other covered parts, or when operative treatment is contra-indicated, the use of tuberculin and exposure to the Röntgen rays have proved beneficial. The induction of passive hyperæmia, by Bier's or by Klapp's apparatus, should also be used, either alone or supplementary to other measures.

No ulcerative process responds so readily to medicinal treatment as the *syphilitic ulcer* does to the intra-venous administration of arsenical preparations of the "606" or "914" groups or to full doses of iodide of potassium and mercury, and the local application of black wash. When the ulceration has lasted for a long time, however, and is widespread and deep, the duration of treatment is materially shortened by a thorough scraping with the sharp spoon.

Treatment in relation to the Condition of the Ulcer.—*Ulcers in a weak condition.*—If the weak condition of the ulcer is due to anæmia or kidney disease, these affections must first be treated. Locally, the imperfect granulations should be scraped away, and some stimulating agent applied to the raw surface to promote the growth of healthy granulations. For this purpose the sore may be covered with gauze smeared with a 6 to 8 per cent. ointment of scarlet-red, the surrounding parts being protected from the irritant action of the scarlet-red by a layer of vaseline. A dressing of gauze moistened with eusol or of boracic lint wrung out of red lotion (2 grains of sulphate of zinc, and 10 minims of compound tincture of lavender, to an ounce of water), and covered with a layer of gutta-percha tissue, is also useful.

When the condition has resulted from the prolonged use of moist dressings, these must be stopped, the redundant granulations clipped away with scissors, the surface rubbed with silver nitrate or sulphate of copper (bluestone), and dry dressings applied.

When the ulcer has assumed the characters of a healing sore, skin-grafts may be applied to hasten cicatrisation.

Ulcers in a callous condition call for treatment in three directions—(1) The infective element must be eliminated. When the ulcer is foul, relays of charcoal poultices (three parts of linseed meal to one of charcoal), maintained for thirty-six to forty-eight hours, are useful as a preliminary step. The base of the ulcer and the thickened edges should then be freely scraped with a sharp spoon, and the resulting raw surface sponged over with undiluted carbolic acid or iodine, after which an antiseptic dressing is applied, and changed daily till healthy granulations appear. (2) The venous return must be facilitated by elevation of the limb and massage. (3) The induration of the surrounding parts must be got rid of before contraction of the sore is possible. For this purpose the free application of blisters, as first recommended by Syme, leaves little to be desired. Liquor epispasticus painted over the parts, or a large fly-blister (emplastrum cantharidis) applied all round the ulcer, speedily disperses the inflammatory products which cause the induration. The use of elastic pressure or of strapping, of hot-air baths, or the making of multiple incisions in the skin around the ulcer, fulfils the same object.

As soon as the ulcer assumes the characters of a healing sore, it should be covered with skin-grafts, which furnish a much better cicatrix than that which forms when the ulcer is allowed to heal without such aid.

A more radical method of treatment consists in excising the whole ulcer, including its edges and about a quarter of an inch of the surrounding tissue, as well as the underlying fibrous tissue, and grafting the raw surface.

Ambulatory Treatment.—When the circumstances of the patient forbid his lying up in bed, the healing of the ulcer is much delayed. He should be instructed to take every possible opportunity of placing the limb in an elevated position, and must constantly wear a firm bandage of *elastic webbing.* This webbing is porous and admits of evaporation of the skin and wound secretions—an advantage it has over Martin's rubber bandage. The bandage should extend from the toes to well above the knee, and should always be applied while the patient is in the recumbent position with the leg elevated, preferably before getting out of bed in the morning. Additional support is given to the veins if the bandage is applied as a figure of eight.

We have found the following method satisfactory in out-patient practice. The patient lying on a couch, the limb is raised about eighteen inches and kept in this position for five minutes—till the excess of blood has left it. With the limb still raised, the ulcer with the surrounding skin is covered with a layer, about half an inch thick, of finely powdered boracic acid, and the leg, from foot to knee, excluding the sole, is enveloped in a thick layer of wood-wool wadding. This is held in position by ordinary cotton bandages, painted over with liquid starch; while the starch is drying the limb is kept elevated. With this appliance the patient may continue to work, and the dressing does not require to be changed oftener than once in three or four weeks (W. G. Richardson).

When an ulcer becomes acutely *inflamed* as a result of superadded infection, antiseptic measures are employed to overcome the infection, and ichthyol or other soothing applications may be used to allay the pain.

The *phagedænic ulcer* calls for more energetic means of disinfection; the whole of the affected surface is touched with the actual cautery at a white heat, or is painted with pure carbolic acid. Relays of charcoal poultices are then applied until the spread of the disease is arrested.

For the *irritable ulcer* the most satisfactory treatment is complete excision and subsequent skin-grafting.

· VI ·

GANGRENE

*Definition · Types: Dry, Moist
Varieties · Gangrene Primarily Due to Interference with Circulation:
Senile Gangrene; Embolic Gangrene;
Gangrene Following Ligation of Arteries;
Gangrene from Mechanical Causes;
Gangrene from Heat, Chemical Agents, and Cold;
Diabetic Gangrene; Gangrene Associated with Spasm of Blood
Vessels; Raynaud's Disease; Angio-sclerotic Gangrene; Gangrene
from Ergot · Bacterial Varieties of Gangrene. Pathology · Clinical
Varieties · Acute Infective Gangrene; Malignant Oedema; Acute
Emphysematous or Gas Gangrene; Cancrum Oris, etc. · Bed-sores:
Acute; Chronic.*

Gangrene or mortification is the process by which a portion of tissue dies *en masse*, as distinguished from the molecular or cellular death which constitutes ulceration. The dead portion is known as a *slough*.

In this chapter we shall confine our attention to the process as it affects the limbs and superficial parts, leaving gangrene of the viscera to be described in regional surgery.

TYPES OF GANGRENE

Two distinct types of gangrene are met with, which, from their most obvious point of difference, are known respectively as *dry* and *moist*, and there are several clinical varieties of each type.

Speaking generally, it may be said that dry gangrene is essentially due to a simple *interference with the blood supply* of a part; while the main factor in the production of moist gangrene is *bacterial infection*.

The cardinal signs of gangrene are: change in the colour of the part, coldness, loss of sensation and motor power, and, lastly, loss of pulsation in the arteries.

Dry Gangrene or **Mummification** is a comparatively slow form of local death due, as a rule, to a diminution in the arterial blood supply of the affected part, resulting from such causes as the gradual narrowing of the lumen of the arteries by disease of their coats, or the blocking of the main vessel by an embolus.

As the fluids in the tissues are lost by evaporation the part becomes dry and shrivelled, and as the skin is usually intact, infection does not take place, or if it does, the want of moisture renders the part an unsuitable soil, and the organisms do not readily find a footing. Any spread of the process that may take place is chiefly influenced by the anatomical distribution of the blocked arteries, and is arrested as soon as it reaches an area rich in anastomotic vessels. The dead portion is then cast off, the irritation resulting from the contact of the dead with the still living tissue inducing the formation of granulations on the proximal side of the junction, and these by slowly eating into the dead portion produce a furrow—the *line of demarcation*—which gradually deepens until complete separation is effected. As the muscles and bones have a richer blood supply than the integument, the death of skin and subcutaneous tissues extends higher than that of muscles and bone, with the result that the stump left after spontaneous separation is conical, the end of the bone projecting beyond the soft parts.

Clinical Features.—The part undergoing mortification becomes colder than normal, the temperature falling to that of the surrounding atmosphere. In many instances, but not in all, the onset of the process is accompanied by severe neuralgic pain in the part, probably due to anæmia of the nerves, to neuritis, or to the irritation of the exposed axis cylinders by the dead and dying tissues around them. This pain soon ceases and gives place to a complete loss of sensation. The dead part becomes dry, horny, shrivelled, and semi-transparent—at first of a dark brown, but finally of a black colour, from the dissemination of blood pigment throughout the tissues. There is no putrefaction, and therefore no putrid odour; and the condition being non-infective, there is not necessarily any constitutional disturbance. In itself, therefore, dry gangrene does not involve immediate risk to life; the danger lies in the fact that the breach of surface at the line of demarcation furnishes a possible means of entrance for bacteria, which may lead to infective complications.

Moist Gangrene is an acute process, the dead part retaining its fluids and so affording a favourable soil for the development of bacteria. The action of the organisms and their toxins on the adjacent tissues leads to a rapid and wide spread of the process. The skin becomes moist and macerated, and bullæ, containing dark-coloured fluid or gases, form under the epidermis. The putrefactive gases evolved cause the skin to become emphysematous and crepitant and produce an offensive odour. The tissues assume a greenish-black colour from the formation in them of a sulphide of iron resulting from decomposition of the blood pigment. Under certain conditions the dead part may undergo changes resembling more closely those of ordinary post-mortem decomposition. Owing to its nature the spread of the gangrene is seldom arrested by the natural protective processes, and it usually continues until the condition proves fatal from the absorption of toxins into the circulation.

The *clinical features* vary in the different varieties of moist gangrene, but the local results of bacterial action and the constitutional disturbance associated with toxin absorption are present in all; the prognosis therefore is grave in the extreme.

From what has been said, it will be gathered that in dry gangrene there is no urgent call for operation to save the patient's life, the primary indication being to prevent the access of bacteria to the dead part, and especially to the surface exposed at the line of demarcation. In moist gangrene, on the contrary, organisms having already obtained a footing, immediate removal of the dead and dying tissues, as a rule, offers the only hope of saving life.

VARIETIES OF GANGRENE

Varieties of Gangrene essentially due to Interference with the Circulation

While the varieties of gangrene included in this group depend primarily on interference with the circulation, it is to be borne in mind that the clinical course of the affection may be profoundly influenced by superadded infection with micro-organisms. Although the bacteria do not play the most important part in producing tissue necrosis, their subsequent introduction is an accident of such importance that it may change the whole aspect of affairs and convert a dry form of gangrene into one of the moist type. Moreover, the low state of vitality of the tissues, and the extreme difficulty of securing and maintaining asepsis, make it a sequel of great frequency.

Senile Gangrene.—Senile gangrene is the commonest example of local death produced by a *gradual* diminution in the quantity of blood passing through the parts, as a result of arterio-sclerosis or other chronic disease of the arteries leading to diminution of their calibre. It is the most characteristic example of the dry type of gangrene. As the term indicates, it occurs in old persons, but the patient's age is to be reckoned by the condition of his arteries rather than by the number of his years. Thus the vessels of a comparatively young man who has suffered from syphilis and been addicted to alcohol are more liable to atheromatous degeneration leading to this form of gangrene than are those of a much older man who has lived a regular and abstemious life. This form of gangrene is much more common in men than in women. While it usually attacks only one foot, it is not uncommon for the other foot to be affected after an interval, and in some cases it is bilateral from the outset. It must clearly be understood that any form of gangrene may occur in old persons, the term senile being here restricted to that variety which results from arterio-sclerosis.

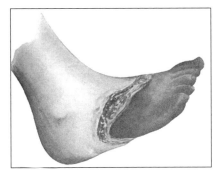

FIG. 20. Senile Gangrene of the Foot, showing line of demarcation.

Clinical Features.—The commonest seat of the disease is in the toes, especially the great toe, whence it spreads up the foot to the heel, or even to the leg (Fig. 20). There is often a history of some slight injury preceding its onset. The vitality of the tissues is so low that the balance between life and death may be turned by the most trivial injury, such as a cut while paring a toe-nail or a corn, a blister caused by an ill-fitting shoe or the contact of a hot-bottle. In some cases the actual gangrene is determined by thrombosis of the popliteal or tibial arteries, which are already narrowed by obliterating endarteritis.

It is common to find that the patient has been troubled for a long time before the onset of definite signs of gangrene, with cold feet, with tingling and loss of feeling, or a peculiar sensation as if walking on cotton wool.

The first evidence of the death of the part varies in different cases. Sometimes a dark-blue spot appears on the medial side of the great toe and gradually increases in size; or a blister containing blood-stained fluid may form. Streaks or patches of dark-blue mottling appear higher up on the foot or leg. In other cases a small sore surrounded by a congested areola forms in relation to the nail and refuses to heal. Such sores on the toes of old persons are always to be looked upon with suspicion and treated with the greatest care; and the urine should be examined for sugar. There is often severe, deep-seated pain of a neuralgic character, with cramps in the limb, and these may persist long after a line of demarcation has formed. The dying part loses sensibility to touch and becomes cold and shrivelled.

All the physical appearances and clinical symptoms associated with dry gangrene supervene, and the dead portion is delimited by a line of demarcation. If this forms slowly and irregularly it indicates a very unsatisfactory condition of the circulation; while, if it forms quickly and decidedly, the presumption is that the circulation in the parts above is fairly good. The separation of the dead part is always attended with the risk of infection taking place, and should this occur, the temperature rises and other evidences of toxæmia appear.

Prophylaxis.—The toes and feet of old people, the condition of whose circulation predisposes them to gangrene, should be protected from slight injuries such as may be received while paring nails, cutting corns, or wearing ill-fitting boots. The patient should also be warned of the risk of exposure to cold, the use of hot-bottles, and of placing the feet near a fire. Attempts have been made to improve the peripheral circulation by establishing an anastomosis between the main artery of a limb and its companion vein, so that arterial blood may reach the peripheral capillaries—reversal of the circulation—but the clinical results have proved disappointing. (See *Op. Surg.*, p. 29.)

Treatment.—When there is evidence that gangrene has occurred, the first indication is to prevent infection by purifying the part, and after careful drying to wrap it in a thick layer of absorbent and antiseptic wool, retained in place by a loosely applied bandage. A slight degree of elevation of the limb is an advantage, but it must not be sufficient to diminish the amount of blood entering the part. Hot-bottles are to be used with the utmost caution. As absolute dryness is essential, ointments or other greasy dressings are to be avoided, as they tend to prevent evaporation from the skin. Opium should be given freely to alleviate pain. Stimulation is to be avoided, and the patient should be carefully dieted.

When the gangrene is limited to the toes in old and feeble patients, some surgeons advocate the expectant method of treatment, waiting for a line of demarcation to form and allowing the dead part to be separated. This takes place so slowly, however, that it necessitates the patient being laid up for many weeks, or even months; and we agree with the majority in advising early amputation.

In this connection it is worthy of note that there are certain points at which gangrene naturally tends to become arrested—namely, at the highly vascular areas in the neighbourhood of joints. Thus gangrene of the great toe often stops when it reaches the metatarso-phalangeal joint; or if it trespasses this limit it may be arrested either at the tarso-metatarsal or at the ankle joint. If these be passed, it usually spreads up the leg to just below the knee before signs of arrestment appear. Further, it is seen from pathological specimens that the spread is greater on the dorsal than on the plantar aspect, and that the death of skin and subcutaneous tissues extends higher than that of bone and muscle.

These facts furnish us with indications as to the seat and method of amputation. Experience has proved that in senile gangrene of the lower extremity the most reliable and satisfactory results are obtained by amputating in the region of the knee, care being taken to perform the operation so as to leave the prepatellar anastomosis intact by retaining the patella in the anterior flap. The most satisfactory operation in these cases is Gritti's supra-condylar amputation. Hæmorrhage is easily controlled by digital pressure, and the use of a tourniquet should be dispensed with, as the constriction of the limb is liable to interfere with the vitality of the flaps.

When the tibial vessels can be felt pulsating at the ankle it may be justifiable, if the patient urgently desires it, to amputate lower than the knee; but there is considerable risk of gangrene recurring in the stump and necessitating a second operation.

That amputation for senile gangrene performed between the ankle and the knee seldom succeeds, is explained by the fact that the vascular obstruction is usually in the upper part of the posterior tibial artery, and the operation is therefore performed through tissues with an inadequate blood supply. It is not uncommon, indeed, on amputating above the knee, to find even the popliteal artery plugged by a clot. This should be removed at the amputation by squeezing the vessel from above downward by a "milking" movement, or by "catheterising the artery" with the aid of a cannula with a terminal aperture.

It is to be borne in mind that the object of amputation in these cases is merely to remove the gangrenous part, and so relieve the patient of the discomfort and the risks from infection which its presence involves. While it is true that in many of these patients the operation is borne remarkably well, it must be borne in mind that those who suffer from senile gangrene are of necessity bad lives, and a guarded opinion should be expressed as to the prospects of survival. The possibility of the disease developing in the other limb has already been referred to.

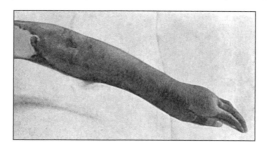

FIG. 21. Embolic Gangrene of Hand and Arm.

Embolic Gangrene (Fig. 21).—This is the most typical form of gangrene resulting from the *sudden* occlusion of the main artery of a part, whether by the impaction of an embolus or the formation of a thrombus in its lumen, when the collateral circulation is not sufficiently free to maintain the vitality of the tissues.

There is sudden pain at the site of impaction of the embolus, and the pulses beyond are lost. The limb becomes cold, numb, insensitive, and powerless. It is often pale at first—hence the term "white gangrene" sometimes applicable to the early appearances, which closely resemble those presented by the limb of a corpse.

If the part is aseptic it shrivels, and presents the ordinary features of dry gangrene. It is liable, however, especially in the lower extremity and when the veins also are obstructed, to become infected and to assume the characters of the moist type.

The extent of the gangrene depends upon the site of impaction of the embolus, thus if the *abdominal aorta* becomes suddenly occluded by an embolus at its bifurcation, the obstruction of the iliacs and femorals induces symmetrical gangrene of both extremities as high as the inguinal ligaments. When gangrene follows occlusion of the *external iliac* or of the *femoral artery* above the origin of its deep branch, the death of the limb extends as high as the middle or upper third of the thigh. When the *femoral* below the origin of its deep branch or the *popliteal artery* is obstructed, the veins remaining pervious, the anastomosis through the profunda is sufficient to maintain the vascular supply, and gangrene does not necessarily follow. The rupture of a popliteal aneurysm, however, by compressing the vein and the articular branches, usually determines gangrene. When an embolus becomes impacted at the *bifurcation of the popliteal*, if gangrene ensues it usually spreads well up the leg.

When the *axillary artery* is the seat of embolic impaction, and gangrene ensues, the process usually reaches the middle of the upper arm. Gangrene following the blocking of the *brachial* at its bifurcation usually extends as far as the junction of the lower and middle thirds of the forearm.

Gangrene due to thrombosis or embolism is sometimes met with in patients recovering from typhus, typhoid, or other fevers, such as that associated with child-bed. It occurs in peripheral parts, such as the toes, fingers, nose, or ears.

Treatment.—The general treatment of embolic gangrene is the same as that for the senile form. Success has followed opening the artery and removing the embolus. The artery is exposed at the seat of impaction and, having been clamped above and below, a longitudinal opening is made and the clot carefully extracted with the aid of forceps; it is sometimes unexpectedly long (one recorded from the femoral artery measured nearly 34 inches); the wound in the artery is then sewn up with fine silk soaked in paraffin. When amputation is indicated, it must be performed sufficiently high to ensure a free vascular supply to the flaps.

Gangrene following Ligation of Arteries.—After the ligation of an artery in its continuity—for example, in the treatment of aneurysm—the limb may for some days remain in a condition verging on gangrene, the distal parts being cold, devoid of sensation, and powerless. As the collateral circulation is established, the vitality of the tissues is gradually restored and these symptoms pass off. In some cases, however,—and especially in the lower extremity—gangrene ensues and presents the same characters as those resulting from embolism. It tends to be of the dry type. The occlusion of the vein as well as the artery is not found to increase the risk of gangrene.

Gangrene from Mechanical Constriction of the Vessels of the part.—The application of a bandage or plaster-of-Paris case too tightly, or of a tourniquet for too long a time, has been known to lead to death of the part beyond; but such cases are rare, as are also those due to the pressure of a fractured bone or of a tumour on a large artery or vein. When gangrene occurs from such causes, it tends to be of the moist type.

Much commoner is it to meet with localised areas of necrosis due to the excessive *pressure of splints* over bony prominences, such as the lateral malleolus, the medial condyle of the humerus, or femur, or over the dorsum of the foot. This is especially liable to occur when the nutrition of the skin is depressed by any interference with its nerve-supply, such as follows injuries to the spine or peripheral nerves, disease of the brain, or acute anterior poliomyelitis. When the splint is removed the skin pressed upon is found to be of a pale yellow or grey colour, and is surrounded by a ring of hyperæmia. If protected from infection, the clinical course is that of dry gangrene.

Bed-sores, which are closely allied to pressure sores, will be described at the end of this chapter.

When a localised portion of tissue, for example, a piece of skin, is so severely *crushed* or *bruised* that its blood vessels are occluded and its structure destroyed, it dies, and, if not infected with bacteria, dries up, and the shrivelled brown skin is slowly separated by the growth of granulation tissue beneath and around it.

Fingers, toes, or even considerable portions of limbs may in the same way be suddenly destroyed by severe trauma, and undergo mummification. If organisms gain access, typical moist gangrene may ensue, or changes similar to those of ordinary post-mortem decomposition may take place.

Treatment.—The first indication is to exclude bacteria by purifying the damaged part and its surroundings, and applying dry, non-irritating dressings.

When these measures are successful, dry gangrene ensues. The raw surface left after the separation of the dead skin may be allowed to heal by granulation, or may be covered by skin-grafts. In the case of a finger or a limb it is not necessary to wait until spontaneous separation takes place, as this is often a slow process. When a well-marked line of demarcation has formed, amputation may be performed just sufficiently far above it to enable suitable flaps to be made.

The end of a stump, after spontaneous separation of the gangrenous portion, requires to be trimmed, sufficient bone being removed to permit of the soft parts coming together.

If moist gangrene supervenes, amputation must be performed without delay, and at a higher level.

Gangrene from Heat, Chemical Agents, and Cold.—Severe **burns** and **scalds** may be followed by necrosis of tissue. So long as the parts are kept absolutely dry—as, for example, by the picric acid method of treatment—the grossly damaged portions of tissue undergo dry gangrene; but when wet or oily dressings are applied and organisms gain access, moist gangrene follows.

Strong **chemical agents**, such as caustic potash, nitric or sulphuric acid, may also induce local tissue necrosis, the general appearances of the lesions produced being like those of severe burns. The resulting sloughs are slow to separate, and leave deep punched-out cavities which are long of healing.

Carbolic Gangrene.—Carbolic acid, even in comparatively weak solution, is liable to induce dry gangrene when applied as a fomentation to a finger, especially in women and children. Thrombosis occurs in the blood vessels of the part, which at first is pale and soft, but later becomes dark and leathery. On account of the anæsthetic action of carbolic acid, the onset of the process is painless, and the patient does not realise his danger. A line of demarcation soon forms, but the dead part separates very slowly.

Gangrene from Frost-bite.—It is difficult to draw the line between the third degree of chilblain and the milder forms of true frost-bite; the difference is merely one of degree. Frost-bite affects chiefly the toes and fingers—especially the great toe and the little finger—the ears, and the nose. In this country it is seldom seen except in members of the tramp class, who, in addition to being exposed to cold by sleeping in the open air, are ill-fed and generally debilitated. The condition usually manifests itself after the parts, having been subjected to extreme cold, are brought into warm surroundings. The first symptom is numbness in the part, followed by a sense of weight, tingling, and finally by complete loss of sensation. The part attacked becomes white and bleached-looking, feels icy cold, and is insensitive to touch. Either immediately, or, it may be, not for several days, it becomes discoloured and swollen, and finally contracts and shrivels. Above the dead area the limb may be the seat of excruciating pain. The dead portion is cast off, as in other forms of dry gangrene, by the formation of a line of demarcation.

To prevent the occurrence of gangrene from frost-bite it is necessary to avoid the sudden application of heat. The patient should be placed in a cold room, and the part rubbed with snow, or put in a cold bath, and have light friction applied to it. As the circulation is restored the general surroundings and the local applications are gradually made warmer. Elevation of the part, wrapping it in cotton wool, and removal to a warmer room, are then permissible, and stimulants and warm drinks may be given with caution. When by these means the occurrence of gangrene is averted, recovery ensues, its onset being indicated by the white parts assuming a livid red hue and becoming the seat of an acute burning sensation.

A condition known as *Trench feet* was widely prevalent amongst the troops in France during the European War. Although allied to frost-bite, cold appears to play a less important part in its causation than humidity and constriction of the limbs producing ischæmia of the feet. Changes were found in the endothelium of the blood vessels, the axis cylinders of nerves, and the muscles. The condition does not occur in civil life.

Diabetic Gangrene.—This form of gangrene is prone to occur in persons over fifty years of age who suffer from glycosuria. The arteries are often markedly diseased. In some cases the existence of the glycosuria is unsuspected before the onset of the gangrene, and it is only on examining the urine that the cause of the condition is discovered. The gangrenous process seldom begins as suddenly as that associated with embolism, and, like senile gangrene, which it may closely simulate in its early stages, it not infrequently begins after a slight injury to one of the toes. It but rarely, however, assumes the dry, shrivelling type, as a rule being attended with swelling, oedema, and dusky redness of the foot, and severe pain. According to Paget, the dead part remains warm longer than in other forms of senile gangrene; there is a greater tendency for patches of skin at some distance from the primary seat of disease to become gangrenous, and for the death of tissue to extend upwards in the subcutaneous planes, leaving the overlying skin unaffected. The low vitality of the tissues favours the growth of bacteria, and if these gain access, the gangrene assumes the characters of the moist type and spreads rapidly.

The rules for amputation are the same as those governing the treatment of senile gangrene, the level at which the limb is removed depending upon whether the gangrene is of the dry or moist type. The general treatment for diabetes must, of course, be employed whether amputation is performed or not. Paget recommended that the dietetic treatment should not be so rigid as in uncomplicated diabetes, and that opium should be given freely.

The *prognosis* even after amputation is unfavourable. In many cases the patient dies with symptoms of diabetic coma within a few days of the operation; or, if he survives this, he may eventually succumb to diabetes. In others there is sloughing of the flaps and death results from toxæmia. Occasionally the other limb becomes gangrenous. On the other hand, the glycosuria may diminish or may even disappear after amputation.

Gangrene associated with Spasm of Blood Vessels.—Raynaud's Disease, or symmetrical gangrene, is supposed to be due to spasm of the arterioles, resulting from peripheral neuritis. It occurs oftenest in women, between the ages of eighteen and thirty, who are the subjects of uterine disorders, anæmia, or chlorosis. Cold is an aggravating factor, as the disease is commonest during the winter months. The digits of both hands or the toes of both feet are simultaneously attacked, and the disease seldom spreads beyond the phalanges or deeper than the skin.

The first evidence is that the fingers become cold, white, and insensitive to touch and pain. These attacks of local *syncope* recur at varying intervals for months or even years. They last for a few minutes or even for some hours, and as they pass off the parts become hyperæmic and painful.

A more advanced stage of the disease is known as *local asphyxia*. The circulation through the fingers becomes exceedingly sluggish, and the parts assume a dull, livid hue. There is swelling and burning or shooting pain. This may pass off in a few days, or may increase in severity, with the formation of bullæ, and end in dry gangrene. As a rule, the slough which forms is comparatively small and superficial, but it may take some months to separate. The condition tends to recur in successive winters.

The *treatment* consists in remedying any nervous or uterine disorder that may be present, keeping the parts warm by wrapping them in cotton wool, and in the use of hot-air or electric baths, the parts being immersed in water through which a constant current is passed. When gangrene occurs, it is treated on the same lines as other forms of dry gangrene, but if amputation is called for it is only with a view to removing the dead part.

Angio-sclerotic Gangrene.—A form of gangrene due to *angio-sclerosis* is occasionally met with in young persons, even in children. It bears certain analogies to Raynaud's disease in that spasm of the vessels plays a part in determining the local death.

The main arteries are narrowed by hyperplastic endarteritis followed by thrombosis, and similar changes are found in the veins. The condition is usually met with in the feet, but the upper extremity may be affected, and is attended with very severe pain, rendering sleep impossible.

The patient is liable to sudden attacks of numbness, tingling and weakness of the limbs which pass off with rest—*intermittent claudication*. During these attacks the large arteries—femoral, brachial, and subclavian—can be felt as firm cords, while pulsation is lost in the peripheral vessels. Gangrene eventually ensues, is attended with great pain and runs a slow course. It is treated on the same lines as Raynaud's disease.

Gangrene from Ergot.—Gangrene may occur from interference with blood supply, the result of tetanic contraction of the minute vessels, such as results in ill-nourished persons who eat large quantities of coarse rye bread contaminated with the *claviceps purpurea* and containing the ergot of rye. It has also occurred in the fingers of patients who have taken ergot medicinally over long periods. The gangrene, which attacks the toes, fingers, ears, or nose, is preceded by formication, numbness, and pains in the parts to be affected, and is of the dry variety.

In this country it is usually met with in sailors off foreign ships, whose dietary largely consists of rye bread. Trivial injuries may be the starting-point, the anæsthesia produced by the ergotin preventing the patient taking notice of them. Alcoholism is a potent predisposing cause.

As it is impossible to predict how far the process will spread, it is advisable to wait for the formation of a line of demarcation before operating, and then to amputate immediately above the dead part.

BACTERIAL VARIETIES OF GANGRENE

The acute bacillary forms of gangrene all assume the moist type from the first, and, spreading rapidly, result in extensive necrosis of tissue, and often end fatally. The infection is usually a mixed one in which anaërobic bacteria predominate. The anaërobe most constantly present is the *bacillus ærogenes capsulatus*, usually in association with other anaërobes, and sometimes with pyogenic diplo- and streptococci. According to the mode of action of the associated organisms and the combined effects of their toxins on the tissues, the gangrenous process presents different pathological and clinical features. Some combinations, for example, result in a rapidly spreading cellulitis with early necrosis of connective tissue accompanied by thrombosis throughout the capillary and venous circulation of the parts implicated; other combinations cause great oedema of the part, and others again lead to the formation of gases in the tissues, particularly in the muscles.

These different effects do not appear to be due to a specific action of any one of the organisms present, but to the combined effect of a particular group living in symbiosis.

According as the cellulitic, the oedematous, or the gaseous characteristics predominate, the clinical varieties of bacillary gangrene may be separately described, but it must be clearly understood that they frequently overlap and cannot always be distinguished from one another.

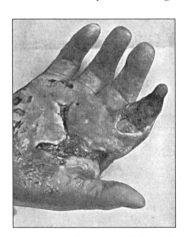

FIG. 22. Gangrene of Terminal Phalanx of Index-Finger, following cellulitis of hand resulting from a scratch on the palm of the hand.

Clinical Varieties of Bacillary Gangrene.—Acute infective gangrene is the form most commonly met with in civil practice. It may follow such trivial injuries as a pin-prick or a scratch, the signs of acute cellulitis rapidly giving place to those of a spreading gangrene. Or it may ensue on a severe railway, machinery, or street accident, when lacerated and bruised tissues are contaminated with gross dirt. Often within a few hours of the injury the whole part rapidly becomes painful, swollen, oedematous, and tense. The skin is at first glazed, and perhaps paler than normal, but soon assumes a dull red or purplish hue, and bullæ form on the surface. Putrefactive gases may be evolved in the tissues, and their presence is indicated by emphysematous crackling when the part is handled. The spread of the disease is so rapid that its progress is quite visible from hour to hour, and may be traced by the occurrence of red lines along the course of the lymphatics of the limb. In the most acute cases the death of the affected part takes place so rapidly that the local changes indicative of gangrene have not time to occur, and the fact that the part is dead may be overlooked.

Rigors may occur, but the temperature is not necessarily raised—indeed, it is sometimes subnormal. The pulse is small, feeble, rapid, and irregular. Unless amputation is promptly performed, death usually follows within thirty-six or forty-eight hours. Even early operation does not always avert the fatal issue, because the quantity of toxin absorbed and its extreme virulence are often more than even a robust subject can outlive.

Treatment.—Every effort must be made to purify all such wounds as are contaminated by earth, street dust, stable refuse, or other forms of gross dirt. Devitalised and contaminated tissue is removed with the knife or scissors and the wound purified with antiseptics of the chlorine group or with hydrogen peroxide. If there is a reasonable prospect that infection has been overcome, the wound may be at once sutured, but if this is doubtful it is left open and packed or irrigated.

When acute gangrene has set in no treatment short of amputation is of any avail, and the sooner this is done, the greater is the hope of saving the patient. The limb must be amputated well beyond the apparent limits of the infected area, and stringent precautions must be taken to avoid discharge from the already gangrenous area reaching the operation wound. An assistant or nurse, who is to take no other part in the operation, is told off to carry out the preliminary purification, and to hold the limb during the operation.

Malignant Oedema.—This form of acute gangrene has been defined as "a spreading inflammatory oedema attended with emphysema, and ultimately followed by gangrene of the skin and adjacent parts." The predominant organism is the *bacillus of malignant oedema* or *vibrion septique* of Pasteur, which is found in garden soil, dung, and various putrefying substances. It is anaërobic, and occurs as long, thick rods with somewhat rounded ends and several laterally placed flagella. Spores, which have a high power of resistance, form in the centre of the rods, and bulge out the sides so as to give the organisms a spindle-shaped outline. Other pathogenic organisms are also present and aid the specific bacillus in its action.

At the bedside it is difficult, if not impossible, to distinguish it from acute infective gangrene. Both follow on the same kinds of injury and run an exceedingly rapid course. In malignant oedema, however, the incidence of the disease is mainly on the superficial parts, which become oedematous and emphysematous, and acquire a marbled appearance with the veins clearly outlined. Early disappearance of sensation is a particularly grave symptom. Bullæ form on the skin, and the tissues have "a peculiar heavy but not putrid odour." The constitutional effects are extremely severe, and death may ensue within a few hours.

Acute Emphysematous or **Gas Gangrene** was prevalent in certain areas at various periods during the European War. It follows infection of lacerated wounds with the *bacillus ærogenes capsulatus*, usually in combination with other anaërobes, and its main incidence is on the muscles, which rapidly become infiltrated with gas that spreads throughout the whole extent of the muscle, disintegrating its fibres and leading to necrosis. The gangrenous process spreads with appalling rapidity, the limb becoming enormously swollen, painful, and crepitant or even tympanitic. Patches of coppery or purple colour appear on the skin, and bullæ containing blood-stained serum form on the surface. The toxæmia is profound, and the face and lips assume a characteristic cyanosis. The condition is attended with a high mortality. Only in the early stages and when the infection is limited are local measures successful in arresting the spread; in more severe cases amputation is the only means of saving life.

Cancrum Oris or Noma.—This disease is believed to be due to a specific bacillus, which occurs in long delicate rods, and is chiefly found at the margin of the gangrenous area. It is prone to attack unhealthy children from two to five years of age, especially during their convalescence from such diseases as measles, scarlet fever, or typhoid, but may attack adults when they are debilitated. It is most common in the mouth, but sometimes occurs on the vulva. In the mouth it begins as an ulcerative stomatitis, more especially affecting the gums or inner aspect of the cheek. The child lies prostrated, and from the open mouth foul-smelling saliva, streaked with blood, escapes; the face is of an ashy-grey colour, the lips dark and swollen. On the inner aspect of the cheek is a deeply ulcerated surface, with sloughy shreds of dark-brown or black tissue covering its base; the edges are irregular, firm, and swollen, and the surrounding mucous membrane is infiltrated and oedematous. In the course of a few hours a dark spot appears on the outer aspect of the cheek, and rapidly increases in size; towards the centre it is black, shading off through blue and grey into a dark-red area which extends over the cheek (Fig. 23). The tissue implicated is at first firm and indurated, but as it loses its vitality it becomes doughy and sodden. Finally a slough forms, and, when it separates, the cheek is perforated.

Meanwhile the process spreads inside the mouth, and the gums, the floor of the mouth, or even the jaws, may become gangrenous and the teeth fall out. The constitutional disturbance is severe, the temperature raised, and the pulse feeble and rapid.

The extremely foetid odour which pervades the room or even the house the patient occupies, is usually sufficient to suggest the diagnosis of cancrum oris. The odour must not be mistaken for that due to decomposition of sordes on the teeth and gums of a debilitated patient.

The *prognosis* is always grave in the extreme, the main risks being general toxæmia and septic pneumonia. When recovery takes place there is serious deformity, and considerable portions of the jaws may be lost by necrosis.

Treatment.—The only satisfactory treatment is thorough removal under an anæsthetic of all the sloughy tissue, with the surrounding zone in which the organisms are active. This is most efficiently accomplished by the knife or scissors, cutting until the tissue bleeds freely, after which the raw surface is painted with undiluted carbolic acid and dressed with iodoform gauze. It may be necessary to remove large pieces of bone when the necrotic process has implicated the jaws. The mouth must be constantly sprayed with peroxide of hydrogen, and washed out with a disinfectant and deodorant lotion, such as Condy's fluid.

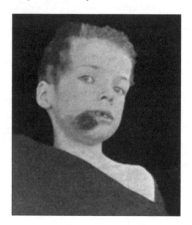

FIG. 23. Cancrum oris. (From a photograph lent by Sir George T. Beatson.)

The patient's general condition calls for free stimulation.

The deformity resulting from these necessarily heroic measures is not so great as might be expected, and can be further diminished by plastic operations, which should be undertaken before cicatricial contraction has occurred.

BED-SORES

Bed-sores are most frequently met with in old and debilitated patients, or in those whose tissues are devitalised by acute or chronic diseases associated with stagnation of blood in the peripheral veins. Any interference with the nerve-supply of the skin, whether from injury or disease of the central nervous system or of the peripheral nerves, strongly predisposes to the formation of bed-sores. Prolonged and excessive pressure over a bony prominence, especially if the parts be moist with skin secretions, urine, or wound discharges, determines the formation of a sore. Excoriations, which may develop into true bed-sores, sometimes form where two skin surfaces remain constantly apposed, as in the region of the scrotum or labium, under pendulous mammæ, or between fingers or toes confined in a splint.

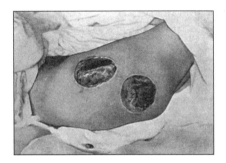

FIG. 24. Acute Bed-Sores over Right Buttock.

Clinical Features.—Two clinical varieties are met with—the acute and the chronic bed-sore.

The *acute* bed-sore usually occurs over the sacrum or buttock. It develops rapidly after spinal injuries and in the course of certain brain diseases. The part affected becomes red and congested, while the surrounding parts are oedematous and swollen, blisters form, and the skin loses its vitality (Fig. 24).

In advanced cases of general paralysis of the insane, a peculiar form of acute bed-sore beginning as a blister, and passing on to the formation of a black, dry eschar, which slowly separates, occurs on such parts as the medial side of the knee, the angle of the scapula, and the heel.

The *chronic* bed-sore begins as a dusky reddish purple patch, which gradually becomes darker till it is almost black. The parts around are oedematous, and a blister may form. This bursts and exposes the papillæ of the skin, which are of a greenish hue. A tough greyish-black slough forms, and is slowly separated. It is not uncommon for the gangrenous area to continue to spread both in width and in depth till it reaches the periosteum or bone. Bed-sores over the sacrum sometimes implicate the vertebral canal and lead to spinal meningitis, which usually proves fatal.

In old and debilitated patients the septic absorption taking place from a bed-sore often proves a serious complication of other surgical conditions. From this cause, for example, old people may succumb during the treatment of a fractured thigh.

The granulating surface left on the separation of the slough tends to heal comparatively rapidly.

Prevention of Bed-sores.—The first essential in the prevention of bed-sores is the regular changing of the patient's position, so that no one part of the body is continuously pressed upon for any length of time. Ring-pads of wool, air-cushions, or water-beds are necessary to remove pressure from prominent parts. Absolute dryness of the skin is all-important. At least once a day, the sacrum, buttocks, shoulder-blades, heels, elbows, malleoli, or other parts exposed to pressure, must be sponged with soap and water, thoroughly dried, and then rubbed with methylated spirit, which is allowed to dry on the skin. Dusting the part with boracic acid powder not only keeps it dry, but prevents the development of bacteria in the skin secretions.

In operation cases, care must be taken that irritating chemicals used to purify the skin do not collect under the patient and remain in contact with the skin of the sacrum and buttocks during the time he is on the operating-table. There is reason to believe that the so-called "post-operation bed-sore" may be due to such causes. A similar result has been known to follow soiling of the sheets by the escape of a turpentine enema.

Treatment.—Once a bed-sore has formed, every effort must be made to prevent its spread. Alcohol is used to cleanse the broken surface, and dry absorbent dressings are applied and frequently changed. It is sometimes found necessary to employ moist or oily substances, such as boracic poultices, eucalyptus ointment, or balsam of Peru, to facilitate the separation of sloughs, or to promote the growth of granulations. In patients who are not extremely debilitated the slough may be excised, the raw surface scraped, and then painted with iodine.

Skin-grafting is sometimes useful in covering in the large raw surface left after separation or removal of sloughs.

⋆ VII ⋆

BACTERIAL AND OTHER WOUND INFECTIONS

Erysipelas ⋆ *Diphtheria* ⋆ *Tetanus*
Hydrophobia ⋆ *Anthrax* ⋆ *Glanders*
Actinomycosis ⋆ *Mycetoma* ⋆ *Delhi Boil*
Chigoe ⋆ *Poisoning by Insects* ⋆ *Snake-bites*

ERYSIPELAS

Erysipelas, popularly known as "rose," is an acute spreading infective disease of the skin or of a mucous membrane due to the action of a streptococcus. Infection invariably takes place through an abrasion of the surface, although this may be so slight that it escapes observation even when sought for. The streptococci are found most abundantly in the lymph spaces just beyond the swollen margin of the inflammatory area, and in the serous blebs which sometimes form on the surface.

Clinical Features.—*Facial erysipelas* is the commonest clinical variety, infection usually occurring through some slight abrasion in the region of the mouth or nose, or from an operation wound in this area. From this point of origin the inflammation may spread all over the face and scalp as far back as the nape of the neck. It stops, however, at the chin, and never extends on to the front of the neck. There is great oedema of the face, the eyes becoming closed up, and the features unrecognisable. The inflammation may spread to the meninges, the intracranial venous sinuses, the eye, or the ear. In some cases the erysipelas invades the mucous membrane of the mouth, and spreads to the fauces and larynx, setting up an oedema of the glottis which may prove dangerous to life.

Erysipelas occasionally attacks an operation wound that has become septic; and it may accompany septic infection of the genital tract in puerperal women, or the separation of the umbilical cord in infants (*erysipelas neonatorum*). After an incubation period, which varies from fifteen to sixty hours, the patient complains of headache, pains in the back and limbs, loss of appetite, nausea, and frequently there is vomiting. He has a chill or slight rigor, initiating a rise of temperature to 103°, 104°, or 105° F.; and a full bounding pulse of about 100 (Fig. 25). The tongue is foul, the breath heavy, and, as a rule, the bowels are constipated. There is frequently albuminuria, and occasionally nocturnal delirium. A moderate degree of leucocytosis (15,000 to 20,000) is usually present.

Around the seat of inoculation a diffuse red patch forms, varying in hue from a bright scarlet to a dull brick-red. The edges are slightly raised above the level of the surrounding skin, as may readily be recognised by gently stroking the part from the healthy towards the affected area. The skin is smooth, tense, and glossy, and presents here and there blisters filled with serous fluid. The local temperature is raised, and the part is the seat of a burning sensation and is tender to the touch, the most tender area being the actively spreading zone which lies about half an inch beyond the red margin.

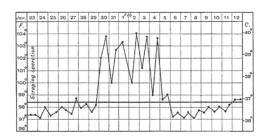

FIG. 25. Chart of Erysipelas occurring in a wound.

The disease tends to spread spasmodically and irregularly, and the direction and extent of its progress may be recognised by mapping out the peripheral zone of tenderness. Red streaks appear along the lines of the superficial lymph vessels, and the deep lymphatics may sometimes be palpated as firm, tender cords. The neighbouring glands, also, are generally enlarged and tender.

The disease lasts for from two or three days to as many weeks, and relapses are frequent. Spontaneous resolution usually takes place, but the disease may prove fatal from absorption of toxins, involvement of the brain or meninges, or from general streptococcal infection.

Complications.—*Diffuse suppurative cellulitis* is the most serious local complication, and results from a mixed infection with other pyogenic bacteria. Small *localised superficial abscesses* may form during the convalescent stage. They are doubtless due to the action of skin bacteria, which attack the tissues devitalised by the erysipelas. A persistent form of *oedema* sometimes remains after recurrent attacks of erysipelas, especially when they affect the face or the lower extremity, a condition which is referred to with elephantiasis.

Treatment.—The first indication is to endeavour to arrest the spread of the process. We have found that by painting with linimentum iodi, a ring half an inch broad, about an inch in front of the peripheral tender zone—not the red margin—an artificial leucocytosis is produced, and the advancing streptococci are thereby arrested. Several coats of the iodine are applied, one after the other, and this is repeated daily for several days, even although the erysipelas has not overstepped the ring. Success depends upon using the liniment of iodine (the tincture is not strong enough), and in applying it well in front of the disease. To allay pain the most useful local applications are ichthyol ointment (1 in 6), or lead and opium fomentations.

The general treatment consists in attending to the emunctories, in administrating quinine in small—two-grain—doses every four hours, or salicylate of iron (2-5 gr. every three hours), and in giving plenty of fluid nourishment. It is worthy of note that the anti-streptococcic serum has proved of less value in the treatment of erysipelas than might have been expected, probably because the serum is not made from the proper strain of streptococcus.

It is not necessary to isolate cases of erysipelas, provided the usual precautions against carrying infection from one patient to another are rigidly carried out.

DIPHTHERIA

Diphtheria is an acute infective disease due to the action of a specific bacterium, the *bacillus diphtheriæ* or *Klebs-Löffler bacillus*. The disease is usually transmitted from one patient to another, but it may be contracted from cats, fowls, or through the milk of infected cows. Cases have occurred in which the surgeon has carried the infection from one patient to another through neglect of antiseptic precautions. The incubation period varies from two to seven days.

Clinical Features.—In *pharyngeal diphtheria*, on the first or second day of the disease, redness and swelling of the mucous membrane of the pharynx, tonsils, and palate are well marked, and small, circular greenish or grey patches of false membrane, composed of necrosed epithelium, fibrin, leucocytes, and red blood corpuscles, begin to appear. These rapidly increase in area and thickness, till they coalesce and form a complete covering to the parts. In the pharynx the false membrane is less adherent to the surface than it is when the disease affects the air-passages. The diphtheritic process may spread from the pharynx to the nasal cavities, causing blocking of the nares, with a profuse ichorous discharge from the nostrils, and sometimes severe epistaxis. The infection may spread along the nasal duct to the conjunctiva. The middle ear also may become involved by spread along the auditory (Eustachian) tube.

The lymph glands behind the angle of the jaw enlarge and become tender, and may suppurate from superadded infection. There is pain on swallowing, and often earache; and the patient speaks with a nasal accent. He becomes weak and anæmic, and loses his appetite. There is often albuminuria. Leucocytosis is usually well marked before the injection of antitoxin; after the injection there is usually a diminution in the number of leucocytes. The false membrane may separate and be cast off, after which the patient gradually recovers. Death may take place from gradual failure of the heart's action or from syncope during some slight exertion.

Laryngeal Diphtheria.—The disease may arise in the larynx, although, as a rule, it spreads thence from the pharynx. It first manifests itself by a short, dry, croupy cough, and hoarseness of the voice. The first difficulty in breathing usually takes place during the night, and once it begins, it rapidly gets worse. Inspiration becomes noisy, sometimes stridulous or metallic or sibilant, and there is marked indrawing of the epigastrium and lower intercostal spaces. The hoarseness becomes more marked, the cough more severe, and the patient restless. The difficulty of breathing occurs in paroxysms, which gradually increase in frequency and severity, until at length the patient becomes asphyxiated. The duration of the disease varies from a few hours to four or five days.

After the acute symptoms have passed off, various localised paralyses may develop, affecting particularly the nerves of the palatal and orbital muscles, less frequently the lower limbs.

Diagnosis.—The finding of the Klebs-Löffler bacillus is the only conclusive evidence of the disease. The bacillus may be obtained by swabbing the throat with a piece of aseptic—not antiseptic—cotton wool or clean linen rag held in a pair of forceps, and rotated so as to entangle portions of the false membrane or exudate. The swab thus obtained is placed in a test-tube, previously sterilised by having had some water boiled in it, and sent to a laboratory for investigation. To identify the bacillus a piece of the membrane from the swab is rubbed on a cover glass, dried, and stained with methylene blue or other basic stain; or cultures may be made on agar or other suitable medium. When a bacteriological examination is impossible, or when the clinical features do not coincide with the results obtained, the patient should always be treated on the assumption that he suffers from diphtheria. So much doubt exists as to the real nature of membranous croup and its relationship to true diphtheria, that when the diagnosis between the two is uncertain the safest plan is to treat the case as one of diphtheria.

In children, diphtheria may occur on the vulva, vagina, prepuce, or glans penis, and give rise to difficulty in diagnosis, which is only cleared up by demonstration of the bacillus.

Treatment.—An attempt may be made to destroy or to counteract the organisms by swabbing the throat with strong antiseptic solutions, such as 1 in 1000 corrosive sublimate or 1 in 30 carbolic acid, or by spraying with peroxide of hydrogen.

The antitoxic serum is our sheet-anchor in the treatment of diphtheria, and recourse should be had to its use as early as possible.

Difficulty of swallowing may be met by the use of a stomach tube passed either through the mouth or nose. When this is impracticable, nutrient enemata are called for.

In laryngeal diphtheria, the interference with respiration may call for intubation of the larynx, or tracheotomy, but the antitoxin treatment has greatly diminished the number of cases in which it becomes necessary to have recourse to these measures.

Intubation consists in introducing through the mouth into the larynx a tube which allows the patient to breathe freely during the period while the membrane is becoming separated and thrown off. This is best done with the apparatus of O'Dwyer; but when this instrument is not available, a simple gum-elastic catheter with a terminal opening (as suggested by Macewen and Annandale) may be employed.

When intubation is impracticable, the operation of tracheotomy is called for if the patient's life is endangered by embarrassment of respiration. Unless the patient is in hospital with skilled assistance available, tracheotomy is the safer of the two procedures.

TETANUS

Tetanus is a disease resulting from infection of a wound by a specific micro-organism, the *bacillus tetani*, and characterised by increased reflex excitability, hypertonus, and spasm of one or more groups of voluntary muscles.

Etiology and Morbid Anatomy.—The tetanus bacillus, which is a perfect anaërobe, is widely distributed in nature and can be isolated from garden earth, dung-heaps, and stable refuse. It is a slender rod-shaped bacillus, with a single large spore at one end giving it the shape of a drum-stick (Fig. 26). The spores, which are the active agents in producing tetanus, are highly resistant to chemical agents, retain their vitality in a dry condition, and even survive boiling for five minutes.

The organism does not readily establish itself in the human body, and seems to flourish best when it finds a nidus in necrotic tissue and is accompanied by aërobic organisms, which, by using up the oxygen in the tissues, provide for it a suitable environment. The presence of a foreign body in the wound seems to favour its action. The infection is for all practical purposes a local one, the symptoms of the disease being due to the toxins produced in the wound of infection acting upon the central nervous system.

The toxin acts principally on the nerve centres in the spinal medulla, to which it travels from the focus of infection by way of the nerve fibres supplying the voluntary muscles. Its first effect on the motor ganglia of the cord is to render them hypersensitive, so that they are excited by mild stimuli, which under ordinary conditions would produce no reaction. As the toxin accumulates the reflex arc is affected, with the result that when a stimulus reaches the ganglia a motor discharge takes place, which spreads by ascending and descending collaterals to the reflex apparatus of the whole cord. As the toxin spreads it causes both motor hyper-tonus and hyper-excitability, which accounts for the tonic contraction and the clonic spasms characteristic of tetanus.

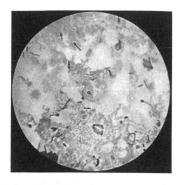

FIG. 26. Bacillus of Tetanus from scraping of a wound of finger, × 1000 diam. Basic fuchsin stain.

Clinical Varieties of Tetanus.—*Acute* or *Fulminating Tetanus.*—This variety is characterised by the shortness of the incubation period, the rapidity of its progress, the severity of its symptoms, and its all but universally fatal issue in spite of treatment, death taking place in from one to four days. The characteristic symptoms may appear within three or four days of the infliction of the wound, but the incubation period may extend to three weeks, and the wound may be quite healed before the disease declares itself—*delayed tetanus.* Usually, however, the wound is inflamed and suppurating, with ragged and sloughy edges. A slight feverish attack may mark the onset of the tetanic condition, or the patient may feel perfectly well until the spasms begin. If careful observations be made, it may be found that the muscles in the immediate neighbourhood of the wound are the first to become contracted; but in the majority of instances the patient's first complaint is of pain and stiffness in the muscles of mastication, notably the masseter, so that he has difficulty in opening the mouth—hence the popular name "lock-jaw." The muscles of expression soon share in the rigidity, and the face assumes a taut, mask-like aspect. The angles of the mouth may be retracted, producing a grinning expression known as the *risus sardonicus.*

The next muscles to become stiff and painful are those of the neck, especially the sterno-mastoid and trapezius. The patient is inclined to attribute the pain and stiffness to exposure to cold or rheumatism. At an early stage the diaphragm and the muscles of the anterior abdominal wall become contracted; later the muscles of the back and thorax are involved; and lastly those of the limbs. Although this is the typical order of involvement of the different groups of muscles, it is not always adhered to.

To this permanent tonic contraction of the muscles there are soon added clonic spasms. These spasms are at first slight and transient, with prolonged intervals between the attacks, but rapidly tend to become more frequent, more severe, and of longer duration, until eventually the patient simply passes out of one seizure into another.

The distribution of the spasms varies in different cases: in some it is confined to particular groups of muscles, such as those of the neck, back, abdominal walls, or limbs; in others all these groups are simultaneously involved.

When the muscles of the back become spasmodically contracted, the body is raised from the bed, sometimes to such an extent that the patient rests only on his heels and occiput—the position of *opisthotonos*. Lateral arching of the body from excessive action of the muscles on one side—*pleurosthotonos*—is not uncommon, the arching usually taking place towards the side on which the wound of infection exists. Less frequently the body is bent forward so that the knees and chin almost meet (*emprosthotonos*). Sometimes all the muscles simultaneously become rigid, so that the body assumes a statuesque attitude (*orthotonos*). When the thoracic muscles, including the diaphragm, are thrown into spasm, the patient experiences a distressing sensation as if he were gripped in a vice, and has extreme difficulty in getting breath. Between the attacks the limbs are kept rigidly extended. The clonic spasms may be so severe as to rupture muscles or even to fracture one of the long bones.

As time goes on, the clonic exacerbations become more and more frequent, and the slightest external stimulus, such as the feeling of the pulse, a whisper in the room, a noise in the street, a draught of cold air, the effort to swallow, a question addressed to the patient or his attempt to answer, is sufficient to determine an attack. The movements are so forcible and so continuous that the nurse has great difficulty in keeping the bedclothes on the patient, or even in keeping him in bed.

The general condition of the patient is pitiful in the extreme. He is fully conscious of the gravity of the disease, and his mind remains clear to the end. The suffering induced by the cramp-like spasms of the muscles keeps him in a constant state of fearful apprehension of the next seizure, and he is unable to sleep until he becomes utterly exhausted.

The temperature is moderately raised (100° to 102° F.), or may remain normal throughout. Shortly before death very high temperatures (110° F.) have been recorded, and it has been observed that the thermometer sometimes continues to rise after death, and may reach as high as 112° F. or more.

The pulse corresponds with the febrile condition. It is accelerated during the spasms, and may become exceedingly rapid and feeble before death, probably from paralysis of the vagus. Sudden death from cardiac paralysis or from cardiac spasm is not uncommon.

The respiration is affected in so far as the spasms of the respiratory muscles produce dyspnoea, and a feeling of impending suffocation which adds to the horrors of the disease.

One of the most constant symptoms is a copious perspiration, the patient being literally bathed in sweat. The urine is diminished in quantity, but as a rule is normal in composition; as in other acute infective conditions, albumen and blood may be present. Retention of urine may result from spasm of the urethral muscles, and necessitate the use of the catheter.

The fits may cease some time before death, or, on the other hand, death may occur during a paroxysm from fixation of the diaphragm and arrest of respiration.

Differential Diagnosis.—There is little difficulty, as a rule, in diagnosing a case of fulminating tetanus, but there are several conditions with which it may occasionally be confused. In *strychnin poisoning*, for example, the spasms come on immediately after the patient has taken a toxic dose of the drug; they are clonic in character, but the muscles are relaxed between the fits. If the dose is not lethal, the spasms soon cease. In *hydrophobia* a history of having been bitten by a rabid animal is usually forthcoming; the spasms, which are clonic in character, affect chiefly the muscles of respiration and deglutition, and pass off entirely in the intervals between attacks. Certain cases of *hæmorrhage into the lateral ventricles* of the brain also simulate tetanus, but an analysis of the symptoms will prevent errors in diagnosis. *Cerebro-spinal meningitis* and *basal meningitis* present certain superficial resemblances to tetanus, but there is no trismus, and the spasms chiefly affect the muscles of the neck and back. *Hysteria and catalepsy* may assume characters resembling those of tetanus, but there is little difficulty in distinguishing between these diseases. Lastly, in the *tetany* of children, or that following operations on the thyroid gland, the spasms are of a jerking character, affect chiefly the hands and fingers, and yield to medicinal treatment.

Chronic Tetanus.—The difference between this and acute tetanus is mainly one of degree. Its incubation period is longer, it is more slow and insidious in its progress, and it never reaches the same degree of severity. Trismus is the most marked and constant form of spasm; and while the trunk muscles may be involved, those of respiration as a rule escape. Every additional day the patient lives adds to the probability of his ultimate recovery. When the disease does prove fatal, it is from exhaustion, and not from respiratory or cardiac spasm. The usual duration is from six to ten weeks.

Delayed Tetanus.—During the European War acute tetanus occasionally developed many weeks or even months after a patient had been injured, and when the original wound had completely healed. It usually followed some secondary operation, *e.g.*, for the removal of a foreign body, or the breaking down of adhesions, which aroused latent organisms.

Local Tetanus.—This term is applied to a form of the disease in which the hypertonus and spasms are localised to the muscles in the vicinity of the wound. It usually occurs in patients who have had prophylactic injections of anti-tetanic serum, the toxins entering the blood being probably neutralised by the antibodies in circulation, while those passing along the motor nerves are unaffected.

When it occurs in the *limbs*, attention is usually directed to the fact by pain accompanying the spasms; the muscles are found to be hard and there are frequent twitchings of the limb. A characteristic reflex is present in the lower extremity, namely, extension of the foot and leg when the sole is tickled.

Cephalic Tetanus is another localised variety which follows injury in the distribution of the facial nerve. It is characterised by the occurrence on the same side as the injury, of facial spasm, rapidly followed by more or less complete paralysis of the muscles of expression, with unilateral trismus and difficulty in swallowing. Other cranial nerves, particularly the oculomotor and the hypoglossal, may also be implicated. A remarkable feature of this condition is that although the muscles are irresponsive to ordinary physiological stimuli, they are thrown into spasm by the abnormal impulses of tetanus.

Trismus.—This term is used to denote a form of tetanic spasm limited to the muscles of mastication. It is really a mild form of chronic tetanus, and the prognosis is favourable. It must not be confused with the fixation of the jaw sometimes associated with a wisdom-tooth gumboil, with tonsillitis, or with affections of the temporo-mandibular articulation.

Tetanus neonatorum is a form of tetanus occurring in infants of about a week old. Infection takes place through the umbilicus, and manifests itself clinically by spasms of the muscles of mastication. It is almost invariably fatal within a few days.

Prophylaxis.—Experience in the European War has established the fact that the routine injection of anti-tetanic serum to all patients with lacerated and contaminated wounds greatly reduces the frequency of tetanus. The sooner the serum is given after the injury, the more certain is its effect; within twenty-four hours 1500 units injected subcutaneously is sufficient for the initial dose; if a longer period has elapsed, 2000 to 3000 units should be given intra-muscularly, as this ensures more rapid absorption. A second injection is given a week after the first.

The wound must be purified in the usual way, and all instruments and appliances used for operations on tetanic patients must be immediately sterilised by prolonged boiling.

Treatment.—When tetanus has developed the main indications are to prevent the further production of toxins in the wound, and to neutralise those that have been absorbed into the nervous system. Thorough purification with antiseptics, excision of devitalised tissues, and drainage of the wound are first carried out. To arrest the absorption of toxins intra-muscular injections of 10,000 units of serum are given daily into the muscles of the affected limb, or directly into the nerve trunks leading from the focus of infection, in the hope of "blocking" the nerves with antitoxin and so preventing the passage of toxins towards the spinal cord.

To neutralise the toxins that have already reached the spinal cord, 5000 units should be injected intra-thecally daily for four or five days, the foot of the bed being raised to enable the serum to reach the upper parts of the cord.

The quantity of toxin circulating in the blood is so small as to be practically negligible, and the risk of anaphylactic shock attending intra-venous injection outweighs any benefit likely to follow this procedure.

Baccelli recommends the injection of 20 c.c. of a 1 in 100 solution of carbolic acid into the subcutaneous tissues every four hours during the period that the contractions persist. Opinions vary as to the efficiency of this treatment. The intra-thecal injection of 10 c.c. of a 15 per cent. solution of magnesium sulphate has proved beneficial in alleviating the severity of the spasms, but does not appear to have a curative effect.

To conserve the patient's strength by preventing or diminishing the severity of the spasms, he should be placed in a quiet room, and every form of disturbance avoided. Sedatives, such as bromides, paraldehyde, or opium, must be given in large doses. Chloral is perhaps the best, and the patient should rarely have less than 150 grains in twenty-four hours. When he is unable to swallow, it should be given by the rectum. The administration of chloroform is of value in conserving the strength of the patient, by abolishing the spasms, and enabling the attendants to administer nourishment or drugs either through a stomach tube or by the rectum. Extreme elevation of temperature is met by tepid sponging. It is necessary to use the catheter if retention of urine occurs.

HYDROPHOBIA

Hydrophobia is an acute infective disease following on the bite of a rabid animal. It most commonly follows the bite or lick of a rabid dog or cat. The virus appears to be communicated through the saliva of the animal, and to show a marked affinity for nerve tissues; and the disease is most likely to develop when the patient is infected on the face or other uncovered part, or in a part richly endowed with nerves.

A dog which has bitten a person should on no account be killed until its condition has been proved one way or the other. Should rabies develop and its destruction become necessary, the head and spinal cord should be retained and forwarded, packed in ice, to a competent observer. Much anxiety to the person bitten and to his friends would be avoided if these rules were observed, because in many cases it will be shown that the animal did not after all suffer from rabies, and that the patient consequently runs no risk. If, on the other hand, rabies is proved to be present, the patient should be submitted to the Pasteur treatment.

Clinical Features.—There is almost always a history of the patient having been bitten or licked by an animal supposed to suffer from rabies. The incubation period averages about forty days, but varies from a fortnight to seven or eight months, and is shorter in young than in old persons. The original wound has long since healed, and beyond a slight itchiness or pain shooting along the nerves of the part, shows no sign of disturbance. A few days of general malaise, with chills and giddiness precede the onset of the acute manifestations, which affect chiefly the muscles of deglutition and respiration. One of the earliest signs is that the patient has periodically a sudden catch in his breathing "resembling what often occurs when a person goes into a cold bath." This is due to spasm of the diaphragm, and is frequently accompanied by a loud-sounding hiccough, likened by the laity to the barking of a dog. Difficulty in swallowing fluids may be the first symptom.

The spasms rapidly spread to all the muscles of deglutition and respiration, so that the patient not only has the greatest difficulty in swallowing, but has a constant sense of impending suffocation. To add to his distress, a copious secretion of viscid saliva fills his mouth. Any voluntary effort, as well as all forms of external stimuli, only serve to aggravate the spasms which are always induced by the attempt to swallow fluid, or even by the sound of running water.

The temperature is raised; the pulse is small, rapid, and intermittent; and the urine may contain sugar and albumen.

The mind may remain clear to the end, or the patient may have delusions, supposing himself to be surrounded by terrifying forms. There is always extreme mental agitation and despair, and the sufferer is in constant fear of his impending fate. Happily the inevitable issue is not long delayed, death usually occurring in from two to four days from the onset. The symptoms of the disease are so characteristic that there is no difficulty in diagnosis. The only condition with which it is liable to be confused is the variety of cephalic tetanus in which the muscles of deglutition are specially involved—the so-called tetanus hydrophobicus.

Prophylaxis.—The bite of an animal suspected of being rabid should be cauterised at once by means of the actual or Paquelin cautery, or by a strong chemical escharotic such as pure carbolic acid, after which antiseptic dressings are applied.

It is, however, to Pasteur's *preventive inoculation* that we must look for our best hope of averting the onset of symptoms. "It may now be taken as established that a grave responsibility rests on those concerned if a person bitten by a mad animal is not subjected to the Pasteur treatment" (Muir and Ritchie).

This method is based on the fact that the long incubation period of the disease admits of the patient being inoculated with a modified virus producing a mild attack, which protects him from the natural disease.

Treatment.—When the symptoms have once developed they can only be palliated. The patient must be kept absolutely quiet and free from all sources of irritation. The spasms may be diminished by means of chloral and bromides, or by chloroform inhalation.

ANTHRAX

Anthrax is a comparatively rare disease, communicable to man from certain of the lower animals, such as sheep, oxen, horses, deer, and other herbivora. In animals it is characterised by symptoms of acute general poisoning, and, from the fact that it produces a marked enlargement of the spleen, is known in veterinary surgery as "splenic fever."

The *bacillus anthracis* (Fig. 27), the largest of the known pathogenic bacteria, occurs in groups or in chains made up of numerous bacilli, each bacillus measuring from 6 to 8 μ in length. The organisms are found in enormous numbers throughout the bodies of animals that have died of anthrax, and are readily recognised and cultivated. Sporulation only takes place outside the body, probably because free oxygen is necessary to the process. In the spore-free condition, the organisms are readily destroyed by ordinary germicides, and by the gastric juice. The spores, on the other hand, have a high degree of resistance. Not only do they remain viable in the dry state for long periods, even up to a year, but they survive boiling for five minutes, and must be subjected to dry heat at 140° C. for several hours before they are destroyed.

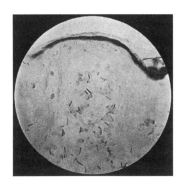

FIG. 27. Bacillus of Anthrax in section of skin, from a case of malignant pustule; shows vesicle containing bacilli. × 400 diam. Gram's stain.

Clinical Varieties of Anthrax.—In man, anthrax may manifest itself in one of three clinical forms.

It may be transmitted by means of spores or bacilli directly from a diseased animal to those who, by their occupation or otherwise, are brought into contact with it—for example, shepherds, butchers, veterinary surgeons, or hide-porters. Infection may occur on the face by the use of a shaving-brush contaminated by spores. The path of infection is usually through an abrasion of the skin, and the primary manifestations are local, constituting what is known as *the malignant pustule*.

In other cases the disease is contracted through the inhalation of the dried spores into the respiratory passages. This occurs oftenest in those who work amongst wool, fur, and rags, and a form of acute pneumonia of great virulence ensues. This affection is known as *wool-sorter's disease*, and is almost universally fatal.

There is reason to believe that infection may also take place by means of spores ingested into the alimentary canal in meat or milk derived from diseased animals, or in infected water.

Clinical Features of Malignant Pustule.—We shall here confine ourselves to the consideration of the local lesion as it occurs in the skin—*the malignant pustule*.

The point of infection is usually on an uncovered part of the body, such as the face, hands, arms, or back of the neck, and the wound may be exceedingly minute. After an incubation period varying from a few hours to several days, a reddish nodule resembling a small boil appears at the seat of inoculation, the immediately surrounding skin becomes swollen and indurated, and over the indurated area there appear a number of small vesicles containing serum, which at first is clear but soon becomes blood-stained (Fig. 28). Coincidently the subcutaneous tissue for a considerable distance around becomes markedly oedematous, and the skin red and tense. Within a few hours, blood is extravasated in the centre of the indurated area, the blisters burst, and a dark brown or black eschar, composed of necrosed skin and subcutaneous tissue and altered blood, forms (Fig. 29). Meanwhile the induration extends, fresh vesicles form and in turn burst, and the eschar increases in size. The neighbouring lymph glands soon become swollen and tender. The affected part is hot and itchy, but the patient does not complain of great pain. There is a moderate degree of constitutional disturbance, with headache, nausea, and sometimes shivering.

If the infection becomes generalised—*anthracæmia*—the temperature rises to 103° or 104° F., the pulse becomes feeble and rapid, and other signs of severe blood-poisoning appear: vomiting, diarrhoea, pains in the limbs, headache and delirium, and the condition proves fatal in from five to eight days.

Differential Diagnosis.—When the malignant pustule is fully developed, the central slough with the surrounding vesicles and the widespread oedema are characteristic. The bacillus can be obtained from the peripheral portion of the slough, from the blisters, and from the adjacent lymph vessels and glands. The occupation of the patient may suggest the possibility of anthrax infection.

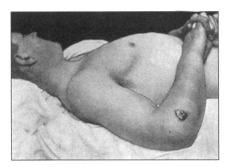

FIG. 28. Malignant Pustule, third day after infection with Anthrax, showing great oedema of upper extremity and pectoral region (cf. Fig. 29).

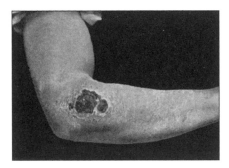

FIG. 29. Malignant Pustule, fourteen days after infection, showing black eschar in process of separation. The œdema has largely disappeared. Treated by Sclavo's serum (cf. Fig. 28).

Prophylaxis.—Any wound suspected of being infected with anthrax should at once be cauterised with caustic potash, the actual cautery, or pure carbolic acid.

Treatment.—The best results hitherto obtained have followed the use of the anti-anthrax serum introduced by Sclavo. The initial dose is 40 c.c., and if the serum is given early in the disease, the beneficial effects are manifest in a few hours. Favourable results have also followed the use of pyocyanase, a vaccine prepared from the bacillus pyocyaneus.

By some it is recommended that the local lesion should be freely excised; others advocate cauterisation of the affected part with solid caustic potash till all the indurated area is softened. Gräf has had excellent results by the latter method in a large series of cases, the oedema subsiding in about twenty-four hours and the constitutional symptoms rapidly improving. Wolff and Wiewiorowski, on the other hand, have had equally good results by simply protecting the local lesion with a mild antiseptic dressing, and relying upon general treatment.

The general treatment consists in feeding and stimulating the patient as freely as possible. Quinine, in 5 to 10 grain doses every four hours, and powdered ipecacuanha, in 40 to 60 grain doses every four hours, have also been employed with apparent benefit.

GLANDERS

Glanders is due to the action of a specific bacterium, the *bacillus mallei*, which resembles the tubercle bacillus, save that it is somewhat shorter and broader, and does not stain by Gram's method. It requires higher temperatures for its cultivation than the tubercle bacillus, and its growth on potato is of a characteristic chocolate-brown colour, with a greenish-yellow ring at the margin of the growth. The bacillus mallei retains its vitality for long periods under ordinary conditions, but is readily killed by heat and chemical agents. It does not form spores.

Clinical Features.—Both in the lower animals and in man the bacillus gives rise to two distinct types of disease—*acute glanders*, and *chronic glanders* or *farcy*.

Acute Glanders is most commonly met with in the horse and in other equine animals, horned cattle being immune. It affects the septum of the nose and adjacent parts, firm, translucent, greyish nodules containing lymphoid and epithelioid cells appearing in the mucous membrane. These nodules subsequently break down in the centre, forming irregular ulcers, which are attended with profuse discharge, and marked inflammatory swelling. The cervical lymph glands, as well as the lungs, spleen, and liver, may be the seat of secondary nodules.

In man, acute glanders is commoner than the chronic variety. Infection always takes place through an abraded surface, and usually on one of the uncovered parts of the body—most commonly the skin of the hands, arms, or face; or on the mucous membrane of the mouth, nose, or eye. The disease has been acquired by accidental inoculation in the course of experimental investigations in the laboratory, and proved fatal. The incubation period is from three to five days.

The *local* manifestations are pain and swelling in the region of the infected wound, with inflammatory redness around it and along the lines of the superficial lymphatics. In the course of a week, small, firm nodules appear, and are rapidly transformed into pustules. These may occur on the face and in the vicinity of joints, and may be mistaken for the eruption of small-pox.

After breaking down, these pustules give rise to irregular ulcers, which by their confluence lead to extensive destruction of skin. Sometimes the nasal mucous membrane becomes affected, and produces a discharge—at first watery, but later sanious and purulent. Necrosis of the bones of the nose may take place, in which case the discharge becomes peculiarly offensive. In nearly every case metastatic abscesses form in different parts of the body, such as the lungs, joints, or muscles.

During the development of the disease the patient feels ill, complains of headache and pains in the limbs, the temperature rises to 104° or even to 106° F., and assumes a pyæmic type. The pulse becomes rapid and weak. The tongue is dry and brown. There is profuse sweating, albuminuria, and often insomnia with delirium. Death may take place within a week, but more frequently occurs during the second or third week.

Differential Diagnosis.—There is nothing characteristic in the site of the primary lesion in man, and the condition may, during the early stages, be mistaken for a boil or carbuncle, or for any acute inflammatory condition. Later, the disease may simulate acute articular rheumatism, or may manifest all the symptoms of acute septicæmia or pyæmia. The diagnosis is established by the recognition of the bacillus. Veterinary surgeons attach great importance to the mallein test as a means of diagnosis in animals, but in the human subject its use is attended with considerable risk and is not to be recommended.

Treatment.—Excision of the primary nodule, followed by the application of the thermo-cautery and sponging with pure carbolic acid, should be carried out, provided the condition is sufficiently limited to render complete removal practicable.

When secondary abscesses form in accessible situations, they must be incised, disinfected, and drained. The general treatment is carried out on the same lines as in other acute infective diseases.

Chronic Glanders.—*In the horse* the chronic form of glanders is known as *farcy*, and follows infection through an abrasion of the skin, involving chiefly the superficial lymph vessels and glands. The lymphatics become indurated and nodular, constituting what veterinarians call *farcy pipes* and *farcy buds*.

In man also the clinical features of the chronic variety of the disease are somewhat different from those of the acute form. Here, too, infection takes place through a broken cutaneous surface, and leads to a superficial lymphangitis with nodular thickening of the lymphatics (*farcy buds*). The neighbouring glands soon become swollen and indurated. The primary lesion meanwhile inflames, suppurates, and, after breaking down, leaves a large, irregular ulcer with thickened edges and a foul, purulent or bloody discharge. The glands break down in the same way, and lead to wide destruction of skin, and the resulting sinuses and ulcers are exceedingly intractable. Secondary deposits in the subcutaneous tissue, the muscles, and other parts, are not uncommon, and the nasal mucous membrane may become involved. The disease often runs a chronic course, extending to four or five months, or even longer. Recovery takes place in about 50 per cent. of cases, but the convalescence is prolonged, and at any time the disease may assume the characters of the acute variety and speedily prove fatal.

The *differential diagnosis* is often difficult, especially in the chronic nodules, in which it may be impossible to demonstrate the bacillus. The ulcerated lesions of farcy have to be distinguished from those of tubercle, syphilis, and other forms of infective granuloma.

Treatment.—Limited areas of disease should be completely excised. The general condition of the patient must be improved by tonics, good food, and favourable hygienic surroundings. In some cases potassium iodide acts beneficially.

ACTINOMYCOSIS

Actinomycosis is a chronic disease due to the action of an organism somewhat higher in the vegetable scale than ordinary bacteria—the *streptothrix actinomyces* or *ray fungus*.

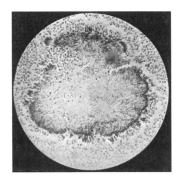

FIG. 30. Section of Actinomycosis Colony in Pus from Abscess of Liver, showing filaments and clubs of streptothrix actinomyces. × 400 diam. Gram's stain.

Etiology and Morbid Anatomy.—The actinomyces, which has never been met with outside the body, gives rise in oxen, horses, and other animals to tumour-like masses composed of granulation tissue; and in man to chronic suppurative processes which may result in a condition resembling chronic pyæmia. The actinomyces is more complex in structure than other pathogenic organisms, and occurs in the tissues in the form of small, round, semi-translucent bodies, about the size of a pin-head or less, and consisting of colonies of the fungus. On account of their yellow tint they are spoken of as "sulphur grains." Each colony is made up of a series of thin, interlacing, and branching *filaments*, some of which are broken up so as to form masses or chains of *cocci*; and around the periphery of the colony are elongated, pear-shaped, hyaline, *club-like bodies* (Fig. 30).

Infection is believed to be conveyed by the husks of cereals, especially barley; and the organism has been found adhering to particles of grain embedded in the tissues of animals suffering from the disease. In the human subject there is often a history of exposure to infection from such sources, and the disease is said to be most common during the harvesting months.

Around each colony of actinomyces is a zone of granulation tissue in which suppuration usually occurs, so that the fungus comes to lie in a bath of greenish-yellow pus. As the process spreads these purulent foci become confluent and form abscess cavities. When metastasis takes place, as it occasionally does, the fungus is transmitted by the blood vessels, as in pyæmia.

Clinical features.—In man the disease may be met with in the skin, the organisms gaining access through an abrasion, and spreading by the formation of new nodules in the same way as tuberculosis.

The region of the mouth and jaws is one of the commonest sites of surgical actinomycosis. Infection takes place, as a rule, along the side of a carious tooth, and spreads to the lower jaw. A swelling is slowly and insidiously developed, but when the loose connective tissue of the neck becomes infiltrated, the spread is more rapid. The whole region becomes infiltrated and swollen, and the skin ultimately gives way and free suppuration occurs, resulting in the formation of sinuses. The characteristic greenish-grey or yellow granules are seen in the pus, and when examined microscopically reveal the colonies of actinomyces.

Less frequently the maxilla becomes affected, and the disease may spread to the base of the skull and brain. The vertebræ may become involved by infection taking place through the pharynx or oesophagus, and leading to a condition simulating tuberculous disease of the spine. When it implicates the intestinal canal and its accessory glands, the lungs, pleura, and bronchial tubes, or the brain, the disease is not amenable to surgical treatment.

Differential Diagnosis.—The conditions likely to be mistaken for surgical actinomycosis are sarcoma, tubercle, and syphilis. In the early stages the differential diagnosis is exceedingly difficult. In many cases it is only possible when suppuration has occurred and the fungus can be demonstrated.

The slow destruction of the affected tissue by suppuration, the absence of pain, tenderness, and redness, simulate tuberculosis, but the absence of glandular involvement helps to distinguish it.

Syphilitic lesions are liable to be mistaken for actinomycosis, all the more that in both diseases improvement follows the administration of iodides. When it affects the lower jaw, in its early stages, actinomycosis may closely simulate a periosteal sarcoma.

The recognition of the fungus is the crucial point in diagnosis.

Prognosis.—Spontaneous cure rarely occurs. When the disease implicates internal organs, it is almost always fatal. On external parts the destructive process gradually spreads, and the patient eventually succumbs to superadded

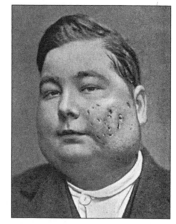

FIG. 31. Actinomycosis of Maxilla. The disease spread to opposite side; finally implicated base of skull, and proved fatal. Treated by radium. (Mr. D. P. D. Wilkie's case.)

septic infection. When, from its situation, the primary focus admits of removal, the prognosis is more favourable.

Treatment.—The surgical treatment is early and free removal of the affected tissues, after which the wound is cauterised by the actual cautery, and sponged over with pure carbolic acid. The cavity is packed with iodoform gauze, no attempt being made to close the wound.

Success has attended the use of a vaccine prepared from cultures of the organism; and the X-rays and radium, combined with the administration of iodides in large doses, or with intra-muscular injections of a 10 per cent. solution of cacodylate of soda, have proved of benefit.

MYCETOMA, OR MADURA FOOT.—Mycetoma is a chronic disease due to an organism resembling that of actinomycosis, but not identical with it. It is endemic in certain tropical countries, and is most frequently met with in India. Infection takes place through an abrasion of the skin, and the disease usually occurs on the feet of adult males who work barefooted in the fields.

Clinical Features.—The disease begins on the foot as an indurated patch, which becomes discoloured and permeated by black or yellow nodules containing the organism. These nodules break down by suppuration, and numerous minute abscesses lined by granulation tissues are thus formed. In the pus are found yellow particles likened to fish-roe, or black pigmented granules like gunpowder. Sinuses form, and the whole foot becomes greatly swollen and distorted by flattening of the sole and dorsiflexion of the toes. Areas of caries or necrosis occur in the bones, and the disease gradually extends up the leg (Fig. 32). There is but little pain, and no glandular involvement or constitutional disturbance. The disease runs a prolonged course, sometimes lasting for twenty or thirty years. Spontaneous cure never takes place, and the risk to life is that of prolonged suppuration.

If the disease is localised, it may be removed by the knife or sharp spoon, and the part afterwards cauterised. As a rule, amputation well above the disease is the best line of treatment. Unlike actinomycosis, this disease does not appear to be benefited by iodides.

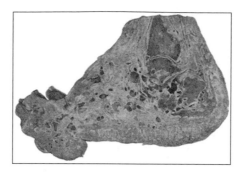

FIG. 32. Mycetoma, or Madura Foot. (Museum of Royal College of Surgeons, Edinburgh.)

DELHI BOIL.—*Synonyms*—Aleppo boil, Biskra button, Furunculus orientalis, Natal sore.

Delhi boil is a chronic inflammatory disease, most commonly met with in India, especially towards the end of the wet season. The disease occurs oftenest on the face, and is believed to be due to an organism, although this has not been demonstrated. The infection is supposed to be conveyed through water used for washing, or by the bites of insects.

Clinical Features.—A red spot, resembling the mark of a mosquito bite, appears on the affected part, and is attended with itching. After becoming papular and increasing to the size of a pea, desquamation takes place, leaving a dull-red surface, over which in the course of several weeks there develops a series of small yellowish-white spots, from which serum exudes, and, drying, forms a thick scab. Under this scab the skin ulcerates, leaving small oval sores with sharply bevelled edges, and an uneven floor covered with yellow or sanious pus. These sores vary in number from one to forty or fifty. They may last for months and then heal spontaneously, or may continue to spread until arrested by suitable treatment. There is no enlargement of adjacent glands, and but little inflammatory reaction in the surrounding tissues; nor is there any marked constitutional disturbance. Recovery is often followed by cicatricial contraction leading to deformity of the face.

The *treatment* consists in destroying the original papule by the actual cautery, acid nitrate of mercury, or pure carbolic acid. The ulcers should be scraped with the sharp spoon, and cauterised.

CHIGOE.—Chigoe or jigger results from the introduction of the eggs of the sand-flea (*Pulex penetrans*) into the tissues. It occurs in tropical Africa,

South America, and the West Indies. The impregnated female flea remains attached to the part till the eggs mature, when by their irritation they cause localised inflammation with pustules or vesicles on the surface. Children are most commonly attacked, particularly about the toe-nails and on the scrotum. The treatment consists in picking out the insect with a blunt needle, special care being taken not to break it up. The puncture is then cauterised. The application of essential oils to the feet acts as a preventive.

POISONING BY INSECTS.—The bites of certain insects, such as mosquitoes, midges, different varieties of flies, wasps, and spiders, may be followed by serious complications. The effects are mainly due to the injection of an irritant acid secretion, the exact nature of which has not been ascertained.

The local lesion is a puncture, surrounded by a zone of hyperæmia, wheals, or vesicles, and is associated with burning sensations and itching which usually pass off in a few hours, but may recur at intervals, especially when the patient is warm in bed. Scratching also reproduces the local signs and symptoms. Where the connective tissue is loose—for example, in the eyelid or scrotum—there is often considerable swelling; and in the mouth and fauces this may lead to oedema of the glottis, which may prove fatal.

The *treatment* consists in the local application of dilute alkalies such as ammonia water, solutions of carbonate or bicarbonate of soda, or sal-volatile. Weak carbolic lotions, or lead and opium lotion, are useful in allaying the local irritation. One of the best means of neutralising the poison is to apply to the sting a drop of a mixture containing equal parts of pure carbolic acid and liquor ammoniæ.

Free stimulation is called for when severe constitutional symptoms are present.

SNAKE-BITES.—We are here only concerned with the injuries inflicted by the venomous varieties of snakes, the most important of which are the hooded snakes of India, the rattle-snakes of America, the horned snakes of Africa, the viper of Europe, and the adder of the United Kingdom.

While the virulence of these creatures varies widely, they are all capable of producing in a greater or less degree symptoms of acute poisoning in man and other animals. By means of two recurved fangs attached to the upper jaw, and connected by a duct with poison-secreting glands, they introduce into their prey a thick, transparent, yellowish fluid, of acid reaction, probably of the nature of an albumose, and known as the *venom.*

The *clinical features* resulting from the injection of the venom vary directly in intensity with the amount of the poison introduced, and the rapidity with which it reaches the circulating blood, being most marked when it immediately enters a large vein. The poison is innocuous when taken into the stomach.

Locally the snake inflicts a double wound, passing vertically into the subcutaneous tissue; the edges of the punctures are ecchymosed, and the adjacent vessels the seat of thrombosis. Immediately there is intense pain, and considerable swelling with congestion, which tends to spread towards the trunk. Extensive gangrene may ensue. There is no special involvement of the lymphatics.

The *general symptoms* may come on at once if the snake is a particularly venomous one, or not for some hours if less virulent. In the majority of viper or adder bites the constitutional disturbance is slight and transient, if it appears at all. Snake-bites in children are particularly dangerous.

The patient's condition is one of profound shock with faintness, giddiness, dimness of sight, and a feeling of great terror. The pupils dilate, the skin becomes moist with a clammy sweat, and nausea with vomiting, sometimes of blood, ensues. High fever, cramps, loss of sensation, hæmaturia, and melæna are among the other symptoms that may be present. The pulse becomes feeble and rapid, the respiratory nerve centres are profoundly depressed, and delirium followed by coma usually precedes the fatal issue, which may take place in from five to forty-eight hours. If the patient survives for two days the prognosis is favourable.

Treatment.—A broad ligature should be tied tightly round the limb above the seat of infection, to prevent the poison passing into the general circulation, and bleeding from the wound should be encouraged. The application of an elastic bandage from above downward to empty the blood out of the infected portion of the limb has been recommended. The whole of the bite should at once be excised, and crystals of permanganate of potash rubbed into the wound until it is black, or peroxide of hydrogen applied with the object of destroying the poison by oxidation.

The general treatment consists in free stimulation with whisky, brandy, ammonia, digitalis, etc. Hypodermic injections of strychnin in doses sufficiently large to produce a slight degree of poisoning by the drug are particularly useful. The most rational treatment, when it is available, is the use of the *antivenin* introduced by Fraser and Calmette.

· VIII ·

TUBERCULOSIS

*Tubercle Bacillus ◆ Methods of Infection
Inherited and Acquired Predisposition
Relationship of Tuberculosis to Injury
Human and Bovine Tuberculosis
Action of the Bacillus Upon the Tissues
Tuberculous Granulation Tissue ◆ Natural Cure
Recrudescence of the Disease ◆ The Tuberculous Abscess
Contents and Wall of the Abscess ◆ Tuberculous Sinuses*

Tuberculosis occurs more frequently in some situations than in others; it is common, for example, in lymph glands, in bones and joints, in the peritoneum, the intestine, the kidney, prostate and testis, and in the skin and subcutaneous cellular tissue; it is seldom met with in the breast or in muscles, and it rarely affects the ovary, the pancreas, the parotid, or the thyreoid.

Tubercle bacilli vary widely in their virulence, and they are more tenacious of life than the common pyogenic bacteria. In a dry state, for example, they can retain their vitality for months; and they can also survive immersion in water for prolonged periods. They resist the action of the products of putrefaction for a considerable time, and are not destroyed by digestive processes in the stomach and intestine. They may be killed in a few minutes by boiling, or by exposure to steam under pressure, or by immersion for less than a minute in 1 in 20 carbolic lotion.

Methods of Infection.—In marked contrast to what obtains in the infective diseases that have already been described, tuberculosis rarely results from the *infection of a wound.* In exceptional instances, however, this does occur, and in illustration of the fact may be cited the case of a servant who cut her finger with a broken spittoon containing the sputum of her consumptive master; the wound subsequently showed evidence of tuberculous infection, which ultimately spread up along the lymph vessels of the arm. Pathologists, too, whose hands, before the days of rubber gloves, were frequently exposed to the contact of tuberculous tissues and pus, were liable to suffer from a form of tuberculosis of the skin of the finger, known as *anatomical tubercle*. Slight wounds of the feet in children who go about barefoot in towns sometimes become infected with tubercle. Operation wounds made with instruments contaminated with tuberculous material have also been known to become infected. It is highly probable that the common form of tuberculosis of the skin known as "lupus" arises by direct infection from without.

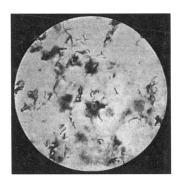

FIG. 33. Tubercle Bacilli in caseous material × 1000 diam.
Z. Neilsen stain.

In the vast majority of cases the tubercle bacillus gains entrance to the body by way of the mucous surfaces, the organisms being either inhaled or swallowed; those inhaled are mostly derived from the human subject, those swallowed, from cattle. Bacilli, whether inhaled or swallowed, are especially apt to lodge about the pharynx and pass to the pharyngeal lymphoid tissue and tonsils, and by way of the lymph vessels to the glands. The glands most frequently infected in this way are the cervical glands, and those within the cavity of the chest—particularly the bronchial glands at the root of the lung. From these, infection extends at any later period in life to the bones, joints, and internal organs.

There is reason to believe that the organisms may lie in a dormant condition for an indefinite period in these glands, and only become active long afterwards, when some depression of the patient's health produces conditions which favour their growth. When the organisms become active in this way, the tuberculous tissue undergoes softening and disintegration, and the infective material, by bursting into an adjacent vein, may enter the blood-stream, in which it is carried to distant parts of the body. In this way a *general tuberculosis* may be set up, or localised foci of tuberculosis may develop in the tissues in which the organisms lodge. Many tuberculous patients are to be regarded as possessing in their bronchial glands, or elsewhere, an internal store of bacilli, to which the disease for which advice is sought owes its origin, and from which similar outbreaks of tuberculosis may originate in the future.

The alimentary mucous membrane, especially that of the lower ileum and cæcum, is exposed to infection by swallowed sputum and by food materials, such as milk, containing tubercle bacilli. The organisms may lodge in the mucous membrane and cause tuberculous ulceration, or they may be carried through the wall of the bowel into the lacteals, along which they pass to the mesenteric glands where they become arrested and give rise to tuberculous disease.

Relationship of Tuberculosis to Trauma.—Any tissue whose vitality has been lowered by injury or disease furnishes a favourable nidus for the lodgment and growth of tubercle bacilli. The injury or disease, however, is to be looked upon as determining the *localisation* of the tuberculous lesion rather than as an essential factor in its causation. In a person, for example, in whose blood tubercle bacilli are circulating and reaching every tissue and organ of the body, the occurrence of tuberculous disease in a particular part may be determined by the depression of the tissues resulting from an injury of that part. There can be no doubt that excessive movement and jarring of a limb aggravates tuberculous disease of a joint; also that an injury may light up a focus that has been long quiescent, but we do not agree with those—Da Costa, for example—who maintain that injury may be a determining cause of tuberculosis. The question is not one of mere academic interest, but one that may raise important issues in the law courts.

Human and Bovine Tuberculosis.—The frequency of the bovine bacillus in the abdominal and in the glandular and osseous tuberculous lesions of children would appear to justify the conclusion that the disease is transmissible from the ox to the human subject, and that the milk of tuberculous cows is probably a common vehicle of transmission.

CHAPTER VIII

Changes in the Tissues following upon the successful Lodgment of Tubercle Bacilli.—The action of the bacilli on the tissues results in the formation of granulation tissue comprising characteristic tissue elements and with a marked tendency to undergo caseation.

The recognition of the characteristic elements, with or without caseation, is usually sufficient evidence of the tuberculous nature of any portion of tissue examined for diagnostic purposes. The recognition of the bacillus itself by appropriate methods of staining makes the diagnosis a certainty; but as it is by no means easy to identify the organism in many forms of surgical tuberculosis, it may be necessary to have recourse to experimental inoculation of susceptible animals such as guinea-pigs.

The changes subsequent to the formation of tuberculous granulation tissue are liable to many variations. It must always be borne in mind that although the bacilli have effected a lodgment and have inaugurated disease, the relation between them and the tissues remains one of mutual antagonism; which of them is to gain and keep the upper hand in the conflict depends on their relative powers of resistance.

If the tissues prevail, there ensues a process of repair. In the immediate vicinity of the area of infection young connective tissue, and later, fibrous tissue, is formed. This may replace the tuberculous tissue and bring about repair—a fibrous cicatrix remaining to mark the scene of the previous contest. Scars of this nature are frequently discovered at the apex of the lung after death in persons who have at one time suffered from pulmonary phthisis. Under other circumstances, the tuberculous tissue that has undergone caseation, or even calcification, is only encapsulated by the new fibrous tissue, like a foreign body. Although this may be regarded as a victory for the tissues, the cure, if such it may be called, is not necessarily a permanent one, for at any subsequent period, if the part affected is disturbed by injury or through some other influence, the encapsulated tubercle may again become active and get the upper hand of the tissues, and there results a relapse or recrudescence of the disease. This *tendency to relapse* after apparent cure is a notable feature of tuberculous disease as it is met with in the spine, or in the hip-joint, and it necessitates a prolonged course of treatment to give the best chance of a lasting cure.

If, however, at the inauguration of the tuberculous disease the bacilli prevail, the infection tends to spread into the tissues surrounding those originally infected, and more and more tuberculous granulation tissue is formed.

Finally the tuberculous tissue breaks down and liquefies, resulting in the formation of a cold abscess. In their struggle with the tissues, tubercle bacilli receive considerable support and assistance from any pyogenic organisms that may be present. A tuberculous infection may exhibit its aggressive qualities in a more serious manner by sending off detachments of bacilli, which are carried by the lymphatics to the nearest glands, or by the blood-stream to more distant, and it may be to all, parts of the body. When the infection is thus generalised, the condition is called *general tuberculosis*. Considering the extraordinary frequency of localised forms of surgical tuberculosis, general dissemination of the disease is rare.

The clinical features of surgical tuberculosis will be described with the individual tissues and organs, as they vary widely according to the situation of the lesion.

The general treatment consists in combating the adverse influences that have been mentioned as increasing the liability to tuberculous infection. Within recent years the value of the "open-air" treatment has been widely recognised. An open-air life, even in the centre of a city, may be followed by marked improvement, especially in the hospital class of patient, whose home surroundings tend to favour the progress of the disease. The purer air of places away from centres of population is still better; and, according to the idiosyncrasies of the individual patient, mountain air or that of the sea coast may be preferred. In view of the possible discomforts and gastric disturbance which may attend a sea-voyage, this should be recommended to patients suffering from tuberculous lesions with more caution than has hitherto been exercised. The diet must be a liberal one, and should include those articles which are at the same time easily digested and nourishing, especially proteids and fats; milk obtained from a reliable source and underdone butcher-meat are among the best. When the ordinary nourishment taken is insufficient, it may be supplemented by such articles as malt extract, stout, and cod-liver oil. The last is specially beneficial in patients who do not take enough fat in other forms. It is noteworthy that many tuberculous patients show an aversion to fat.

For *the use of tuberculin in diagnosis* and for the *vaccine treatment of tuberculosis* the reader is referred to text-books on medicine.

In addition to increasing the resisting power of the patient, it is important to enable the fluids of the body, so altered, to come into contact with the tuberculous focus. One of the obstacles to this is that the focus is often surrounded by tissues or fluids which have been almost entirely deprived of bactericidal substances. In the case of caseated glands in the neck, for example, it is obvious that the removal of this inert material is necessary before the tissues can be irrigated with fluids of high bactericidal value. Again, in tuberculous ascites the abdominal cavity is filled with a fluid practically devoid of anti-bacterial substances, so that the bacilli are able to thrive and work their will on the tissues. When the stagnant fluid is got rid of by laparotomy, the parts are immediately douched with lymph charged with protective substances, the bactericidal power of which may be many times that of the fluid displaced.

It is probable that the beneficial influence of *counter-irritants*, such as blisters, and exposure to the *Finsen light* and other forms of *rays*, is to be attributed in part to the increased flow of blood to the infected tissues.

Artificial Hyperæmia.—As has been explained, the induction of hyperæmia by the method devised by Bier, constitutes one of our most efficient means of combating bacterial infection. The treatment of tuberculosis on this plan has been proved by experience to be a valuable addition to our therapeutic measures, and the simplicity of its application has led to its being widely adopted in practice. It results in an increase in the reactive changes around the tuberculous focus, an increase in the immigration of leucocytes, and infiltration with the lymphocytes.

The constricting bandage should be applied at some distance above the seat of infection; for instance, in disease of the wrist, it is put on above the elbow, and it must not cause pain either where it is applied or in the diseased part. The bandage is only applied for a few hours each day, either two hours at a time or twice a day for one hour, and, while it is on, all dressings are removed save a piece of sterile gauze over any wound or sinus that may be present. The process of cure takes a long time—nine or even twelve months in the case of a severe joint affection.

In cases in which a constricting bandage is inapplicable, for example, in cold abscesses, tuberculous glands or tendon sheaths, Klapp's suction bell is employed. The cup is applied for five minutes at a time and then taken off for three minutes, and this is repeated over a period of about three-quarters of an hour. The pus is allowed to escape by a small incision, and no packing or drain should be introduced.

It has been found that tuberculous lesions tend to undergo cure when the infected tissues are exposed to the rays of the sun—*heliotherapy*—therefore whenever practicable this therapeutic measure should be had recourse to.

Since the introduction of the methods of treatment described above, and especially by their employment at an early stage in the disease, the number of cases of tuberculosis requiring operative interference has greatly diminished. There are still circumstances, however, in which an operation is required; for example, in disease of the lymph glands for the removal of inert masses of caseous material, in disease of bone for the removal of sequestra, or in disease of joints to improve the function of the limb. It is to be understood, however, that operative treatment must always be preceded by and combined with other therapeutic measures.

TUBERCULOUS ABSCESS

The caseation of tuberculous granulation tissue and its liquefaction is a slow and insidious process, and is unattended with the classical signs of inflammation—hence the terms "cold" and "chronic" applied to the tuberculous abscess.

In a cold abscess, such as that which results from tuberculous disease of the vertebræ, the clinical appearances are those of a soft, fluid swelling without heat, redness, pain, or fever. When toxic symptoms are present, they are usually due to a mixed infection.

A tuberculous abscess results from the disintegration and liquefaction of tuberculous granulation tissue which has undergone caseation. Fluid and cells from the adjacent blood vessels exude into the cavity, and lead to variations in the character of its contents. In some cases the contents consist of a clear amber-coloured fluid, in which are suspended fragments of caseated tissue; in others, of a white material like cream-cheese. From the addition of a sufficient number of leucocytes, the contents may resemble the pus of an ordinary abscess.

The wall of the abscess is lined with tuberculous granulation tissue, the inner layers of which are undergoing caseation and disintegration, and present a shreddy appearance; the outer layers consist of tuberculous tissue which has not yet undergone caseation. The abscess tends to increase in size by progressive liquefaction of the inner layers, caseation of the outer layers, and the further invasion of the surrounding tissues by tubercle bacilli. In this way a tuberculous abscess is capable of indefinite extension and increase in size until it reaches a free surface and ruptures externally. The direction in which it spreads is influenced by the anatomical arrangement of the tissues, and possibly to some extent by gravity, and the abscess may reach the surface at a considerable distance from its seat of origin. The best illustration of this is seen in the psoas abscess, which may originate in the dorsal vertebræ, extend downwards within the sheath of the psoas muscle, and finally appear in the thigh.

Clinical Features.—The insidious development of the tuberculous abscess is one of its characteristic features. The swelling may attain a considerable size without the patient being aware of its existence, and, as a matter of fact, it is often discovered accidentally. The absence of toxæmia is to be associated with the incapacity of the wall of the abscess to permit of absorption; this is shown also by the fact that when even a large quantity of iodoform is inserted into the cavity of the abscess, there are no symptoms of poisoning. The abscess varies in size from a small cherry to a cavity containing several pints of pus. Its shape also varies; it is usually that of a flattened sphere, but it may present pockets or burrows running in various directions. Sometimes it is hour-glass or dumb-bell shaped, as is well illustrated in the region of the groin in disease of the spine or pelvis, where there may be a large sac occupying the venter ilii, and a smaller one in the thigh, the two communicating by a narrow channel under Poupart's ligament. By pressing with the fingers the pus may be displaced from one compartment to the other. The usual course of events is that the abscess progresses slowly, and finally reaches a free surface—generally the skin. As it does so there may be some pain, redness, and local elevation of temperature. Fluctuation becomes evident and superficial, and the skin becomes livid and finally gives way. If the case is left to nature, the discharge of pus continues, and the track opening on the skin remains as a *sinus*. The persistence of suppuration is due to the presence in the wall of the abscess and of the sinus, of tuberculous granulation tissue, which, so long as it remains, continues to furnish discharge, and so prevents healing. Sooner or later pyogenic organisms gain access to the sinus, and through it to the wall of the abscess. They tend further to depress the resisting power of the tissues, and thereby aggravate and perpetuate the tuberculous disease. This superadded infection with pyogenic organisms exposes the patient to the further risks of septic intoxication, especially in the form of hectic fever and septicæmia, and increases the liability to general tuberculosis, and to waxy degeneration of the internal organs. The mixed infection is chiefly responsible for the pyrexia, sweating, and emaciation which the laity associate with consumptive disease. A tuberculous abscess may in one or other of these ways be a cause of death.

Residual abscess is the name given to an abscess that makes its appearance months, or even years, after the apparent cure of tuberculous disease—as, for example, in the hip-joint or spine. It is called residual because it has its origin in the remains of the original disease.

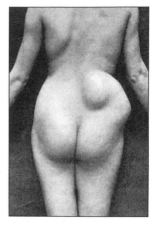

Diagnosis.—A cold abscess is to be diagnosed from a syphilitic gumma, a cyst, and from lipoma and other soft tumours. The differential diagnosis of these affections will be considered later; it is often made easier by recognising the presence of a lesion that is likely to cause a cold abscess, such as tuberculous disease of the spine or of the

FIG. 34. Tuberculous Abscess in right lumbar region in a woman aged thirty.

sacro-iliac joint. When it is about to burst externally, it may be difficult to distinguish a tuberculous abscess from one due to infection with pyogenic organisms. Even when the abscess is opened, the appearances of the pus may not supply the desired information, and it may be necessary to submit it to bacteriological examination. When the pus is found to be sterile, it is usually safe to assume that the condition is tuberculous, as in other forms of suppuration the causative organisms can usually be recognised. Experimental inoculation will establish a definite diagnosis, but it implies a delay of two to three weeks.

Treatment.—The tuberculous abscess may recede and disappear under general treatment. Many surgeons advise that so long as the abscess is quiescent it should be left alone. All agree, however, that if it shows a tendency to spread, to increase in size, or to approach the skin or a mucous membrane, something should be done to avoid the danger of its bursting and becoming infected with pyogenic organisms. Simple evacuation of the abscess by a hollow needle may suffice, or bismuth or iodoform may be introduced after withdrawal of the contents.

Evacuation of the Abscess and Injection of Iodoform.—The iodoform is employed in the form of a 10 per cent. solution in ether or the same proportion suspended in glycerin. Either form becomes sterile soon after it is prepared. Its curative effects would appear to depend upon the liberation of iodine, which restrains the activity of the bacilli, and upon its capacity for irritating the tissues and so inducing a protective leucocytosis, and also of stimulating the formation of scar tissue. An anæsthetic is rarely called for, except in children. The abscess is first evacuated by means of a large trocar and cannula introduced obliquely through the overlying soft parts, avoiding any part where the skin is thin or red. If the cannula becomes blocked with caseous material, it may be cleared with a probe, or a small quantity of saline solution is forced in by the syringe. The iodoform is injected by means of a glass-barrelled syringe, which is firmly screwed on to the cannula. The amount injected varies with the size of the abscess and the age of the patient; it may be said to range from two or three drams in the case of children to several ounces in large abscesses in adults. The cannula is withdrawn, the puncture is closed by a Michel's clip, and a dressing applied so as to exert a certain amount of compression. If the abscess fills up again, the procedure should be repeated; in doing so, the contents show the coloration due to liberated iodine. When the contents are semi-solid, and cannot be withdrawn even through a large cannula, an incision must be made, and, after the cavity has been emptied, the iodoform is introduced through a short rubber tube attached to the syringe. Experience has shown that even large abscesses, such as those associated with spinal disease, may be cured by iodoform injection, and this even when rupture of the abscess on the skin surface has appeared to be imminent.

Another method of treatment which is less popular now than it used to be, and which is chiefly applicable in abscesses of moderate size, is by *incision of the abscess and removal of the tuberculous tissue in its wall* with the sharp spoon. An incision is made which will give free access to the interior of the abscess, so that outlying pockets or recesses may not be overlooked. After removal of the pus, the wall of the abscess is scraped with the Volkmann spoon or with Barker's flushing spoon, to get rid of the tuberculous tissue with which it is lined. In using the spoon, care must be taken that its sharp edge does not perforate the wall of a vein or other important structure. Any debris which may adhere to the walls is removed by rubbing with dry gauze. The oozing of blood is arrested by packing the cavity for a few minutes with gauze. After the packing is removed, iodoform powder is rubbed into the raw surface. The soft parts divided by the incision are sutured in layers so as to ensure primary union. If, on the other hand, there is fear of a mixed infection, especially in abscesses near the rectum or anus, it is safer to treat it by the open method, packing the cavity with iodoform worsted or bismuth gauze, which is renewed at intervals of a week or ten days as the cavity heals from the bottom.

Another method is to incise the abscess, cleanse the cavity with gauze, irrigate with Carrel-Dakin solution and pack with gauze smeared with the dilute non-toxic B.I.P.P. (bismuth and iodoform 2 parts, vaseline 12 parts, hard paraffin, sufficient to give the consistence of butter). The wound is closed with "bipped" silk sutures; one of these—the "waiting suture"—is left loose to permit of withdrawal of the gauze after forty-eight hours; the waiting suture is then tied, and delayed primary union is thus effected.

When the skin over the abscess is red, thin, and about to give way, as is frequently the case when the abscess is situated in the subcutaneous cellular tissue, any skin which is undermined and infected with tubercle should be removed with the scissors at the same time that the abscess is dealt with.

In abscesses treated by the open method, when the cavity has become lined with healthy granulations, it may be closed by secondary suture, or, if the granulating surface is flush with the skin, healing may be hastened by skin-grafting.

If the tuberculous abscess has burst and left a *sinus*, this is apt to persist because of the presence of tuberculous tissue in its wall, and of superadded pyogenic infection, or because it serves as an avenue for the escape of discharge from a focus of tubercle in a bone or a lymph gland.

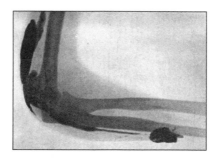

FIG. 35. Tuberculous Sinus injected through its opening in the forearm with bismuth paste. Mr. Pirie Watson's case— Radiogram by Dr. Hope Fowler.)

The treatment varies with the conditions present, and must include measures directed to the lesion from which the sinus has originated. The extent and direction of any given sinus may be demonstrated by the use of the probe, or, more accurately, by injecting the sinus with a paste consisting of white vaseline containing 10 to 30 per cent. of bismuth subcarbonate, and following its track with the X-rays (Fig. 35).

It was found by Beck of Chicago that the injection of bismuth paste is frequently followed by healing of the sinus, and that, if one injection fails to bring about a cure, repeating the injection every second day may be successful. Some caution must be observed in this treatment, as symptoms of poisoning have been observed to follow its use. If they manifest themselves, an injection of warm olive oil should be given; the oil, left in for twelve hours or so, forms an emulsion with the bismuth, which can be withdrawn by aspiration. Iodoform suspended in glycerin may be employed in a similar manner. When these and other non-operative measures fail, and the whole track of the sinus is accessible, it should be laid open, scraped, and packed with bismuth or iodoform gauze until it heals from the bottom.

The *tuberculous ulcer* is described in the chapter on ulcers.

· IX ·

SYPHILIS

Syphilis is an infective disease due to the entrance into the body of a specific virus. It is nearly always communicated from one individual to another by contact infection, the discharge from a syphilitic lesion being the medium through which the virus is transmitted, and the seat of inoculation is almost invariably a surface covered by squamous epithelium. The disease was unknown in Europe before the year 1493, when it was introduced into Spain by Columbus' crew, who were infected in Haiti, where the disease had been endemic from time immemorial (Bloch).

The granulation tissue which forms as a result of the reaction of the tissues to the presence of the virus is chiefly composed of lymphocytes and plasma cells, along with an abundant new formation of capillary blood vessels. Giant cells are not uncommon, but the endothelioid cells, which are so marked a feature of tuberculous granulation tissue, are practically absent.

When syphilis is communicated from one individual to another by contact infection, the condition is spoken of as *acquired syphilis*, and the first visible sign of the disease appears at the site of inoculation, and is known as *the primary lesion*. Those who have thus acquired the disease may transmit it to their offspring, who are then said to suffer from *inherited syphilis*.

The Virus of Syphilis.—The cause of syphilis, whether acquired or inherited, is the organism, described by Schaudinn and Hoffman, in 1905, under the name of *spirochæta pallida* or *spironema pallidum*. It is a delicate, thread-like spirilla, in length averaging from 8 to 10 μ and in width about 0.25 μ, and is distinguished from other spirochætes by its delicate shape, its dead-white appearance, together with its closely twisted spiral form, with numerous undulations (10 to 26), which are perfectly regular, and are characteristic in that they remain the same during rest and in active movement (Fig. 36). In a fresh specimen, such as a scraping from a hard chancre suspended in a little salt solution, it shows active movements. The organism is readily destroyed by heat, and perishes in the absence of moisture. It has been proved experimentally that it remains infective only up to six hours after its removal from the body. Noguchi has succeeded in obtaining pure cultures from the infected tissues of the rabbit.

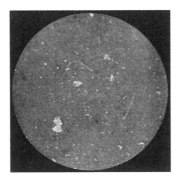

FIG. 36. Spirochæta pallida from scraping of hard Chancre of Prepuce. × 1000 diam. Burri method.

The spirochæte may be recognised in films made by scraping the deeper parts of the primary lesion, from papules on the skin, or from blisters artificially raised on lesions of the skin or on the immediately adjacent portion of healthy skin. It is readily found in the mucous patches and condylomata of the secondary period. It is best stained by Giemsa's method, and its recognition is greatly aided by the use of the ultra-microscope.

The spirochæte has been demonstrated in every form of syphilitic lesion, and has been isolated from the blood—with difficulty—and from lymph withdrawn by a hollow needle from enlarged lymph glands. The saliva of persons suffering from syphilitic lesions of the mouth also contains the organism.

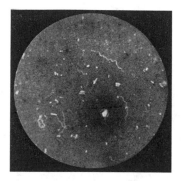

FIG. 37. Spirochæta refrigerans from scraping of Vagina. × 1000 diam. Burri method.

In tertiary lesions there is greater difficulty in demonstrating the spirochæte, but small numbers have been found in the peripheral parts of gummata and in the thickened patches in syphilitic disease of the aorta. Noguchi and Moore have discovered the spirochæte in the brain in a number of cases of general paralysis of the insane. The spirochæte may persist in the body for a long time after infection; its presence has been demonstrated as long as sixteen years after the original acquisition of the disease.

In inherited syphilis the spirochæte is present in enormous numbers throughout all the organs and fluids of the body.

Considerable interest attaches to the observations of Metchnikoff, Roux, and Neisser, who have succeeded in conveying syphilis to the chimpanzee and other members of the ape tribe, obtaining primary and secondary lesions similar to those observed in man, and also containing the spirochæte. In animals the disease has been transmitted by material from all kinds of syphilitic lesions, including even the blood in the secondary and tertiary stages of the disease. The primary lesion is in the form of an indurated papule, in every respect resembling the corresponding lesion in man, and associated with enlargement and induration of the lymph glands. The primary lesion usually appears about thirty days after inoculation, to be followed, in about half the cases, by secondary manifestations, which are usually of a mild character; in no instance has any tertiary lesion been observed. The severity of the affection amongst apes would appear to be in proportion to the nearness of the relationship of the animal to the human subject. The eye of the rabbit is also susceptible to inoculation from syphilitic lesions; the material in a finely divided state is introduced into the anterior chamber of the eye.

Attempts to immunise against the disease have so far proved negative, but Metchnikoff has shown that the inunction of the part inoculated with an ointment containing 33 per cent. of calomel, within one hour of infection, suffices to neutralise the virus in man, and up to eighteen hours in monkeys. He recommends the adoption of this procedure in the prophylaxis of syphilis.

Noguchi has made an emulsion of dead spirochætes which he calls *luetin*, and which gives a specific reaction resembling that of tuberculin in tuberculosis, a papule or a pustule forming at the site of the intra-dermal injection. It is said to be most efficacious in the tertiary and latent forms of syphilis, which are precisely those forms in which the diagnosis is surrounded with difficulties.

ACQUIRED SYPHILIS

In the vast majority of cases, infection takes place during the congress of the sexes. Delicate, easily abraded surfaces are then brought into contact, and the discharge from lesions containing the virus is placed under favourable conditions for conveying the disease from one person to the other. In the male the possibility of infection taking place is increased if the virus is retained under cover of a long and tight prepuce, and if there are abrasions on the surface with which it comes in contact. The frequency with which infection takes place on the genitals during sexual intercourse warrants syphilis being considered a venereal disease, although there are other ways in which it may be contracted.

Some of these imply direct contact—such, for example, as kissing, the digital examination of syphilitic patients by doctors or nurses, or infection of the surgeon's fingers while operating upon a syphilitic patient. In suckling, a syphilitic wet nurse may infect a healthy infant, or a syphilitic infant may infect a healthy wet nurse. In other cases the infection is by indirect contact, the virus being conveyed through the medium of articles contaminated by a syphilitic patient—such, for example, as surgical instruments, tobacco pipes, wind instruments, table utensils, towels, or underclothing. Physiological secretions, such as saliva, milk, or tears, are not capable of communicating the disease unless contaminated by discharge from a syphilitic sore. While the saliva itself is innocuous, it can be, and often is, contaminated by the discharge from mucous patches or other syphilitic lesions in the mouth and throat, and is then a dangerous medium of infection. Unless these extra-genital sources of infection are borne in mind, there is a danger of failing to recognise the primary lesion of syphilis in unusual positions, such as the lip, finger, or nipple. When the disease is thus acquired by innocent transfer, it is known as *syphilis insontium*.

Stages or Periods of Syphilis.—Following the teaching of Ricord, it is customary to divide the life-history of syphilis into three periods or stages, referred to, for convenience, as primary, secondary, and tertiary. This division is to some extent arbitrary and artificial, as the different stages overlap one another, and the lesions of one stage merge insensibly into those of another. Wide variations are met with in the manifestations of the secondary stage, and histologically there is no valid distinction to be drawn between second-ary and tertiary lesions.

The primary period embraces the interval that elapses between the initial infection and the first constitutional manifestations,—roughly, from four to eight weeks,—and includes the period of incubation, the development of the primary sore, and the enlargement of the nearest lymph glands.

The secondary period varies in duration from one to two years, during which time the patient is liable to suffer from manifestations which are for the most part superficial in character, affecting the skin and its appendages, the mucous membranes, and the lymph glands.

The tertiary period has no time-limit except that it follows upon the sec-ondary, so that during the remainder of his life the patient is liable to suffer from manifestations which may affect the deeper tissues and internal organs as well as the skin and mucous membranes.

Primary Syphilis.—*The period of incubation* represents the interval that elapses between the occurrence of infection and the appearance of the pri-mary lesion at the site of inoculation. Its limits may be stated as varying from two to six weeks, with an average of from twenty-one to twenty-eight days. While the disease is incubating, there is nothing to show that infection has occurred.

The Primary Lesion.—The incubation period having elapsed, there appears at the site of inoculation a circumscribed area of infiltration which represents the reaction of the tissues to the entrance of the virus. The first appearance is that of a sharply defined papule, rarely larger than a split pea. Its surface is at first smooth and shiny, but as necrosis of the tissue elements takes place in the centre, it becomes concave, and in many cases the epithelium is shed, and an ulcer is formed. Such an ulcer has an elevated border, sharply cut edges, an indurated base, and exudes a scanty serous discharge; its surface is at first occupied by yellow necrosed tissue, but in time this is replaced by smooth, pale-pink granulation tissue; finally, epithelium may spread over the surface, and the ulcer heals. As a rule, the patient suffers little discomfort, and may even be ignorant of the existence of the lesion, unless, as a result of exposure to mechanical or septic irritation, ulceration ensues, and the sore becomes painful and tender, and yields a purulent discharge. The primary lesion may persist until the secondary manifestations make their appearance, that is, for several weeks.

It cannot be emphasised too strongly that the induration of the primary lesion, which has obtained for it the name of "hard chancre," is its most important characteristic. It is best appreciated when the sore is grasped from side to side between the finger and thumb. The sensation on grasping it has been aptly compared to that imparted by a nodule of cartilage, or by a button felt through a layer of cloth. The evidence obtained by touch is more valuable than that obtained by inspection, a fact which is made use of in the recognition of *concealed chancres*—that is, those which are hidden by a tight prepuce. The induration is due not only to the dense packing of the connective-tissue spaces with lymphocytes and plasma cells, but also to the formation of new connective-tissue elements. It is most marked in chancres situated in the furrow between the glans and the prepuce.

In the male, the primary lesion specially affects certain *situations*, and the appearances vary with these: (1) On the inner aspect of the prepuce, and in the fold between the prepuce and the glans; in the latter situation the induration imparts a "collar-like" rigidity to the prepuce, which is most apparent when it is rolled back over the corona. (2) At the orifice of the prepuce the primary lesion assumes the form of multiple linear ulcers or fissures, and as each of these is attended with infiltration, the prepuce cannot be pulled back—a condition known as *syphilitic phimosis*. (3) On the glans penis the infiltration may be so superficial that it resembles a layer of parchment, but if it invades the cavernous tissue there is a dense mass of induration. (4) On the external aspect of the prepuce or on the skin of the penis itself. (5) At either end of the torn frænum, in the form of a diamond-shaped ulcer raised above the surroundings. (6) In relation to the meatus and canal of the urethra, in either of which situations the swelling and induration may lead to narrowing of the urethra, so that the urine is passed with pain and difficulty and in a minute stream; stricture results only in the exceptional cases in which the chancre has ulcerated and caused destruction of tissue. A chancre within the orifice of the urethra is rare, and, being concealed from view, it can only be recognised by the discharge from the meatus and by the induration felt between the finger and thumb on palpating the urethra.

In the female, the primary lesion is not so typical or so easily recognised as in men; it is usually met with on the labia; the induration is rarely characteristic and does not last so long. The primary lesion may take the form of condylomata. Indurated oedema, with brownish-red or livid discoloration of one or both labia, is diagnostic of syphilis.

The hard chancre is usually solitary, but sometimes there are two or more; when there are several, they are individually smaller than the solitary chancre.

It is the exception for a hard chancre to leave a visible scar, hence, in examining patients with a doubtful history of syphilis, little reliance can be placed on the presence or absence of a scar on the genitals. When the primary lesion has taken the form of an open ulcer with purulent discharge, or has sloughed, there is a permanent scar.

Infection of the adjacent lymph glands is usually found to have taken place by the time the primary lesion has acquired its characteristic induration. Several of the glands along Poupart's ligament, on one or on both sides, become enlarged, rounded, and indurated; they are usually freely movable, and are rarely sensitive unless there is superadded septic infection. The term *bullet-bubo* has been applied to them, and their presence is of great value in diagnosis. In a certain number of cases, one of the main *lymph vessels* on the dorsum of the penis is transformed into a fibrous cord easily recognisable on palpation, and when grasped between the fingers appears to be in size and consistence not unlike the vas deferens.

Concealed chancre is the term applied when one or more chancres are situated within the sac of a prepuce which cannot be retracted. If the induration is well marked, the chancre can be palpated through the prepuce, and is tender on pressure. As under these conditions it is impossible for the patient to keep the parts clean, septic infection becomes a prominent feature, the prepuce is oedematous and inflamed, and there is an abundant discharge of pus from its orifice. It occasionally happens that the infection assumes a virulent character and causes sloughing of the prepuce—a condition known as *phagedæna*. The discharge is then foul and blood-stained, and the prepuce becomes of a dusky red or purple colour, and may finally slough, exposing the glans.

Extra-genital or Erratic Chancres (Fig. 38).—Erratic chancre is the term applied by Jonathan Hutchinson to the primary lesion of syphilis when it appears on parts of the body other than the genitals. It differs in some respects from the hard chancre as met with on the penis; it is usually larger, the induration is more diffused, and the enlarged glands are softer and more sensitive. The glands in nearest relation to the sore are those first affected, for example, the epitrochlear or axillary glands in chancre of the finger; the sub-maxillary glands in chancre of the lip or mouth; or the pre-auricular gland in chancre of the eyelid or forehead. In consequence of their divergence from the typical chancre, and of their being often met with in persons who, from age, surroundings, or moral character, are unlikely subjects of venereal disease, the true nature of erratic chancres is often overlooked until the persistence of the lesion, its want of resemblance to anything else, or the onset of constitutional symptoms, determines the diagnosis of syphilis. A solitary, indolent sore occurring on the lip, eyelid, finger, or nipple, which does not heal but tends to increase in size, and is associated with induration and enlargement of the adjacent glands, is most likely to be the primary lesion of syphilis.

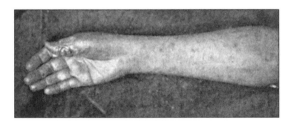

FIG. 38. Primary Lesion on Thumb, with Secondary Eruption on Forearm [1].

The Soft Sore, Soft Chancre, or Chancroid.—The differential diagnosis of syphilis necessitates the consideration of the *soft sore*, *soft chancre*, or *chancroid*, which is also a common form of venereal disease, and is due to infection with a virulent pus-forming bacillus, first described by Ducrey in 1889. Ducrey's bacillus occurs in the form of minute oval rods measuring about

[1] From *A System of Syphilis*, vol. ii., edited by D'Arcy Power and J. Keogh Murphy, Oxford Medical Publications.

1.5 μ in length, which stain readily with any basic aniline dye, but are quickly decolorised by Gram's method. They are found mixed with other organisms in the purulent discharge from the sore, and are chiefly arranged in small groups or in short chains. Soft sores are always contracted by direct contact from another individual, and the incubation period is a short one of from two to five days. They are usually situated in the vicinity of the frænum, and, in women, about the labia minora or fourchette; they probably originate in abrasions in these situations. They appear as pustules, which are rapidly converted into small, acutely inflamed ulcers with sharply cut, irregular margins, which bleed easily and yield an abundant yellow purulent discharge. They are devoid of the induration of syphilis, are painful, and nearly always multiple, reproducing themselves in successive crops by auto-inoculation. Soft sores are often complicated by phimosis and balanitis, and they frequently lead to infection of the glands in the groin. The resulting bubo is ill-defined, painful, and tender, and suppuration occurs in about one-fourth of the cases. The overlying skin becomes adherent and red, and suppuration takes place either in the form of separate foci in the interior of the individual glands, or around them; in the latter case, on incision, the glands are found lying bathed in pus. Ducrey's bacillus is found in pure culture in the pus. Sometimes other pyogenic organisms are superadded. After the bubo has been opened the wound may take on the characters of a soft sore.

Treatment.—Soft sores heal rapidly when kept clean. If concealed under a tight prepuce, an incision should be made along the dorsum to give access to the sores. They should be washed with eusol, and dusted with a mixture of one part iodoform and two parts boracic or salicylic acid, or, when the odour of iodoform is objected to, of equal parts of boracic acid and carbonate of zinc. Immersion of the penis in a bath of eusol for some hours daily is useful. The sore is then covered with a piece of gauze kept in position by drawing the prepuce over it, or by a few turns of a narrow bandage. Sublimed sulphur frequently rubbed into the sore is recommended by C. H. Mills. If the sores spread in spite of this, they should be painted with cocaine and then cauterised. When the glands in the groin are infected, the patient must be confined to bed, and a dressing impregnated with ichthyol and glycerin (10 per cent.) applied; the repeated use of a suction bell is of great service. Harrison recommends aspiration of a bubonic abscess, followed by injection of 1 in 20 solution of tincture of iodine into the cavity; this is in turn aspirated, and then

1 or 2 c.c. of the solution injected and left in. This is repeated as often as the cavity refills. It is sometimes necessary to let the pus out by one or more small incisions and continue the use of the suction bell.

Diagnosis of Primary Syphilis.—In cases in which there is a history of an incubation period of from three to five weeks, when the sore is indurated, persistent, and indolent, and attended with bullet-buboes in the groin, the diagnosis of primary syphilis is not difficult. Owing, however, to the great importance of instituting treatment at the earliest possible stage of the infection, an effort should be made to establish the diagnosis without delay by demonstrating the spirochæte. Before any antiseptic is applied, the margin of the suspected sore is rubbed with gauze, and the serum that exudes on pressure is collected in a capillary tube and sent to a pathologist for microscopical examination. A better specimen can sometimes be obtained by puncturing an enlarged lymph gland with a hypodermic needle, injecting a few minims of sterile saline solution and then aspirating the blood-stained fluid.

The Wassermann test must not be relied upon for diagnosis in the early stage, as it does not appear until the disease has become generalised and the secondary manifestations are about to begin. The practice of waiting in doubtful cases before making a diagnosis until secondary manifestations appear is to be condemned.

Extra-genital chancres, *e.g.* sores on the fingers of doctors or nurses, are specially liable to be overlooked, if the possibility of syphilis is not kept in mind.

It is important to bear in mind *the possibility of a patient having acquired a mixed infection* with the virus of soft chancre, which will manifest itself a few days after infection, and the virus of syphilis, which shows itself after an interval of several weeks. This occurrence was formerly the source of much confusion in diagnosis, and it was believed at one time that syphilis might result from soft sores, but it is now established that syphilis does not follow upon soft sores unless the virus of syphilis has been introduced at the same time. The practitioner must be on his guard, therefore, when a patient asks his advice concerning a venereal sore which has appeared within a few days of exposure to infection. Such a patient is naturally anxious to know whether he has contracted syphilis or not, but neither a positive nor a negative answer can be given—unless the spirochæte can be identified.

Syphilis is also to be diagnosed from *epithelioma*, the common form of cancer of the penis. It is especially in elderly patients with a tight prepuce that the induration of syphilis is liable to be mistaken for that associated with epithelioma. In difficult cases the prepuce must be slit open.

Difficulty may occur in the diagnosis of primary syphilis from *herpes*, as this may appear as late as ten days after connection; it commences as a group of vesicles which soon burst and leave shallow ulcers with a yellow floor; these disappear quickly on the use of an antiseptic dusting powder.

Apprehensive patients who have committed sexual indiscretions are apt to regard as syphilitic any lesion which happens to be located on the penis—for example, acne pustules, eczema, psoriasis papules, boils, balanitis, or venereal warts.

The local treatment of the primary sore consists in attempting to destroy the organisms *in situ*. An ointment made up of calomel 33 parts, lanoline 67 parts, and vaseline 10 parts (Metchnikoff's cream) is rubbed into the sore several times a day. If the surface is unbroken, it may be dusted lightly with a powder composed of equal parts of calomel and carbonate of zinc. A gauze dressing is applied, and the penis and scrotum should be supported against the abdominal wall by a triangular handkerchief or bathing-drawers; if there is inflammatory oedema the patient should be confined to bed.

In *concealed chancres* with phimosis, the sac of the prepuce should be slit up along the dorsum to admit of the ointment being applied. If phagedæna occurs, the prepuce must be slit open along the dorsum, or if sloughing, cut away, and the patient should have frequent sitz baths of weak sublimate lotion. When the chancre is within the meatus, iodoform bougies are inserted into the urethra, and the urine should be rendered bland by drinking large quantities of fluid.

General treatment is considered on p. 149.

Secondary Syphilis.—The following description of secondary syphilis is based on the average course of the disease in untreated cases. The onset of constitutional symptoms occurs from six to twelve weeks after infection, and the manifestations are the result of the entrance of the virus into the general circulation, and its being carried to all parts of the body. The period during which the patient is liable to suffer from secondary symptoms ranges from six months to two years.

In some cases the general health is not disturbed; in others the patient is feverish and out of sorts, losing appetite, becoming pale and anæmic, complaining of lassitude, incapacity for exertion, headache, and pains of a rheumatic type referred to the bones. There is a moderate degree of leucocytosis, but the increase is due not to the polymorpho-nuclear leucocytes but to lymphocytes. In isolated cases the temperature rises to 101° or 102° F. and the patient loses flesh. The lymph glands, particularly those along the posterior border of the sterno-mastoid, become enlarged and slightly tender. The hair comes out, eruptions appear on the skin and mucous membranes, and the patient may suffer from sore throat and affections of the eyes. The local lesions are to be regarded as being of the nature of reactions against accumulations of the parasite, lymphocytes and plasma cells being the elements chiefly concerned in the reactive process.

Affections of the Skin are among the most constant manifestations. An evanescent macular rash, not unlike that of measles—*roseola*—is the first to appear, usually in from six to eight weeks from the date of infection; it is widely diffused over the trunk, and the original dull rose-colour soon fades, leaving brownish stains, which in time disappear. It is usually followed by a *papular eruption*, the individual papules being raised above the surface of the skin, smooth or scaly, and as they are due to infiltration of the skin they are more persistent than the roseoles. They vary in size and distribution, being sometimes small, hard, polished, and closely aggregated like lichen, sometimes as large as a shilling-piece, with an accumulation of scales on the surface like that seen in psoriasis. The co-existence of scaly papules and faded roseoles is very suggestive of syphilis.

Other types of eruption are less common, and are met with from the third month onwards. A *pustular* eruption, not unlike that of acne, is sometimes a prominent feature, but is not characteristic of syphilis unless it affects the scalp and forehead and is associated with the remains of the papular eruption. The term *ecthyma* is applied when the pustules are of large size, and, after breaking on the surface, give rise to superficial ulcers; the discharge from the ulcer often dries up and forms a scab or crust which is continually added to from below as the ulcer extends in area and depth. The term *rupia* is applied when the crusts are prominent, dark in colour, and conical in shape, roughly resembling the shell of a limpet. If the crust is detached, a sharply defined ulcer is exposed, and when this heals it leaves a scar which is usually circular, thin, white, shining like satin, and the surrounding skin is darkly pigmented; in the case of deep ulcers, the scar is depressed and adherent (Fig. 39).

In the later stages there may occur a form of creeping or *spreading ulceration of the skin* of the face, groin, or scrotum, healing at one edge and spreading at another like tuberculous lupus, but distinguished from this by its more rapid progress and by the pigmentation of the scar.

Condylomata are more characteristic of syphilis than any other type of skin lesion. They are papules occurring on those parts of the body where the skin is habitually moist, and especially where two skin surfaces are in contact. They are chiefly met with on the exter-nal genitals, especially in women, around the

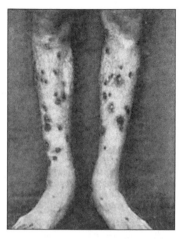

FIG. 39. Syphilitic Rupia, showing the limpet-shaped crusts or scabs.

anus, beneath large pendulous mammæ, between the toes, and at the angles of the mouth, and in these situations their development is greatly favoured by neglect of cleanliness. They present the appearance of well-defined circular or ovoid areas in which the skin is thickened and raised above the surface; they are covered with a white sodden epidermis, and furnish a scanty but very infective discharge. Under the influence of irritation and want of rest, as at the anus or at the angle of the mouth, they are apt to become fissured and superficially ulcerated, and the discharge then becomes abundant and may crust on the surface, forming yellow scabs. At the angle of the mouth the condylomatous patches may spread to the cheek, and when they ulcerate may leave fissure-like scars radiating from the mouth—an appearance best seen in inherited syphilis (Fig. 44).

The Appendages of the Skin.—The *hair* loses its gloss, becomes dry and brittle, and readily falls out, either as an exaggeration of the normal shedding of the hair, or in scattered areas over the scalp (*syphilitic alopoecia*). The hair is not re-formed in the scars which result from ulcerated lesions of the scalp. The *nail-folds* occasionally present a pustular eruption and superficial ulceration, to which the name *syphilitic onychia* has been applied; more commonly the nails become brittle and ragged, and they may even be shed.

The Mucous Membranes, and especially those of the *mouth* and *throat*, suffer from lesions similar to those met with on the skin. On a mucous surface the papular eruption assumes the form of *mucous patches*, which are areas with a congested base covered with a thin white film of sodden epithelium like wet tissue-paper. They are best seen on the inner aspect of the cheeks, the soft palate, uvula, pillars of the fauces, and tonsils. In addition to mucous patches, there may be a number of small, *superficial, kidney-shaped ulcers*, especially along the margins of the tongue and on the tonsils. In the absence of mucous patches and ulcers, the sore throat may be characterised by a bluish tinge of the inflamed mucous membrane and a thin film of shed epithelium on the surface. Sometimes there is an elongated sinuous film which has been likened to the track of a snail. In the *larynx* the presence of congestion, oedema, and mucous patches may be the cause of persistent hoarseness. The *tongue* often presents a combination of lesions, including ulcers, patches where the papillæ are absent, fissures, and raised white papules resembling warts, especially towards the centre of the dorsum. These lesions are specially apt to occur in those who smoke, drink undiluted alcohol or spirits, or eat hot condiments to excess, or who have irregular, sharp-cornered teeth. At a later period, and in those who are broken down in health from intemperance or other cause, the sore throat may take the form of rapidly spreading, penetrating ulcers in the soft palate and pillars of the fauces, which may lead to extensive destruction of tissue, with subsequent scars and deformity highly characteristic of previous syphilis.

In the *Bones*, lesions occur which assume the clinical features of an evanescent periostitis, the patient complaining of nocturnal pains over the frontal bone, sternum, tibiæ, and ulnæ, and localised tenderness on tapping over these bones.

In the *Joints*, a serous synovitis or hydrops may occur, chiefly in the knee, on one or on both sides.

The Affections of the Eyes, although fortunately rare, are of great importance because of the serious results which may follow if they are not recognised and treated. *Iritis* is the commonest of these, and may occur in one or in both eyes, one after the other, from three to eight months after infection. The patient complains of impairment of sight and of frontal or supraorbital pain. The eye waters and is hypersensitive, the iris is discoloured and reacts sluggishly to light, and there is a zone of ciliary congestion around the cornea. The appearance of minute white nodules or flakes of lymph at the margin of the pupil is especially characteristic of syphilitic iritis. When adhesions have formed between the iris and the structures in relation to it, the pupil dilates irregularly under atropin. Although complete recovery is to be expected under early and energetic treatment, if neglected, *iritis* may result in occlusion of the pupil and permanent impairment or loss of sight.

The other lesions of the eye are much rarer, and can only be discovered on ophthalmoscopic examination.

The virus of syphilis exerts a special influence upon the *Blood Vessels*, exciting a proliferation of the endothelial lining which results in narrowing of their lumen, *endarteritis*, and a perivascular infiltration in the form of accumulations of plasma cells around the vessels and in the lymphatics that accompany them.

In the *Brain*, in the later periods of secondary and in tertiary syphilis, changes occur as a result of the narrowing of the lumen of the arteries, or of their complete obliteration by thrombosis. By interfering with the nutrition of those parts of the brain supplied by the affected arteries, these lesions give rise to clinical features of which severe headache and paralysis are the most prominent.

Affections of the *Spinal Cord* are extremely rare, but paraplegia from myelitis has been observed.

Lastly, attention must be directed to the remarkable variations observed in different patients. Sometimes the virulent character of the disease can only be accounted for by an idiosyncrasy of the patient. Constitutional symptoms, particularly pyrexia and anæmia, are most often met with in young women. Patients over forty years of age have greater difficulty in overcoming the infection than younger adults. Malarial and other infections, and the conditions attending life in tropical countries, from the debility which they cause, tend to aggravate and prolong the disease, which then assumes the characters of what has been called *malignant syphilis*. All chronic ailments have a similar influence, and alcoholic intemperance is universally regarded as a serious aggravating factor.

Diagnosis of Secondary Syphilis.—A routine examination should be made of the parts of the body which are most often affected in this disease—the scalp, mouth, throat, posterior cervical glands, and the trunk, the patient being stripped and examined by daylight. Among the *diagnostic features of the skin affections* the following may be mentioned: They are frequently, and sometimes to a marked degree, symmetrical; more than one type of eruption—papules and pustules, for example—are present at the same time; there is little itching; they are at first a dull-red colour, but later present a brown pigmentation which has been likened to the colour of raw ham; they exhibit a predilection for those parts of the forehead and neck which are close to the roots of the hair; they tend to pass off spontaneously; and they disappear rapidly under treatment.

Serum Diagnosis—Wassermann Reaction.—Wassermann found that if an extract of syphilitic liver rich in spirochætes is mixed with the serum from a syphilitic patient, a large amount of complement is fixed. The application of the test is highly complicated and can only be carried out by an expert pathologist. For the purpose he is supplied with from 5 c.c. to 10 c.c. of the patient's blood, withdrawn under aseptic conditions from the median basilic vein by means of a serum syringe, and transferred to a clean and dry glass tube. There is abundant evidence that the Wassermann test is a reliable means of establishing a diagnosis of syphilis.

A definitely positive reaction can usually be obtained between the fifteenth and thirtieth day after the appearance of the primary lesion, and as time goes on it becomes more marked. During the secondary period the reaction is practically always positive. In the tertiary stage also it is positive except in so far as it is modified by the results of treatment. In para-syphilitic lesions such as general paralysis and tabes a positive reaction is almost always present. In inherited syphilis the reaction is positive in every case. A positive reaction may be present in other diseases, for example, frambesia, trypano-somiasis, and leprosy.

As the presence of the reaction is an evidence of the activity of the spiro-chætes, repeated applications of the test furnish a valuable means of estimating the efficacy of treatment. The object aimed at is to change a persistently positive reaction to a permanently negative one.

Treatment of Syphilis.—In the treatment of syphilis the two main objects are to maintain the general health at the highest possible standard, and to introduce into the system therapeutic agents which will inhibit or destroy the invading parasite.

The second of these objects has been achieved by the researches of Ehrlich, who, in conjunction with his pupil, Hata, has built up a compound, the dihydrochloride of dioxydiamido-arseno-benzol, popularly known as salvarsan or "606." Other preparations, such as kharsivan, arseno-billon, and diarsenol, are chemically equivalent to salvarsan, containing from 27 to 31 per cent. of arsenic, and are equally efficient. The full dose is 0.6 grm. All these members of the "606" group form an acid solution when dissolved in water, and must be rendered alkaline before being injected. As subcutaneous and intra-muscular injections cause considerable pain, and may cause sloughing of the tissues, "606" preparations must be injected intravenously. Ehrlich has devised a preparation—neo-salvarsan, or "914," which is more easily prepared and forms a neutral solution. It contains from 18 to 20 per cent. of arsenic. Neo-kharsivan, novo-arseno-billon, and neo-diarsenol belong to the "914" group, the full dosage of which is 0.9 grm. As subcutaneous and intra-muscular injections of the "914" group are not painful, and even more efficient than intravenous injections, the administration is simpler.

Galyl, luargol, and other preparations act in the same way as the "606" and "914" groups.

The "606" preparations may be introduced into the veins by injection or by means of an apparatus which allows the solution to flow in by gravity. The left median basilic vein is selected, and a platino-iridium needle with a short point and a bore larger than that of the ordinary hypodermic syringe is used. The needle is passed for a few millimetres along the vein, and the solution is then slowly introduced; before withdrawing the needle some saline is run in to diminish the risk of thrombosis.

The "914" preparations may be injected either into the subcutaneous tissue of the buttock or into the substance of the gluteus muscle. The part is then massaged for a few minutes, and the massage is repeated daily for a few days.

No hard-and-fast rules can be laid down as to what constitutes a complete course of treatment. Harrison recommends as a minimum course of one of the "914" preparations in *early primary cases* an initial dose of 0.45 grm. given intra-muscularly or into the deep subcutaneous tissue; the same dose a week later; 0.6 grm. the following week; then miss a week and give 9.6 grms. on two successive weeks; then miss two weeks and give 0.6 grm. on two more successive weeks.

When a *positive Wassermann reaction* is present before treatment is commenced, the above course is prolonged as follows: for three weeks is given a course of potassium iodide, after which four more weekly injections of 0.6 grm. of "914" are given.

With each injection of "914" after the first, throughout the whole course 1 grain of mercury is injected intra-muscularly.

In the course of a few hours, there is usually some indisposition, with a feeling of chilliness and slight rise of temperature; these symptoms pass off within twenty-four hours, and in a few days there is a decided improvement of health. Three or four days after an intra-muscular injection there may be pain and stiffness in the gluteal region.

These preparations are the most efficient therapeutic agents that have yet been employed in the treatment of syphilis.

The manifestations of the disease disappear with remarkable rapidity. Observations show that the spirochætes lose their capacity for movement within an hour or two of the administration, and usually disappear altogether in from twenty-four to thirty-six hours. Wassermann's reaction usually yields a negative result in from three weeks to two months, but later may again become positive. Subsequent doses of the arsenical preparation are therefore usually indicated, and should be given in from 7 to 21 days according to the dose.

When syphilis occurs in a *pregnant woman*, she should be given in the early months an ordinary course of "914," followed by 10-grain doses of potassium iodide twice daily. The injections may be repeated two months later, and during the remainder of the pregnancy 2-grain mercury pills are given twice daily (A. Campbell). The presence of albumen in the urine contra-indicates arsenical treatment.

It need scarcely be pointed out that the use of powerful drugs like "606" and "914" is not free from risk; it may be mentioned that each dose contains nearly three grains of arsenic. Before the administration the patient must be overhauled; its administration is contra-indicated in the presence of disease of the heart and blood vessels, especially a combination of syphilitic aortitis and sclerosis of the coronary arteries, with degeneration of the heart muscle; in affections of the central nervous system, especially advanced paralysis, and in such disturbances of metabolism as are associated with diabetes and Bright's disease. Its use is not contra-indicated in any lesion of active syphilis.

The administration is controlled by the systematic examination of the urine for arsenic.

The Administration of Mercury.—The success of the arsenical preparations has diminished the importance of mercury in the treatment of syphilis, but it is still used to supplement the effect of the injections. The amount of mercury to be given in any case must be proportioned to the idiosyncrasies of the patient, and it is advisable, before commencing the treatment, to test his urine and record his body-weight. The small amount of mercury given at the outset is gradually increased. If the body-weight falls, or if the gums become

sore and the breath foul, the mercury should be stopped for a time. If saliva-
tion occurs, the drinking of hot water and the taking of hot baths should be
insisted upon, and half-dram doses of the alkaline sulphates prescribed.

Methods of Administering Mercury.—(1) *By the Mouth.*—This was for long
the most popular method in this country, the preparation usually employed
being grey powder, in pills or tablets, each of which contains one grain of the
powder. Three of these are given daily in the first instance, and the daily dose
is increased to five or even seven grains till the standard for the individual
patient is arrived at. As the grey powder alone sometimes causes irritation
of the bowels, it should be combined with iron, as in the following formula:
Hydrarg. c. cret. gr. 1; ferri sulph. exsiccat. gr. 1 or 2.

(2) *By Inunction.*—Inunction consists in rubbing into the pores of the
skin an ointment composed of equal parts of 20 per cent. oleate of mercury
and lanolin. Every night after a hot bath, a dram of the ointment (made up
by the chemist in paper packets) is rubbed for fifteen minutes into the skin
where it is soft and comparatively free from hairs. When the patient has
been brought under the influence of the mercury, inunction may be replaced
by one of the other methods, of administering the drug.

(3) *By Intra-muscular Injection.*—This consists in introducing the drug
by means of a hypodermic syringe into the substance of the gluteal muscles.
The syringe is made of glass, and has a solid glass piston; the needle of platino-iridium should be 5 cm. long and of a larger calibre than the ordinary
hypodermic needle. The preparation usually employed consists of: metallic
mercury or calomel 1 dram, lanolin and olive oil each 2 drams; it must be
warmed to allow of its passage through the needle. Five minims—containing
one grain of metallic mercury—represent a dose, and this is injected into the
muscles above and behind the great trochanter once a week. The contents of
the syringe are slowly expressed, and, after withdrawing the needle, gentle
massage of the buttock should be employed. Four courses each of ten injections are given the first year, three courses of the same number during the
second and third years, and two courses during the fourth year (Lambkin).

The General Health.—The patient must lead a regular life and cultivate the
fresh-air habit, which is as beneficial in syphilis as in tuberculosis. Anæmia,
malaria, and other sources of debility must receive appropriate treatment.
The diet should be simple and easily digested, and should include a full supply of milk. Alcohol is prohibited. The excretory organs are encouraged to act

by the liberal drinking of hot water between meals, say five or six tumbler-fuls in the twenty-four hours. The functions of the skin are further aided by frequent hot baths, and by the wearing of warm underclothing. While the patient should avoid exposure to cold, and taxing his energies by undue exertion, he should be advised to take exercise in the open air. On account of the liability to lesions of the mouth and throat, he should use tobacco in moderation, his teeth should be thoroughly overhauled by the dentist, and he should brush them after every meal, using an antiseptic tooth powder or wash. The mouth and throat should be rinsed out night and morning with a solution of chlorate of potash and alum, or with peroxide of hydrogen.

Treatment of the Local Manifestations.—*The skin lesions* are treated on the same lines as similar eruptions of other origin. As local applications, preparations of mercury are usually selected, notably the ointments of the red oxide of mercury, ammoniated mercury, or oleate of mercury (5 per cent.), or the mercurial plaster introduced by Unna. In the treatment of condylomata the greatest attention must be paid to cleanliness and dryness. After washing and drying the affected patches, they are dusted with a powder consisting of equal parts of calomel and carbonate of zinc; and apposed skin surfaces, such as the nates or labia, are separated by sublimate wool. In the ulcers of later secondary syphilis, crusts are got rid of in the first instance by means of a boracic poultice, after which a piece of lint or gauze cut to the size of the ulcer and soaked in black wash is applied and covered with oil-silk. If the ulcer tends to spread in area or in depth, it should be scraped with a sharp spoon, and painted over with acid nitrate of mercury, or a local hyperæmia may be induced by Klapp's suction apparatus.

In lesions of the mouth and throat, the teeth should be attended to; the best local application is a solution of chromic acid—10 grains to the ounce—painted on with a brush once daily. If this fails, the lesions may be dusted with calomel the last thing at night. For deep ulcers of the throat the patient should gargle frequently with chlorine water or with perchloride of mercury (1 in 2000); if the ulcer continues to spread it should be painted with acid nitrate of mercury.

In the treatment of *iritis* the eyes are shaded from the light and completely rested, and the pupil is well dilated by atropin to prevent adhesions. If there is much pain, a blister may be applied to the temple.

The Relations of Syphilis to Marriage.—Before the introduction of the Ehrlich-Hata treatment no patient was allowed to marry until three years had elapsed after the disappearance of the last manifestation. While marriage might be entered upon under these conditions without risk of the husband infecting the wife, the possibility of his conveying the disease to the offspring cannot be absolutely excluded. It is recommended, as a precautionary measure, to give a further mercurial course of two or three months' duration before marriage, and an intravenous injection of an arsenical preparation.

Intermediate Stage.—After the dying away of the secondary manifestations and before the appearance of tertiary lesions, the patient may present certain symptoms which Hutchinson called *reminders*. These usually consist of relapses of certain of the affections of the skin, mouth, or throat, already described. In the skin, they may assume the form of peeling patches in the palms, or may appear as spreading and confluent circles of a scaly papular eruption, which if neglected may lead to the formation of fissures and superficial ulcers. Less frequently there is a relapse of the eye affections, or of paralytic symptoms from disease of the cerebral arteries.

Tertiary Syphilis.—While the manifestations of primary and secondary syphilis are common, those of the tertiary period are by comparison rare, and are observed chiefly in those who have either neglected treatment or who have had their powers of resistance lowered by privation, by alcoholic indulgence, or by tropical disease.

It is to be borne in mind that in a certain proportion of men and in a larger proportion of women, the patient has no knowledge of having suffered from syphilis. Certain slight but important signs may give the clue in a number of cases, such as irregularity of the pupils or failure to react to light, abnormality of the reflexes, and the discovery of patches of leucoplakia on the tongue, cheek, or palate.

The *general character of tertiary manifestations* may be stated as follows: They attack by preference the tissues derived from the mesoblastic layer of the embryo—the cellular tissue, bones, muscles, and viscera. They are often localised to one particular tissue or organ, such, for example, as the subcutaneous cellular tissue, the bones, or the liver, and they are rarely symmetrical. They are usually aggressive and persistent, with little tendency to natural cure, and they may be dangerous to life, because of the destructive changes produced in such organs as the brain or the larynx. They are remarkably amenable to treatment if instituted before the stage which is attended with destruction of tissue is reached. Early tertiary lesions may be infective, and the disease may be transmitted by the discharges from them; but the later the lesions the less is the risk of their containing an infective virus.

The most prominent feature of tertiary syphilis consists in the formation of granulation tissue, and this takes place on a scale considerably larger than that observed in lesions of the secondary period. The granulation tissue frequently forms a definite swelling or tumour-like mass (syphiloma), which, from its peculiar elastic consistence, is known as a *gumma*. In its early stages a gumma is a firm, semi-translucent greyish or greyish-red mass of tissue; later it becomes opaque, yellow, and caseous, with a tendency to soften and liquefy. The gumma does harm by displacing and replacing the normal tissue elements of the part affected, and by involving these in the degenerative changes, of the nature of caseation and necrosis, which produce the destructive lesions of the skin, mucous membranes, and internal organs. This is true not only of the circumscribed gumma, but of the condition known as *gummatous infiltration* or *syphilitic cirrhosis*, in which the granulation tissue is diffused throughout the connective-tissue framework of such organs as the tongue or liver. Both the gummatous lesions and the fibrosis of tertiary syphilis are directly excited by the spirochætes.

The life-history of an untreated gumma varies with its environment. When protected from injury and irritation in the substance of an internal organ such as the liver, it may become encapsulated by fibrous tissue, and persist in this condition for an indefinite period, or it may be absorbed and leave in its place a fibrous cicatrix. In the interior of a long bone it may replace the rigid framework of the shaft to such an extent as to lead to pathological fracture. If it is near the surface of the body—as, for example, in the subcutaneous or submucous cellular tissue, or in the periosteum of a superficial bone, such as the palate, the skull, or the tibia—the tissue of which it is composed is apt to undergo necrosis, in which the overlying skin or mucous membrane frequently participates, the result being an ulcer—the tertiary syphilitic ulcer (Figs. 40 and 41).

Tertiary Lesions of the Skin and Subcutaneous Cellular Tissue.—The clinical features of a *subcutaneous gumma* are those of an indolent, painless, elastic swelling, varying in size from a pea to an almond or walnut. After a variable period it usually softens in the centre, the skin over it becomes livid and dusky, and finally separates as a slough, exposing the tissue of the gumma, which sometimes appears as a mucoid, yellowish, honey-like substance, more frequently as a sodden, caseated tissue resembling wash-leather. The caseated tissue of a gumma differs from that of a tuberculous lesion in being tough and firm, of a buff colour like wash-leather, or whitish, like boiled fish. The degenerated tissue separates slowly and gradually, and in untreated cases may be visible for weeks in the floor of the ulcer.

The tertiary ulcer may be situated anywhere, but is most frequently met with on the leg, especially in the region of the knee (Fig. 42) and over the calf. There may be one or more ulcers, and also scars of antecedent ulcers. The edges are sharply cut, as if punched out; the margins are rounded in outline, firm, and congested; the base is occupied by gummatous tissue, or, if this has already separated and sloughed out, by unhealthy granulations and a thick purulent discharge. When the ulcer has healed it leaves a scar which is depressed, and if over a bone, is adherent to it. The features of the tertiary ulcer, however, are

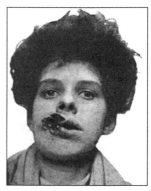

FIG. 40. Ulcerating Gumma of Lips. From a photograph lent by Dr. Stopford Taylor and Dr. R. W. Mackenna.)

not always so characteristic as the above description would imply. It is to be diagnosed from the "leg ulcer," which occurs almost exclusively on the lower third of the leg; from Bazin's disease (p. 74); from the ulcers that result from certain forms of malignant disease, such as rodent cancer, and from those met with in chronic glanders.

Gummatous Infiltration of the Skin ("Syphilitic Lupus").—This is a lesion, met with chiefly on the face and in the region of the external genitals, in which the skin becomes infiltrated with granulation tissue so that it is thickened, raised above the surface, and of a brownish-red colour. It appears as isolated nodules, which may fuse together; the epidermis becomes scaly and is shed, giving rise to superficial ulcers which are usually covered by crusted discharge. The disease tends to spread, creeping over the skin with a serpiginous, crescentic, or horse-shoe margin, while the central portion may heal and leave a scar. From the fact of its healing in the centre while it spreads at the margin, it may resemble tuberculous disease of the skin. It can usually be differentiated by observing that the infiltration is on a larger scale; the progress is much more rapid, involving in the course of months an area which in the case of tuberculosis would require as many years; the scars are sounder and are less liable to break down again; and the disease rapidly yields to anti-syphilitic treatment.

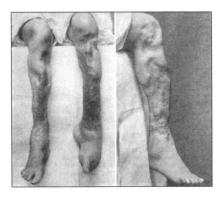

FIG. 41. Ulceration of nineteen year's duration in a woman æt. 24, the subject of inherited syphilis, showing active ulceration, cicatricial contraction, and sabre-blade deformity of tibiæ.

Tertiary lesions of mucous membrane and of the submucous cellular tissue are met with chiefly in the tongue, nose, throat, larynx, and rectum. They originate as gummata or as gummatous infiltrations, which are liable to break down and lead to the formation of ulcers which may prove locally destructive, and, in such situations as the larynx, even dangerous to life. In the tongue the tertiary ulcer may prove the starting-point of cancer; and in the larynx or rectum the healing of the ulcer may lead to cicatricial stenosis.

Tertiary lesions of the *bones and joints*, of the *muscles*, and of the *internal organs*, will be described under these heads. The part played by syphilis in the production of disease of arteries and of aneurysm will be referred to along with diseases of blood vessel

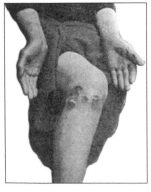

FIG. 42. Tertiary Syphilitic Ulceration in region of Knee and on both Thumbs of woman æt. 37.

Treatment.—The most valuable drugs for the treatment of the manifestations of the tertiary period are the arsenical preparations and the iodides of sodium and potassium. On account of their depressing effects, the latter are frequently prescribed along with carbonate of ammonium. The dose is usually a matter of experiment in each individual case; 5 grains three times a day may suffice, or it may be necessary to increase each dose to 20 or 25 grains. The symptoms of iodism which may follow from the smaller doses usually disappear on giving a larger amount of the drug. It should be taken after meals, with abundant water or other fluid, especially if given in tablet form. It is advisable to continue the iodides for from one to three months after the lesions for which they are given have cleared up. If the potassium salt is not tolerated, it may be replaced by the ammonium or sodium iodide.

Local Treatment.—The absorption of a subcutaneous gumma is often hastened by the application of a fly-blister. When a gumma has broken on the surface and caused an ulcer, this is treated on general principles, with a preference, however, for applications containing mercury or iodine, or both. If a wet dressing is required to cleanse the ulcer, black wash may be used; if a powder to promote dryness, one containing iodoform; if an ointment is indicated, the choice lies between the red oxide of mercury or the dilute nitrate of mercury ointment, and one consisting of equal parts of lanolin and vaselin with 2 per cent. of iodine. Deep ulcers, and obstinate lesions of the bones, larynx, and other parts may be treated by excision or scraping with the sharp spoon.

Second Attacks of Syphilis.—Instances of re-infection of syphilis have been recorded with greater frequency since the more general introduction of arsenical treatment. A remarkable feature in such cases is the shortness of the interval between the original infection and the alleged re-infection; in a recent series of twenty-eight cases, this interval was less than a year. Another feature of interest is that when patients in the tertiary stage of syphilis are inoculated with the virus from lesions from these in the primary and secondary stage lesions of the tertiary type are produced.

Reference may be made to the **relapsing false indurated chancre**, described by Hutchinson and by Fournier, as it may be the source of difficulty in diagnosis. A patient who has had an infecting chancre one or more years before, may present a slightly raised induration on the penis at or close to the site of his original sore. This relapsed induration is often so like that of a primary chancre that it is impossible to distinguish between them, except by the history. If there has been a recent exposure to venereal infection, it is liable to be regarded as the primary lesion of a second attack of syphilis, but the further progress shows that neither bullet-buboes nor secondary manifestations develop. These facts, together with the disappearance of the induration under treatment, make it very likely that the lesion is really gummatous in character.

INHERITED SYPHILIS

One of the most striking features of syphilis is that it may be transmitted from infected parents to their offspring, the children exhibiting the manifestations that characterise the acquired form of the disease.

The more recent the syphilis in the parent, the greater is the risk of the disease being communicated to the offspring; so that if either parent suffers from secondary syphilis the infection is almost inevitably transmitted.

While it is certain that either parent may be responsible for transmitting the disease to the next generation, the method of transmission is not known. In the case of a syphilitic mother it is most probable that the infection is conveyed to the foetus by the placental circulation. In the case of a syphilitic father, it is commonly believed that the infection is conveyed to the ovum through the seminal fluid at the moment of conception. If a series of children, one after the other, suffer from inherited syphilis, it is almost invariably the case that the mother has been infected.

In contrast to the acquired form, inherited syphilis is remarkable for the absence of any primary stage, the infection being a general one from the outset. The spirochæte is demonstrated in incredible numbers in the liver, spleen, lung, and other organs, and in the nasal secretion, and, from any of these, successful inoculations in monkeys can readily be made. The manifestations differ in degree rather than in kind from those of the acquired disease; the difference is partly due to the fact that the virus is attacking developing instead of fully formed tissues.

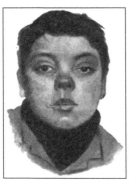

FIG. 43. Facies of Inherited Syphilis. (From Dr. Byrom Bramwell's Atlas of Clinical Medicine.)

The virus exercises an injurious influence on the foetus, which in many cases dies during the early months of intra-uterine life, so that miscarriage results, and this may take place in repeated pregnancies, the date at which the miscarriage occurs becoming later as the virus in the mother becomes attenuated. Eventually a child is carried to full term, and it may be still-born, or, if born alive, may suffer from syphilitic manifestations. It is difficult to explain such vagaries of syphilitic inheritance as the infection of one twin and the escape of the other.

Clinical Features.—We are not here concerned with the severe forms of the disease which prove fatal, but with the milder forms in which the infant is apparently healthy when born, but after from two to six weeks begins to show evidence of the syphilitic taint.

The usual phenomena are that the child ceases to thrive, becomes thin and sallow, and suffers from eruptions on the skin and mucous membranes. There is frequently a condition known as *snuffles*, in which the nasal passages are obstructed by an accumulation of thin muco-purulent discharge which causes the breathing to be noisy. It usually begins within a month after birth and before the eruptions on the skin appear. When long continued it is liable to interfere with the development of the nasal bones, so that when the child grows up there results a condition known as the "saddle-nose" deformity (Figs. 43 and 44).

Affections of the Skin.—Although all types of skin affection are met with in the inherited disease, the most important is a *papular* eruption, the papules being of large size, with a smooth shining top and of a reddish-brown colour. It affects chiefly the buttocks and thighs, the genitals, and other parts which are constantly moist. It is necessary to distinguish this specific eruption from a form of eczema which occurs in these situations in non-syphilitic children, the points that characterise the syphilitic condition being the infiltration of the skin and the coppery colour of the eruption. At the anus the papules acquire the characters of *condylomata*, also at the angles of the mouth, where they often ulcerate and leave radiating scars.

Affections of the Mucous Membranes.—The inflammation of the nasal mucous membrane that causes snuffles has already been referred to. There may be mucous patches in the mouth, or a stomatitis which is of importance, because it results in interference with the development of the permanent teeth. The mucous membrane of the larynx may be the seat of mucous patches or of catarrh, and as a result the child's cry is hoarse.

Affections of the Bones.—Swellings at the ends of the long bones, due to inflammation at the epiphysial junctions, are most often observed at the upper end of the humerus and in the bones in the region of the elbow. Partial displacement and mobility at the ossifying junction may be observed. The infant cries when the part is touched; and as it does not move the limb voluntarily, the condition is spoken of as *the pseudo-paralysis of syphilis*. Recovery takes place under anti-syphilitic treatment and immobilisation of the limb.

Diffuse thickening of the shafts of the long bones, due to a deposit of new bone by the periosteum, is sometimes met with.

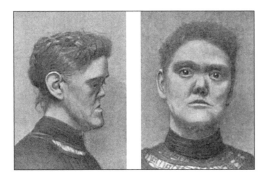

FIG. 44. Facies of Inherited Syphilis.

The conditions of the skull known as Parrot's nodes or bosses, and craniotabes, were formerly believed to be characteristic of inherited syphilis, but they are now known to occur, particularly in rickety children, from other causes. The *bosses* result from the heaping up of new spongy bone beneath the pericranium, and they may be grouped symmetrically around the anterior fontanelle, or may extend along either side of the sagittal suture, which appears as a deep groove—the "natiform skull." The bosses disappear in time, but the skull may remain permanently altered in shape, the frontal and parietal eminences appearing unduly prominent. The term *craniotabes* is applied when the bone becomes thin and soft, reverting to its original membranous condition, so that the affected areas dimple under the finger like parchment or thin cardboard; its localisation in the posterior parts of the skull suggests that the disappearance of the osseous tissue is influenced by the pressure of the head on the pillow. Craniotabes is recovered from as the child improves in health.

Between the ages of three and six months, certain other phenomena may be met with, such as *effusion into the joints*, especially the knees; *iritis*, in one or in both eyes, and enlargement of the spleen and liver.

In the majority of cases the child recovers from these early manifestations, especially when efficiently treated, and may enjoy an indefinite period of good health. On the other hand, when it attains the age of from two to four years, it may begin to manifest lesions which correspond to those of the tertiary period of acquired syphilis.

Later Lesions.—In the skin and subcutaneous tissue, the later manifestations may take the form of localised gummata, which tend to break down and form ulcers, on the leg for example, or of a spreading gummatous infiltration which is also liable to ulcerate, leaving disfiguring scars, especially on the face. The palate and fauces may be destroyed by ulceration. In the nose, especially when the ulcerative process is associated with a putrid discharge—ozæna—the destruction of tissue may be considerable and result in unsightly deformity. The entire palatal portions of the upper jaws, the vomer, turbinate, and other bones bounding the nasal and oral cavities, may disappear, so that on looking into the mouth the base of the skull is readily seen. Gummatous disease is frequently observed also in the flat bones of the skull, in the bones of the hand, as syphilitic dactylitis, and in the bones of the forearm and leg. When the tibia is affected the disease is frequently bilateral, and may assume the form of gummatous ulcers and sinuses. In later years the tibia may present alterations in shape resulting from antecedent gummatous disease—for example, nodular thickenings of the shaft, flattening of the crest, or a more uniform increase in thickness and length of the shaft of the bone, which, when it is curved in addition, is described as the "sabre-blade" deformity. Among lesions of the viscera, mention should be made of gumma of the testis, which causes the organ to become enlarged, uneven, and indurated. This has even been observed in infants a few months old.

Occasionally a syphilitic child suffers from a succession of these gummatous lesions with resulting ill-health, and, it may be, waxy disease of the internal organs; on the other hand, it may recover and present no further manifestations of the inherited taint.

Affections of the Eyes.—At or near puberty there is frequently observed an affection of the eyes, known as *chronic interstitial keratitis*, the relationship of which to inherited syphilis was first established by Hutchinson. It occurs between the ages of six and sixteen years, and usually affects one eye before the other. It commences as a diffuse haziness or steaminess near the centre of the cornea, and as it spreads the entire cornea assumes the appearance of ground glass. The chief complaint is of dimness of sight, which may almost amount to blindness, but there is little pain or photophobia; a certain amount of conjunctival and ciliary congestion is usually present, and there may be *iritis* in addition. The cornea, or parts of it, may become of a deep pink or salmon colour from the formation in it of new blood vessels. The affection may last for from eighteen months to two years. Complete recovery usually takes place, but slight opacities, especially in the site of former salmon patches, may persist, and the disease occasionally relapses. *Choroiditis* and *retinitis* may also occur, and leave permanent changes easily recognised on examination with the ophthalmoscope.

Among the rarer and more serious lesions of the inherited disease may be mentioned gummatous disease in the *larynx and trachea*, attended with ulceration and resulting in stenosis; and lesions of the *nervous system* which may result in convulsions, paralysis, or dementia.

In a limited number of cases, about the period of puberty there may develop *deafness*, which is usually bilateral and may become absolute.

Changes in the Permanent Teeth.—These affect specially the upper central incisors, which are dwarfed and stand somewhat apart in the gum, with their free edges converging towards one another. They are tapering or peg-shaped, and present at their cutting margin a deep semilunar notch. These appearances are commonly associated with the name of Hutchinson, who first described them. Affecting as they do the permanent teeth, they are not available for diagnosis until the child is over eight years of age. Henry Moon drew attention to a change in the first molars; these are reduced in size and dome-shaped through dwarfing of the central tubercle of each cusp.

Diagnosis of Inherited Syphilis.—When there is a typical eruption on the buttocks and snuffles there is no difficulty in recognising the disease. When, however, the rash is scanty or is obscured by co-existing eczema, most reliance should be placed on the distribution of the eruption, on the brown stains which are left after it has passed off, on the presence of condylomata, and of fissuring and scarring at the angles of the mouth. The history of the mother relative to repeated miscarriages and still-born children may afford confirmatory evidence. In doubtful cases, the diagnosis may be aided by the Wassermann test and by noting the therapeutic effects of grey powder, which, in syphilitic infants, usually effects a marked and rapid improvement both in the symptoms and in the general health.

While a considerable number of syphilitic children grow up without showing any trace of their syphilitic inheritance, the majority retain throughout life one or more of the following characteristics, which may therefore be described as *permanent signs of the inherited disease*: Dwarfing of stature from interference with growth at the epiphysial junctions; the forehead low and vertical, and the parietal and frontal eminences unduly prominent; the bridge of the nose sunken and rounded; radiating scars at the angles of the mouth; perforation or destruction of the hard palate; Hutchinson's teeth; opacities of the cornea from antecedent keratitis; alterations in the fundus oculi from choroiditis; deafness; depressed scars or nodes on the bones from previous gummata; "sabre-blade" or other deformity of the tibiæ.

The Contagiousness of Inherited Syphilis.—In 1837, Colles of Dublin stated his belief that, while a syphilitic infant may convey the disease to a healthy wet nurse, it is incapable of infecting its own mother if nursed by her, even although she may never have shown symptoms of the disease. This doctrine, which is known as *Colles' law*, is generally accepted in spite of the alleged occurrence of occasional exceptions. The older the child, the less risk there is of its communicating the disease to others, until eventually the tendency dies out altogether, as it does in the tertiary period of acquired syphilis. It should be added, however, that the contagiousness of inherited syphilis is denied by some observers, who affirm that, when syphilitic infants prove infective, the disease has been really acquired at or soon after birth.

There is general agreement that the subjects of inherited syphilis cannot transmit the disease by inheritance to their offspring, and that, although they very rarely acquire the disease *de novo*, it is possible for them to do so.

Prognosis of Inherited Syphilis.—Although inherited syphilis is responsible for a large but apparently diminishing mortality in infancy, the subjects of this disease may grow up to be as strong and healthy as their neighbours. Hutchinson insisted on the fact that there is little bad health in the general community that can be attributed to inherited syphilis.

Treatment.—Arsenical injections are as beneficial in the inherited as in the acquired disease. An infant the subject of inherited syphilis should, if possible, be nursed by its mother, and failing this it should be fed by hand. In infants at the breast, the drug may be given to the mother; in others, it is administered in the same manner as already described—only in smaller doses. On the first appearance of syphilitic manifestations it should be given 0.05 grm, novarsenbillon, injected into the deep subcutaneous tissues every week for six weeks, followed by one year's mercurial inunction—a piece of mercurial ointment the size of a pea being inserted under the infant's binder. In older children the dose is proportionately increased. The general health should be improved in every possible direction; considerable benefit may be derived from the use of cod-liver oil, and from preparations containing iron and calcium. Surgical interference may be required in the destructive gummatous lesions of the nose, throat, larynx, and bones, either with the object of arresting the spread of the disease, or of removing or alleviating the resulting deformities. In children suffering from keratitis, the eyes should be protected from the light by smoked or coloured glasses, and the pupils should be dilated with atropin from time to time, especially in cases complicated with iritis.

Acquired Syphilis in Infants and Young Children.—When syphilis is met with in infants and young children, it is apt to be taken for granted that the disease has been inherited. It is possible, however, for them to acquire the disease—as, for example, while passing through the maternal passages during birth, through being nursed or kissed by infected women, or through the rite of circumcision. The risk of infection which formerly existed by the arm-to-arm method of vaccination has been abolished by the use of calf lymph.

The clinical features of the acquired disease in infants and young children are similar to those observed in the adult, with a tendency, however, to be more severe, probably because the disease is often late in being recognised and treated.

TUMOURS[2]

Definition ⋄ *Etiology* ⋄ *General Characters of Innocent and Malignant Tumours* ⋄ *Classification of Tumours: I. Connective-tissue Tumours: (1) Innocent: Lipoma, Xanthoma, Chondroma, Osteoma, Odontoma, Fibroma, Myxoma, Endothelioma, etc.; (2) Malignant: Sarcoma II. Epithelial Tumours: (1) Innocent: Papilloma, Adenoma, Cystic Adenoma; (2) Malignant: Epithelioma, Glandular Cancer, Rodent Cancer, Melanotic Cancer III. Dermoids* ⋄ *IV. Teratoma. Cysts: Retention, Exudation, Implantation, Parasitic, Lymphatic or Serous* ⋄ *Ganglion*

A tumour or neoplasm is a localised swelling composed of newly formed tissue which fulfils no physiological function. Tumours increase in size quite independently of the growth of the body, and there is no natural termination to their growth. They are to be distinguished from such over-growths as are of the nature of simple hypertrophy or local giantism, and also from inflammatory swellings, which usually develop under the influence of a definite cause, have a natural termination, and tend to disappear when the cause ceases to act.

The *etiology of tumours* is imperfectly understood. Various factors, acting either singly or in combination, may be concerned in their development. Certain tumours, for example, are the result of some congenital malformation of the particular tissue from which they take origin. This would appear to be the case in many tumours of blood vessels (angioma), of cartilage (chondroma), of bone (osteoma), and of secreting gland tissue (adenoma). The theory that tumours originate from foetal residues or "rests," is associated with the name of Cohnheim. These rests are supposed to be undifferentiated embryonic cells which remain embedded amongst fully formed tissue elements, and lie

[2] For the histology of tumours the reader is referred to a text-book of pathology.

dormant until they are excited into active growth and give rise to a tumour. This mode of origin is illustrated by the development of dermoids from sequestrated portions of epidermis.

Among the local factors concerned in the development of tumours, reference must be made to the influence of irritation. This is probably an important agent in the causation of many of the tumours met with in the skin and in mucous membranes—for example, cancer of the skin, of the lip, and of the tongue. The part played by injury is doubtful. It not infrequently happens that the development of a tumour is preceded by an injury of the part in which it grows, but it does not necessarily follow that the injury and the tumour are related as cause and effect. It is possible that an injury may stimulate into active growth undifferentiated tissue elements or "rests," and so determine the growth of a tumour, or that it may alter the characters of a tumour which already exists, causing it to grow more rapidly.

The popular belief that there is some constitutional peculiarity concerned in the causation of tumours is largely based on the fact that certain forms of new growth—for example, cancer—are known to occur with undue frequency in certain families. The same influence is more striking in the case of certain innocent tumours—particularly multiple osteomas and lipomas—which are hereditary in the same sense as supernumerary or webbed fingers, and appear in members of the same family through several generations.

INNOCENT AND MALIGNANT TUMOURS

For clinical purposes, tumours are arbitrarily divided into two classes—the innocent and the malignant. The outstanding difference between them is, that while the evil effects of innocent tumours are entirely local and depend for their severity on the environment of the growth, malignant tumours wherever situated, in addition to producing similar local effects, injure the general health and ultimately cause death.

Innocent, benign, or simple tumours present a close structural resemblance to the normal tissues of the body. They grow slowly, and are usually definitely circumscribed by a fibrous capsule, from which they are easily enucleated, and they do not tend to recur after removal. In their growth they merely push aside and compress adjacent parts, and they present no tendency to ulcerate and bleed unless the overlying skin or mucous membrane is injured. Although usually solitary, some are multiple from the outset—for example, fatty, fibrous, and bony tumours, warts, and fibroid tumours of the uterus. They produce no constitutional disturbance. They only threaten life when growing in the vicinity of vital organs, and then only in virtue of their situation—for example, death may result from an innocent tumour in the air-passage causing suffocation, in the intestine causing obstruction of the bowels, or in the vertebral canal causing pressure on the spinal medulla.

Malignant tumours usually show a marked departure from the structure and arrangement of the normal tissues of the body. Although the cells of which they are composed are derived from normal tissue cells, they tend to take on a lower, more vegetative form; they may be regarded as parasites living at the expense of the organism, multiplying indefinitely and destroying everything with which they come in contact.

Malignant tumours grow more rapidly than innocent tumours, and tend to infiltrate their surroundings by sending out prolongations or offshoots; they are therefore liable to recur after an operation which is restricted to the removal of the main tumour. They are not encapsulated, although they may appear to be circumscribed by condensation of the surrounding tissues; they are rarely multiple at the outset, but show a marked tendency to spread to other parts of the body. Fragments of the parent tumour may become separated and be carried off in the lymph or blood-stream and deposited in other parts of the body, where they give rise to secondary growths. Malignant tumours tend to invade and destroy the overlying skin or mucous membrane, and thus give rise to bleeding ulcers; if the tumour tissue protrudes through the gap in the skin, it is said to *fungate*. In course of time they give rise to a condition of ill-health or *cachexia*, the patient becoming pale, sallow, feverish, and emaciated, probably as a result of chronic poisoning from the absorption of toxic products from the tumour. They ultimately destroy life, it may be by their local effects, such as ulceration and hæmorrhage, by favouring the entrance of septic infection, by interfering with the function of organs which are essential to life, by cachexia, or by a combination of these effects.

The situation of a malignant tumour exercises considerable influence on the rapidity, as well as on the mode, in which it causes death. Some cancers, such as that known as "rodent," show malignant features which are entirely local, while others, such as melanotic cancer, exhibit a malignancy characterised by rapid generalisation of growths throughout the body. Tumours that are structurally alike may show variations in malignancy, according to their situation and to the age of the patient, as well as to other factors which are as yet unknown.

In attempting to arrive at a conclusion as to the innocence or malignancy of any tumour, too much reliance must not be placed on its histological features; its situation, rate of growth, and other clinical features must also be taken into consideration. It cannot be too emphatically stated that there is no hard-and-fast line between innocent and malignant growths; there is an indefinite transition from one to the other. The possibility of the transformation of a benign into a malignant tumour must be admitted. Such a transformation implies a change in the structure of the growth, and has been observed especially in fibrous and cartilaginous tumours, in tumours of the thyreoid gland, and in uterine fibroids. The alteration in character may take place under the influence of injury, prolonged or repeated irritation, incomplete removal of the benign tumour by operation, or the altered physiological conditions of the tissues which attend upon advancing years.

After a tumour has been removed by operation it should as a routine measure be subjected to microscopical examination; the results are often instructive and sometimes other than what was expected.

Varieties of Tumours.—In the following description, tumours are classified on an anatomical basis, taking in order first the connective-tissue group and subsequently those that originate in epithelium.

INNOCENT CONNECTIVE-TISSUE TUMOURS

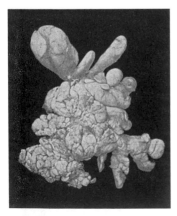

FIG. 45. Subcutaneous Lipoma showing lobulation.

Lipoma.—A lipoma is composed of fat resembling that normally present in the body. The commonest variety is the *subcutaneous lipoma*, which grows from the subcutaneous fat, and forms a soft, irregularly lobulated tumour (Fig. 45). The fat is arranged in lobules separated by connective-tissue septa, which are continuous with the capsule surrounding the tumour and with the overlying skin, which becomes dimpled or puckered when an attempt is made to pinch it up. As the fat is almost fluid at the body temperature, fluctuation can usually be detected. These tumours vary greatly in size, occur at all ages, grow slowly, and, while generally solitary, are sometimes multiple. They are most commonly met with on the shoulder, buttock, or back. In certain situations, such as the thigh and perineum, they tend to become pedunculated (Fig. 46).

A fatty tumour is to be diagnosed from a cold abscess and from a cyst. The distinguishing features of the lipoma are the tacking down and dimpling of the overlying skin, the lobulation of the tumour, which is recognised when it is pressed upon with the flat of the hand, and, more reliable than either of these, the mobility, the tumour slipping away when pressed upon at its margin.

The prognosis is more favourable than in any other tumour as it never changes its characters; the only reasons for its removal by operation are its unsightliness and its probable increase in size in the course of years. The oper-

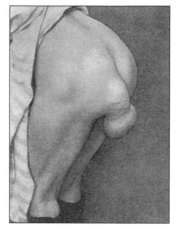

FIG. 46. Pedunculated Lipoma of Buttock of forty years' duration in a woman æt. 68.

ation consists in dividing the skin and capsule over the tumour and shelling it out. Care must be taken that none of the outlying lobules are left behind. If the overlying skin is damaged or closely adherent, it should be removed along with the tumour.

Multiple subcutaneous lipomas are frequently symmetrical, and in a certain group of cases, met with chiefly in women, pain is a prominent symptom, hence the term *adiposis dolorosa* (Dercum). These multiple tumours show little or no tendency to increase in size, and the pain which attends their development does not persist.

In the neck, axilla, and pubes a diffuse overgrowth of the subcutaneous fat is sometimes met with, forming symmetrical tumour-like masses, known as *diffuse lipoma*. As this is not, strictly speaking, a tumour, the term diffuse *lipomatosis* is to be preferred. A similar condition was described by Jonathan Hutchinson as being met with in the domestic animals. If causing disfigurement, the mass of fat may be removed by operation.

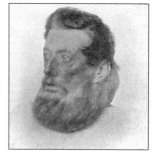

FIG. 47. Diffuse Lipomatosis of Neck.

177

Lipoma in other Situations.—The *periosteal lipoma* is usually congenital, and is most often met with in the hand; it forms a projecting lobulated tumour, which, when situated in the palm, resembles an angioma or a lymphangioma. The *subserous lipoma* arises from the extra-peritoneal fat in the posterior abdominal wall, in which case it tends to grow forwards between the layers of the mesentery and to give rise to an abdominal tumour; or it may grow from the extra-peritoneal fat in the anterior abdominal wall and protrude from one of the hernial openings or through an abnormal opening in the parietes, constituting a *fatty hernia.* A *subsynovial lipoma* grows from the fat surrounding the synovial membrane of a joint, and projects into its interior, giving rise to the symptoms of loose body. Lipomas are also met with growing from the adipose connective tissue *between or in the substance of muscles*, and, when situated beneath the deep fascia, such as the fascia lata of the thigh, the characteristic signs are obscured and a differential diagnosis is difficult. It may be differentiated from a cold abscess by puncture with an exploring needle.

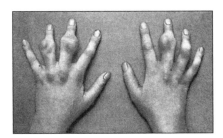

FIG. 48. Zanthoma of Hands in a girl æt. 14, showing multiple subcutaneous tumours (cf. Fig. 49). (Sir H. J. Stiles' case.)

Zanthoma is a rare but interesting form of tumour, composed of a fibrous and fatty tissue, containing a granular orange-yellow pigment, resembling that of the corpus luteum. It originates in the corium and presents two clinical varieties. In the first of these, it occurs in the form of raised yellow patches, usually in the skin of the eyelids of persons after middle life, and in many instances is associated with chronic jaundice; the patches are often symmetrical, and as they increase in size they tend to fuse with another.

The second form occurs in children and adolescents; it may affect several generations of the same family, and is often multiple, there being a combination of thickened yellow patches of skin and projecting tumours, some of which may attain a considerable size (Figs. 48 and 49). On section, the tumour tissue presents a brilliant orange or saffron colour.

There is no indication for removing the tumours unless for the deformity which they cause; exposure to the X-rays is to be preferred to operation.

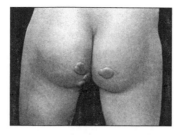

FIG. 49. Zanthoma showing Subcutaneous Tumours on Buttocks. From same patient as Fig. 48.

Chondroma.—A chondroma is mainly composed of cartilage. Processes of vascular connective tissue pass in between the nodules of cartilage composing the tumour from the fibrous capsule which surrounds it. On section it is of a greyish-blue colour and semi-translucent. The tumour is firm and elastic in consistence, but certain portions may be densely hard from calcification or ossification, while other portions may be soft and fluctuating as a result of myxomatous degeneration and liquefaction. These tumours grow slowly and painlessly, and may surround nerves and arteries without injuring them. They may cause a deep hollow in the bone from which they originate. All intermediate forms between the innocent chondroma and the malignant chondro-sarcoma are met with. Chondroma may occur in a multiple form, especially in relation to the phalanges and metacarpal bones. When growing in the interior of a bone it causes a spindle-shaped enlargement of the shaft, which in the case of a phalanx or metacarpal bone may resemble the dactylitis resulting from tubercle or syphilis. A chondroma appears as a clear area in a skiagram.

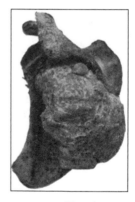

FIG. 50. Chondroma growing from infraspinous fossa of Scapula.

A *skiagram* of a bone in which there is a chondroma shows a clear rounded area in the position of the tumour, which must be differentiated from similar clear areas due to other kinds of tumour, especially the myeloma; when it has undergone calcification or ossification, it gives a shadow as dark as bone.

Treatment.—In view of the unstable quality of the chondroma, especially of its liability to become malignant, it should be removed as soon as it is recognised. In those projecting from the surface of a bone, both the tumour and its capsule should be removed. If in the interior, a sufficient amount of the cortex should be removed to allow of the tumour being scraped out, and care must be taken that no nodules of cartilage are left behind. In multiple chondromas of the hand, when the fingers are crippled and useless, exposure to the X-rays should be given a trial, and in extreme cases the question of amputation may have to be considered. When a cartilaginous tumour takes on active growth, it must be treated as malignant.

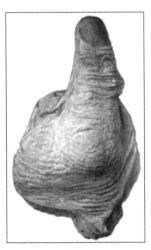

FIG. 51. Chondroma of Metacarpal Bone of Thumb.

The chondromas that are met with at the ends of the long bones in children and young adults form a group by themselves. They are usually related to the epiphysial cartilage, and it was suggested by Virchow that they take origin from islands of cartilage which have not been used up in the process of ossification. They are believed to occur more frequently in those who have suffered from rickets. They have no malignant tendencies and tend to undergo ossification concurrently with the epiphysial cartilage from which they take origin, and constitute what are known as *cartilaginous exostoses*. These are sometimes met with in a multiple form, and may occur in several generations of the same family. They are considered in greater detail in the chapter dealing with tumours of bone.

Minute nodules of cartilage sometimes form in the synovial membrane of joints and lining of tendon sheaths and bursæ: they tend to become detached from the membrane and constitute loose bodies; they also undergo a variable amount of calcification and ossification, so as to be visible in skiagrams. They are further considered with loose bodies in joints.

Cartilaginous tumours in the parotid, submaxillary gland, and testicle belong to a class of "mixed tumours" that will be referred to later.

Osteoma.—The true osteoma is composed of bony tissue, and originates from the skeleton. Two varieties are recognised—the spongy or cancellous, and the ivory or compact. The *spongy* or *cancellous osteoma* is really an ossified chondroma, and is met with at the ends of the long bones (Fig. 52). From the fact that it projects from the surface of the bone it is often spoken of as an *exostosis*. It grows slowly, and rarely causes any discomfort unless it presses upon a nerve-trunk or upon a bursa which has developed over it. The Röntgen rays show a dark shadow corresponding to the ossified portion of the tumour, and continuous with that of the bone from which it is growing (Fig. 138). Operative interference is only indicated when the tumour is giving rise to inconvenience. It is then removed, its base or neck being divided by means of the chisel. The multiple variety of osteoma is considered with the diseases of bone.

The bony outgrowth from the terminal phalanx of the great toe—known as the *subungual exostosis*—is described and figured on p. 404. Bony projections or "spurs" sometimes occur on the under surface of the calcaneus, and, projecting downwards and forwards from the greater process, cause pain on putting the heel to the ground.

The *ivory* or *compact osteoma* is composed of dense bone, and usually grows from the skull. It is generally sessile and solitary, and may grow into the interior of the skull, into the frontal sinus, into the cavity of the orbit or nose, or may fill up the external auditory meatus, causing most unsightly deformity and interference with sight, breathing, and hearing.

Bony formations occur in *muscles and tendons*, especially at their points of attachment to the skeleton, and are known as false exostoses; they are described with the diseases of muscles.

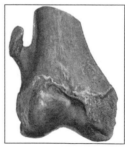

FIG. 52. Cancellous Osteoma of lower end of Femur.

Odontoma.—An odontoma is composed of dental tissues in varying proportions and different degrees of development, arising from tooth-germs or from teeth still in process of growth (Bland Sutton). Odontomas resemble teeth in so far that during their development they remain hidden below the mucous membrane and give no evidence of their existence. There then succeeds, usually between the twentieth and twenty-fifth years, an eruptive stage, which is often attended with suppuration, and this may be the means of drawing attention to the tumour. Following Bland Sutton, several varieties of odontoma may be distinguished according to the part of the tooth-germ concerned in their formation.

The *epithelial odontoma* is derived from persistent portions of the epithelium of the enamel organ, and constitutes a multilocular cystic tumour which is chiefly met with in the mandible. The cystic spaces of the tumour contain a brownish glairy fluid. These tumours have been described by Eve under the name of multilocular cystic epithelial tumours of the jaw.

The *follicular odontoma*, also known as a *dentigerous cyst*, is derived from the distension of a tooth follicle. It constitutes a cyst containing a viscid fluid, and an imperfectly formed tooth is often found embedded in its wall. The cyst usually forms in relation to one of the permanent molars, and may attain considerable dimensions.

The *fibrous odontoma* is the result of an overgrowth of fibrous tissue surrounding the tooth sac, which encapsulates the tooth and prevents its eruption. The thickened tooth sac is usually mistaken for a fibrous tumour, until, after removal, the tooth is recognised in its interior.

Composite Odontoma.—This is a convenient term to apply to certain hard dental tumours which are met with in the jaws, and consist of enamel, dentine, and cement. The tumour is to be regarded as being derived from an abnormal growth of all the elements of a tooth germ, or of two or more tooth germs, indiscriminately fused with one another. It may appear in childhood, and form a smooth unyielding tumour, often of considerable size, replacing the corresponding permanent tooth. It may cause a purulent discharge, and in some cases it has been extruded after sloughing of the overlying soft parts. Many examples of this variety of odontoma, growing in the nasal cavity or in the maxillary sinus, have been erroneously regarded as osteomas even after removal.

On section, the tumour is usually laminated, and is seen to consist mainly of dentine with a partial covering of enamel and cement.

Diagnosis.—Odontomas are often only diagnosed after removal. When attended with suppuration, the condition has been mistaken for disease of the jaw. Fibrous odontomas have been mistaken for sarcoma, and portions of the maxilla removed unnecessarily. Any circumscribed tumour of the jaw, particularly when met with in a young adult, should suggest the possibility of an odontoma. Skiagrams often give useful information both for diagnosis and for treatment.

Treatment.—The solid varieties of odontoma can usually be shelled out after dividing the overlying soft parts. In the follicular variety, it is usually sufficient to excise a portion of the wall, scrape out the interior, and remove any tooth that may be present. The cavity is then packed and allowed to heal from the bottom.

Fibroma.—A fibroma is a tumour composed of fibrous connective tissue. A distinction may be made between the *soft fibroma*, which is comparatively rich in cells and blood vessels, and in which the fibres are arranged loosely; and the *hard fibroma*, which is composed of closely packed bundles of fibres often arranged in a concentric fashion around the blood vessels. The cut surface of the soft fibroma presents a pinkish-white, fleshy appearance, resembling the slowly growing forms of sarcoma; that of a hard fibroma presents a dry, glistening appearance, aptly compared to watered silk. The soft variety grows much more rapidly than the hard. In certain fibromas—in those, for example, which grow from the periosteum of the base of the skull and project into the naso-pharynx—the blood vessels are dilated into sinuses and have no proper sheaths; they therefore tend to remain open when divided, and to bleed excessively. Transition forms between soft fibroma and sarcoma are met with, so that in operating for their removal it is safer to take away the capsule along with the tumour, and the patient should be kept under observation in view of the risk of recurrence.

The skin—especially the skin of the buttock—is one of the favourite seats of fibroma, and it may occur in a multiple form. It is met with also in the subcutaneous and intermuscular cellular tissue, and in the abdominal wall, where it sometimes attains considerable dimensions. Various forms of fibroma are met with in the mamma and are described with diseases of that organ. The fibrous overgrowths in the skin, known as *keloid* and *molluscum fibrosum*, and those met with in the *sheaths of nerves*, are described elsewhere. Fibroid tumours of the uterus are described with myoma.

Diffuse fibroma or *Fibromatosis*, analogous to lipomatosis, is met with in the connective tissue of the skin and sheaths of nerves, and constitutes one form of neuro-fibromatosis; a similar change is also met with in the stomach and colon.

Myxoma.—A myxoma is composed of tissue of a soft gelatinous, semifluid consistence. The pure myxoma is extremely rare, and clinically resembles the lipoma. Myxomatous tissue is, however, frequently found in other connective-tissue tumours as a result of degeneration, for example, in carti-laginous tumours and in sarcomas. Myxomatous tissue is also a prominent constituent of the "innocent parotid tumour." Mucous polypus of the nose, which is often described as a myxoma, is merely a pendulous process of oedematous mucous membrane.

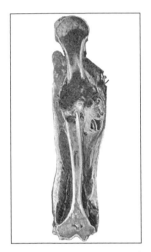

FIG. 53. Myeloma of Shaft of Humerus, caus-ing pathological fracture. (Mr. J. W. Struthers' case.) (The unusual site of the tumour is to be noted.)

Myeloma.—A myeloma is composed of large mul-tinuclear giant cells surrounded by round and spin-dle cells. The cut surface of the tumour presents a deep red or maroon colour. While occasionally met with in tendon sheaths and bursæ, and is then of an orange-yellow colour, the myeloma occurs most frequently in the cancellous tissue at the ends of the long bones, its favourite site being the upper end of the tibia. Although formerly classified as a sarcoma, it is the exception for it to present malig-nant features, and it can usually be extirpated by local measures without fear of recurrence. The diagnosis, X-ray appearances, and the method of removal are considered with the diseases of bone. Sometimes the myeloma is met with in multiple form in the skeleton, in association with an unusual form of protein in the urine (Bence Jones).

Myoma.—A myoma is composed of non-striped muscle fibres. A pure myoma is very rare, and is met with in organs possessed of non-striped muscle, such as the stomach, intestine, urinary bladder, and prostate. In the uterus, which is the most common situation, these tumours contain a consid-erable admixture of fibrous tissue, and arc known as *fibroids* or *fibro-myomas*. They present on section a fasciculated appearance, which may resemble that of a section of balls of cotton (Fig. 54). They are encapsulated and vascular, frequently attain a large size, and may be single or multiple. While they may occasion neither inconvenience nor suffering, they frequently give rise to profuse hæmorrhage from the uterus, and may cause serious symptoms by pressing injuriously on the ureters or the intestine, or by complicating preg-nancy and parturition.

The **Rhabdomyoma** is an extremely rare form of tumour, met with in the kidney, uterus, and testicle. It contains striped muscle fibres, and is supposed to originate from a residue of muscular tissue which has become sequestrated during development.

Glioma.—A glioma is a tumour composed of neuroglia. It is met with exclusively in the central nervous system, retina, and optic nerve. It is a slowly growing, soft, ill-defined tumour, which displaces the adjacent nerve centres and nerve tracts, and is liable to become the seat of hæmorrhage and thus to give rise to pressure symptoms resembling apoplexy. The glioma of the retina tends to grow into the vitreous humour and to perforate the globe. It is usually of the nature of a glio-sarcoma and is highly malignant.

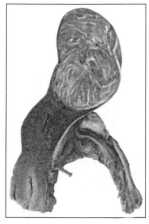

FIG. 54. Fibro-myoma of Uterus. (Anatomical Museum, University of Edinburgh.)

Endotheliomas take origin from the endothelium of lymph vessels and blood vessels, and serous cavities. They show great variation in type, partly because of the number of different kinds of endothelium from which they are derived, and partly because the new connective tissue which is formed is liable to undergo transformation into other tissues. They may be soft or hard, solid or cystic, diffuse or circumscribed; they grow very slowly, and are almost always innocent, although recurrence has been occasionally observed. Cases of multiple endotheliomata of the skin have recently been described by Wise.

Angioma, lymphangioma, and *neuroma* are described with the disease of the individual tissues.

MALIGNANT CONNECTIVE-TISSUE TUMOURS—SARCOMA

The term sarcoma is applied to any connective-tissue tumour which exhibits malignant characters. The essential structural feature is the predominance of the cellular elements over the intercellular substance or stroma, in which respect a sarcoma resembles the connective tissue of the embryo. The typical sarcoma consists chiefly of immature or embryonic connective tissue. It most frequently originates from fascia, intermuscular connective tissue, periosteum, bone-marrow, and skin, and forms a rounded or nodulated tumour which appears to be encapsulated, but the capsule merely consists of the condensed surrounding tissues, and usually contains sarcomatous elements. The consistence of the tumour depends on the nature and amount of the stroma, and on the presence of degenerative changes. The softer medullary forms are composed almost exclusively of cells; while the harder forms—such as the fibro-, chondro-, and osteo-sarcoma—are provided with an abundant stroma and are relatively poor in cells. Degenerative changes may produce areas of softening or liquefaction which result in the formation of cystic cavities in the interior of the tumour. The colour depends on the amount of blood in the tumour, and on the presence of the products of degeneration.

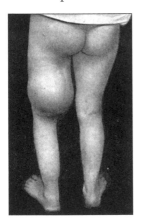

FIG. 55. Recurrent Sarcoma of Sciatic Nerve in a woman æt. 27. Recurrence twenty months after removal of primary growth.

The blood vessels are usually represented by mere chinks or spaces between the cells. This peculiarity accounts for the facility with which hæmorrhage takes place into the substance of the tumour, the persistence of the bleeding when it is incised or ulcerates through the skin, and the readiness with which the sarcomatous cells are carried off and infect distant parts through the blood-stream. Sarcomas are devoid of lymphatics, and unless originating in lymphatic structures—for example, in the tonsil—they rarely infect the lymph glands. Minute portions of the tumour grow into the small veins, and, becoming detached, are transported by the blood-current to distant organs, where they are arrested in the capillaries and give rise to secondary growths. These are most frequently situated in the lungs, except when the primary growth lies within the territory of the portal circulation, in which case they occur in the liver. The secondary growths closely resemble the parent tumour. Sarcoma may invade an adjacent vein on such a scale that if the invading portion becomes detached it may constitute a dangerous embolus. This may be observed in sarcoma of the kidney, the growth taking place along the renal vein until it projects into the vena cava.

In its growth, a sarcoma compresses and destroys neighbouring parts, surrounds vessels and nerves, and may lead to destruction of the skin, either by invading it, or more commonly by causing sloughing from pressure. Inflammatory and suppurative changes may take place as a result of pyogenic infection following upon sloughing of the overlying skin or upon an explor-atory incision. Once the skin is broken the tumour fungates through the opening. Sarcomas vary in malignancy, especially as regards rapidity of growth and capacity for dissemination. Certain of them, such as the so-called "recurrent fibroid of Paget," grow comparatively slowly, and are only malig-nant in the sense that they tend to recur locally after removal; others—espe-cially the more cellular ones—grow with extreme rapidity, and are early disseminated throughout the body, resembling in these respects the most malignant forms of cancer. They are usually solitary in the first instance, although primary multiple growths are occasionally met with in the skin and in the bones.

Many varieties of sarcoma are recognised, according to its structural peculiarities. Thus, in vir-tue of the size and character of the cells, we have the *small round-celled* and the *large round-celled* sarcoma, the *small* and the *large spindle-celled*, the *giant-celled* and the *mixed-celled* sarcoma. The *lympho-sarcoma* presents a structure similar to that of lymph-follicu-lar tissue, and the *alveolar sarcoma* an arrangement of cells in alveoli resembling that seen in cancers. When there is a considerable amount of intercellular fibrous tissue, the tumour is called a *fibro-sarcoma*.

The term *lymphangio-sarcoma* is applied when the cells of the tumour are derived from the endothelium of lymph spaces and vessels. The *angio-sarcomas* are those in which blood vessels form a prominent ele-ment in the structure of the tumour. They are some-times derived from innocent angiomas, and they

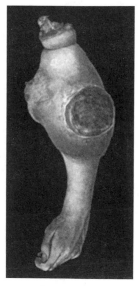

FIG. 56. Fungating Sarcoma of Arm. (Dr. J. M'Watt's case.)

may be so vascular as to pulsate and on auscultation yield a blowing mur-mur like an aneurysm. The *glio-sarcoma, myxo-sarcoma, chondro-sarcoma,* and *myo-sarcoma* are mixed forms which usually develop in pre-existing innocent tumours. The *osteo-sarcoma* is characterised by the formation in the tumour of bone, the medullary spaces being occupied by sarcomatous cells in place of marrow. The *osteoid sarcoma* is characterised by the formation of a tissue resembling bone but deficient in lime salts, and the *petrifying sarcoma* by the formation of calcified areas in the stroma. These varieties, although met with chiefly in the bones, may occur in soft tissues such as muscle, and in such organs as the mamma. The pigmented varieties include the *chloroma*, which is of a light-green colour, and the *melanotic sarcoma*, which is brown or black. The *psammoma* is a sarcoma containing a material resembling sand; it is chiefly met with in the membranes of the brain. The *chordoma* is a rare form of tumour originating from the remains of the notochord in the region of the spheno-occipital synchondrosis or in the sacro-coccygeal region.

Diagnosis of Sarcoma.—A sarcoma is to be differentiated from an inflammatory swelling such as results from tubercle, actinomycosis, or syphilis, from an innocent tumour, and from a cancer. The points on which the diagnosis is founded arc discussed with the different tissues and organs.

Treatment.—The removal of the tumour by operation is the most reliable method of treatment; in order to be successful it must be undertaken before dissemination has taken place, and a considerable area of healthy tissue beyond the apparent margin of the growth must be removed, and in tumours near the surface of the body, the overlying skin also.

In order to prevent recurrence, a tube of *radium*, to which a silk thread is attached, is inserted into the space from which the tumour was removed; the thread is brought out at the drain-opening, and at the end of a week or ten days the tube of radium is removed by pulling on the thread. Radium causes a reaction in the tissues attended with exudation from the vessels, for the escape of which provision must be made. If radium is not available, the affected area is repeatedly exposed to the action of the *X-rays* as soon as the wound has healed. The employment of these measures has diminished to a remarkable degree the recurrence of sarcoma after operation.

It will readily be understood that the less thoroughly or radically the growth has been removed, the more do we depend upon radium or the X-rays for bringing about a permanent cure, and that in advanced cases of sarcoma and in cases in which, on account of their anatomical situation, removal by operation is necessarily incomplete, the prospect of cure is still more dependent on the use of radium or of the X-rays. Finally, there are cases in which removal by operation is impossible, the so-called *inoperable sarcoma*; a tube of radium, to which a silk thread is attached, is inserted into the substance of the tumour, either through an opening made by a large trocar, or, when necessary, by open dissection. A second tube of radium is placed upon the skin over the tumour and is secured there by a stitch or by a strip of plaster, thus securing a cross-fire action of the radium rays, both from within and without, as this is found to be much more efficacious in destroying or inhibiting the cellular elements of the growth. The tubes of radium are left *in situ* for from eight to fourteen days, according to the power of the radium employed, but are moved about every second day or so in order that every part of the tumour may be efficiently radiated. If the tumour shrinks in size after the use of radium and becomes operable, it should be removed before time is given it to resume its growth. It will depend upon the subsequent course of the disease, whether or not a second, or it may be even a third, application of radium will be required.

Where neither radium nor X-rays is available or applicable, recourse may be had to the injection of Coley's fluid, a preparation containing the mixed toxins of the streptococcus of erysipelas and the bacillus prodigiosus; or of selenium.

EPITHELIAL TUMOURS

An excessive and erratic growth of epithelium is the essential and distinguishing feature of these tumours. The innocent forms are the papilloma and the adenoma; the malignant, the carcinoma or cancer.

Papilloma.—A papilloma is a tumour which projects from a cutaneous or mucous surface, and consists of a central axis of vascular fibrous tissue with a covering of epithelium resembling that of the surface from which the tumour grows. In the papillomas of the skin—commonly known as *warts*—the covering consists of epidermis; in those growing from mucous surfaces it consists of the epithelium covering the mucous membrane. When the surface epithelium projects as filiform processes, the tumour is called a *villous papilloma*, the best-known example of which is met with in the urinary bladder. Papillomatous growths are also met with in the larynx, in the ducts of the breast, and in the interior of certain cystic tumours of the breast and of the ovary. Although papillomas are primarily innocent, they may become the starting-point of cancer, especially in persons past middle life and if the papilloma has been subjected to irritation and has ulcerated. The clinical features and treatment of the various forms of papilloma are considered with the individual tissues and organs.

Adenoma.—An adenoma is a tumour constructed on the type of, and growing in connection with, a secreting gland. In the substance of such glands as the mamma, parotid, thyreoid, and prostate, adenomas are met with as encapsulated tumours. When they originate from the glands of the skin or of a mucous membrane, they tend to project from the surface, and form pedunculated tumours or polypi.

Adenomas may be single or multiple, and they vary greatly in size. The tumour is seldom composed entirely of gland tissue; it usually contains a considerable proportion of fibrous tissue, and is then called a *fibro-adenoma*. When it contains myxomatous tissue it is called a *myxo-adenoma*, and when the gland spaces of the tumour become distended with accumulated secretion, a *cystic adenoma*, the best examples of which are met with in the mamma and ovary. A characteristic feature of the cystic variety is the tendency the tumour tissue exhibits to project into the interior of the cysts, constituting what are known as *intracystic growths*. They are essentially innocent, but intracystic growths, especially in the mamma of women over fifty, should be regarded with suspicion and therefore should be removed on radical lines. Transition forms between adenoma and carcinoma are also met with in the rectum and large intestine, and these should be treated on the same lines as cancer.

CARCINOMA OR CANCER

A cancer is a malignant tumour which originates in epithelium. The cancer cells are derived by proliferation from already existing epithelium, and they invade the sub-epithelial connective tissue in the form of simple or branching columns. These columns are enclosed in spaces—termed alveoli—which are probably dilated lymph spaces, and which communicate freely with the lymph vessels. The cells composing the columns and filling the alveoli vary with the character of the epithelium in which the cancer originates. The malignancy of cancer depends on the tendency which the epithelium has of invading the tissues in its neighbourhood, and on the capacity of the cells, when transported elsewhere by the lymph or blood-stream, of giving rise to secondary growths.

Cancer may arise on any surface covered by epithelium or in any of the secreting glands of the body, but it is much more common in some situations than in others. It is frequently met with, for example, in the skin, in the stomach and large intestine, in the breast, the uterus, and the external genitals; less frequently in the gall-bladder, larynx, thyreoid, prostate, and urinary bladder.

Tissues appear to be most liable to cancer when, having attained maturity, they enter upon the phase of decadence or involution, and this phase is reached by different tissues at different periods. It is not so much, therefore, the age of the person in whom it occurs, as the age of the tissue in which it arises, that determines the maximum incidence of cancer. Cancer of the stomach appears and attains a maximum frequency earlier than cancer of the skin; cancer of the uterus and mamma is more frequent towards the decline of reproductive activity than in the later years of life; rectal cancer is not infrequently met with during the second and third decades. There is evidence that the irritation caused by alcohol and tobacco plays a part in the causation of cancer, in the fact that a large proportion of those who become the subjects of cancer of the mouth are excessive drinkers and smokers.

A cancer may appear as a papillary growth on a mucous or a skin surface, as a nodule in the substance of an organ, or as a diffuse thickening of a tubular organ such as the stomach or intestine. The absence of definition in cancerous tumours explains the difficulty of completely removing them by surgical measures, and has led to the practice of complete extirpation of cancerous organs wherever this is possible. The boundaries of the affected organ, moreover, are frequently transgressed by the disease, and the epithelial infiltration implicates the surrounding parts. In cancer of the breast, for example, the disease often extends to the adjacent skin, fat, and muscle; in cancer of the lip or tongue, to the mandible; in cancer of the uterus or intestine, to the investing peritoneum.

In addition to its tendency to infiltrate adjacent tissues and organs, cancer is also liable to give rise to *secondary growths*. These are most often met with in the nearest lymph glands; those in the neck, for example, becoming infected from cancer of the lip, tongue, or throat; those in the axilla, from cancer of the breast; those along the curvatures of the stomach, from cancer of the pylorus; and those in the groin, from cancer of the external genitals. In lymph vessels the cancer cells may merely accumulate so as to fill the lumen and form indurated cords, or they may proliferate and give rise to secondary nodules along the course of the vessels. When the lymphatic network in the skin is diffusely infected, the appearance is either that of a multitude of secondary nodules or of a diffuse thickening, so that the skin comes to resemble coarse leather. On the wall of the chest this condition is known as *cancer en cuirasse*. Although the cancer cells constantly attack the walls of the adjacent veins and spread into their interior at a comparatively early period, secondary growths due to dissemination by the blood-stream rarely show themselves clinically until late in the course of the disease. It is probable that many of the cancer cells which are carried away in the blood or lymph stream undergo necrosis and fail to give rise to secondary growths. Secondary growths present a faithful reproduction of the structure of the primary tumour. Apart from the lymph glands, the chief seats of secondary growths are the liver, lungs, serous membranes, and bone marrow.

It is generally believed that the secondary growths in cancer that develop at a distance from the primary tumour, those, for example, in the medullary canal of the femur or in the diploë of the skull occurring in advanced cases of cancer of the breast, are the result of dissemination of cancer cells by way of the blood-stream and are to be regarded as emboli. Sampson Handley disagrees with this view; he believes that the dissemination is accomplished in a more subtle way, namely, by the actual growth of cancer cells along the finer vessels of the lymph plexuses that ramify in the deep fascia, a method of spread which he calls *permeation*. It is maintained also that permeation occurs as readily against the lymph stream as with it. He compares the spread of cancer to that of an invisible annular ringworm. The growing edge extends in a wider and wider circle, within which a healing process may occur, so that the area of permeation is a ring, rather than a disc. Healing occurs by a process of "peri-lymphatic fibrosis," but as the natural process of healing may fail at isolated points, nodules of cancer appear, which, although apparently separate from the primary growth, have developed in continuity with it, peri-lymphatic fibrosis having destroyed the cancer chain connecting the nodule with the primary growth. This centrifugal spread of cancer is clearly seen in the distribution of the subcutaneous secondary nodules so frequently met with in the late stages of mammary cancer. The area within which the secondary nodules occur is a circle of continually increasing diameter with the primary growth in the centre.

In the rare cases in which the skin of the greater part of the body is affected, the nodules rarely appear below the level of the deltoid or the middle third of the thigh, the patient dying before the spread can reach the distal portions of the limbs.

Handley argues against the embolic origin of the metastases in the bones because of the rarity of these in the bones of the distal parts of the limbs, because of the fact that secondary cancer of the femur nearly always commences in the upper third of the shaft, which harmonises with the intimate connection of the deep fascia with the periosteum over the great trochanter, thus favouring invasion of the bone marrow when permeation has spread thus far. He claims support for the permeation theory from the fact that the humerus is rarely involved below the insertion of the deltoid, and that spontaneous fracture of the femur is three times more common on the side on which the breast cancer is situated.

The tumour tissue may undergo necrosis, and when the overlying skin or mucous membrane gives way an ulcer is formed. The margins of a *cancerous ulcer* (Fig. 57) are made up of tumour tissue which has not broken down. Usually they are irregular, nodularly thickened or indurated; sometimes they are raised and crater-like. The floor of the ulcer is smooth and glazed, or occupied by necrosed tissue, and the discharge is watery and blood-stained, and as a result of putrefactive changes may become offensive. Hæmorrhage is rarely a prominent feature, but discharge of blood may constitute a symptom of considerable diagnostic importance in cancer of internal organs such as the rectum, the bladder, or the uterus.

The Contagiousness of Cancer.—A limited number of cases are on record in which a cancer appears to have been transferred by contact, as from the lower to the upper lip, from one labium majus to the other, from the tongue to the cheek, and from one vocal cord to the other; these being all examples of cancer involving surfaces which are constantly or frequently in contact. The transference of cancer from one human being to another, whether by accident, as in the case of a surgeon wounding his finger while operating for cancer, or by the deliberate introduction of a portion of cancerous tumour into the tissues, has never been known to occur.

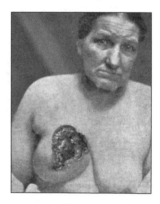

FIG. 57. Carcinoma of Breast with Cancerous Ulcer.

It is by no means infrequent, however, that when recurrence takes place after an operation for the removal of cancer, the recurrent nodules make their appearance in the main scar or in the scars of stitches in its neighbourhood. In the lower animals the grafting of cancer only succeeds in animals of the same species; for example, a cancer taken from a mouse will not grow in the tissues of a rat, but only in a mouse of the same variety as that from which the graft was taken.

While cancer cannot be regarded as either contagious or infectious, it is important to bear in mind the possibility of infection of a wound with cancer when operating for the disease. A cancer should not be cut into unless this is essential for purposes of diagnosis, and the wound made for exploration should be tightly closed by stitches before the curative operation is proceeded with; the instruments used for the exploration must not be used again until they have been boiled. The greatest care should be taken that a cancer which has softened or broken down is not opened into during the operation.

Investigations regarding the cause of cancer have been prosecuted with great energy during recent years, but as yet without positive result. It is recognised that there are a number of conditions which favour the development of cancer, such as prolonged irritation, and a considerable number of cases have been recorded in which cancer of the skin of the hands has followed prolonged and repeated exposure to the Röntgen rays.

The Alleged Increase of Cancer.—Regarding the alleged increase of cancer, it may be pointed out that it is impossible to ascertain how much of the apparent increase is due to more accurate diagnosis and improved registration. It is probable also that some increase has taken place in consequence of the increased average duration of life; a larger proportion of persons now reach the age at which cancer is frequent.

The prognosis largely depends on the variety of cancer and on its situation. Certain varieties—such as the atrophic cancer of the breast which occurs in old people, and some forms of cancer in the rectum—are so indolent in their progress that they can scarcely be said to shorten life; while others—such as the softer varieties of mammary cancer occurring in young women—are among the most malignant of tumours. The mode in which cancer causes death depends to a large extent upon its situation. In the gullet, for example, it usually causes death by starvation; in the larynx or thyreoid, by suffocation; in the intestine, by obstruction of the bowels; in the uterus, prostate, and bladder, by hæmorrhage or by implication of the ureters and kidneys. Independently of their situation, however, cancers frequently cause death by giving rise to a progressive impairment of health known as the *cancerous cachexia*, a condition which is due to the continued absorption of poisonous products from the tumour. The patient loses appetite, becomes emaciated, pale, and feverish, and gradually loses strength until he dies. In many cases, especially those in which ulceration has occurred, the addition of pyogenic infection may also be concerned in the failure of health.

Treatment.—Removal by surgical means affords the best prospect of cure. If carcinomatous disease is to be rooted out, its mode of spread by means of the lymph vessels must be borne in mind, and as this occurs at an early stage, and is not evident on examination, a wide area must be included in the operation. The organ from which the original growth springs should, if practicable, be altogether removed, because its lymph vessels generally communicate freely with each other, and secondary deposits have probably already taken place in various parts of it. In addition, the nearest chain of lymph glands must also be removed, even though they may not be noticeably enlarged, and in some cases—in cancer of the breast, for example—the intervening lymph vessels should be removed at the same time.

The treatment of cancer by other than operative methods has received a great deal of attention within recent years, and many agents have been put to the test, *e.g.* colloidal suspensions of selenium, but without any positive results. Most benefit has resulted from the use of radium and of the X-rays, and one or other should be employed as a routine measure after every operation for cancer.

It has been demonstrated that cancer cells are more sensitive to radium and to the Röntgen rays than the normal cells of the body, and are more easily killed. The effect varies a good deal with the nature and seat of the tumour. In rodent cancers of the skin, for example, both radium and X-ray treatment are very successful, and are to be preferred to operation because they yield a better cosmetic result. While small epitheliomas of the skin may be cured by means of the rays, they are not so amenable as rodent cancers.

Cancers of mucous membranes are less amenable to ray treatment because they are less circumscribed and are difficult of access. In cancers under the skin, the Röntgen rays are less efficient; if radium is employed, the tube containing it should be inserted into the substance of the tumour after the method described in connection with sarcoma—and another tube should be placed on the overlying skin.

In the employment of X-rays and of radium in the treatment of cancer, experience is required, not only to obtain the maximum effect of the rays, but to avoid damage to the adjacent and overlying tissues.

Ray treatment is not to be looked upon as a rival but as a powerful supplement to the operative treatment of cancer.

VARIETIES OF CANCER

The varieties of cancer are distinguished according to the character and arrangement of the epithelial cells.

The *squamous epithelial cancer* or *epithelioma* originates from a surface covered by squamous epithelium, such as the skin, or the mucous membrane of the mouth, gullet, or larynx. The cancer cells retain the characters of squamous epithelium, and, being confined within the lymph spaces of the sub-epithelial connective tissue, become compressed and undergo a horny change. This results in the formation of concentrically laminated masses known as cell nests.

The clinical features are those of a slowly growing indurated tumour, which nearly always ulcerates; there is a characteristic induration of the edges and floor of the ulcer, and its surface is often covered with warty or cauliflower-like outgrowths (Fig. 58). The infection of the lymph glands is early and constant, and constitutes the most dangerous feature of the disease; the secondary growths in the glands exhibit the characteristic induration, and may themselves break down and lead to the formation of ulcers.

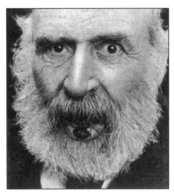

FIG. 58. Epithelioma of Lip.

Epithelioma frequently originates in long-standing ulcers or sinuses, and in scars, and probably results from the displacement and sequestration of epithelial cells during the process of cicatrisation.

The *columnar epithelial cancer* or *columnar epithelioma* originates in mucous membranes covered with columnar epithelium, and is chiefly met with in the stomach and intestine. As it resembles an adenoma in structure it is sometimes described as a *malignant adenoma*. Its malignancy is shown by the proliferating epithelium invading the other coats of the stomach or intestine, and by the development of secondary growths.

Glandular carcinoma originates in organs such as the breast, and in the glands of mucous membranes and skin. The epithelial cells are not arranged on any definite plan, but are closely packed in irregularly shaped alveoli. If the alveoli are large and the intervening stroma is scanty and delicate, the tumour is soft and brain-like, and is described as a *medullary* or *encephaloid cancer*. If the alveoli are small and the intervening stroma is abundant and composed of dense fibrous tissue, the tumour is hard, and is known as a *scirrhous cancer*—a form which is most frequently met with in the breast. If the cells undergo degeneration and absorption and the stroma contracts, the tumour becomes still harder, and tends to shrink and to draw in the surrounding parts, leading, in the breast, to retraction of the nipple and overlying skin, and in the stomach and colon to narrowing of the lumen. When the cells of the tumour undergo colloid degeneration, a *colloid cancer* results; if the degeneration is complete, as may occur in the breast, the malignancy is thereby greatly diminished; if only partial, as is more common in rectal cancer, the malignancy is not appreciably affected. Melanin pigment is formed in relation to the cells and stroma of certain epithelial tumours, giving rise to *melanotic cancer*, one of the most malignant of all new growths. Cyst-like spaces may form in the tumour by the accumulation of the secretion of the epithelial cells, or as a result of their degeneration—*cystic carcinoma*. This is met with chiefly in the breast and ovary, and the tumour resembles the cystic adenoma, but it tends to infect its surroundings and gives rise to secondary growths.

Rodent cancer originates in the glands of the skin, and presents a special tendency to break down and ulcerate on the surface (Figs. 102 and 103). It almost never infects the lymph glands.

DERMOIDS

A dermoid is a tumour containing skin or mucous membrane, occurring in a situation where these tissues are not met under normal conditions.

The *skin dermoid*, or *derma-cyst* as it has been called by Askanazy, arises from a portion of epiblast, which has become sequestrated during the process of coalescence of two cutaneous surfaces in development. This form is therefore most frequently met with on the face and neck in the situations which correspond to the various clefts and fissures of the embryo. It occurs also on the trunk in situations where the lateral halves of the body coalesce during development. Such a dermoid usually takes the form of a globular cyst, the wall of which consists of skin, and the contents of turbid fluid containing desquamated epithelium, fat droplets, cholestrol crystals, and detached hairs. Delicate hairs may also be found projecting from the epithelial lining of the cyst.

Faulty coalescence of the cutaneous covering of the back occurs most frequently over the lower sacral vertebræ, giving rise to small congenital recesses, known as post-anal dimples and coccygeal sinuses. These recesses are lined with skin, which is furnished with hairs, sebaceous and sweat glands. If the external orifice becomes occluded, there results a dermoid cyst.

Tubulo-dermoids arise from embryonic ducts and passages that are normally obliterated at birth, for example, *lingual dermoids* develop in relation to the thyreo-glossal duct; *rectal and post-rectal* dermoids to the post-anal gut; and *branchial dermoids* in relation to the branchial clefts. Tubulo-dermoids present the same structure as skin dermoids, save that mucous membrane takes the place of skin in the wall of the cyst, and the contents consist of the pent-up secretion of mucous glands.

Clinical Features.—Although dermoids are of congenital origin, they are rarely evident at birth, and may not give rise to visible tumours until puberty, when the skin and its appendages become more active, or not till adult life. Superficial dermoids, such as those met with at the outer angle of the orbit, form rounded, definitely limited tumours over which the skin is freely movable. They are usually adherent to the deeper parts, and when situated over the skull may be lodged in a depression or actual gap in the bone. Sometimes the cyst becomes infected and suppurates, and finally ruptures on the surface. This may lead to a natural cure, or a persistent sinus may form. Dermoids more deeply placed, such as those within the thorax, or those situated between the rectum and sacrum, give rise to difficulty in diagnosis, even with the help of the X-rays, and their nature is seldom recognised until the escape of the contents—particularly hairs—supplies the clue. The literature of dermoid cysts is full of accounts of puzzling tumours met with in all sorts of situations.

The treatment is to remove the cyst. When it is impossible to remove the whole of the lining membrane by dissection, the portion that is left should be destroyed with the cautery.

Ovarian Dermoids.—Dermoids are not uncommon in the ovary (Fig. 59). They usually take the form of unilocular or multilocular cysts, the wall of which contains skin, mucous membrane, hair follicles, sebaceous, sweat, and mucous glands, nails, teeth, nipples, and mammary glands. The cavity of the cyst usually contains a pultaceous mixture of shed epithelium, fluid fat, and hair. If the cyst ruptures, the epithelial elements are diffused over the peritoneum, and may give rise to secondary dermoids.

The ovarian dermoid appears clinically as an abdominal or pelvic tumour provided with a pedicle; if the pedicle becomes twisted, the tumour undergoes strangulation, an event which is attended with urgent symptoms, not unlike those of strangulated hernia.

The treatment consists in removing the tumour by laparotomy.

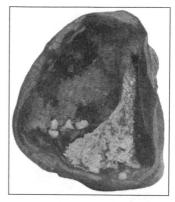

FIG. 59. Dermoid Cyst of Ovary showing Teeth in its interior.

Teratoma.—A teratoma is believed to result from partial dichotomy or cleavage of the trunk axis of the embryo, and is found exclusively in connection with the skull and vertebral column. It may take the form of a monstrosity such as conjoined twins or a parasitic foetus, but more commonly it is met with as an irregularly shaped tumour, usually growing from the sacrum. On dissection, such a tumour is found to contain a curious mixture of tissues—bones, skin, and portions of viscera, such as the intestine or liver. The question of the removal of the tumour requires to be considered in relation to the conditions present in each individual case.

CYSTS[3]

Cysts are rounded sacs, the wall being composed of fibrous tissue lined by epithelium or endothelium; the contents are fluid or semi-solid, and vary in character according to the tissue in which the cyst has originated.

Retention and Exudation Cysts.—*Retention cysts* develop when the duct of a secreting gland is partly obstructed; the secretion accumulates, and the gland and its duct become distended into a cyst. They are met with in the mamma and in the salivary glands. Sebaceous cysts or wens are described with diseases of the skin. *Exudation cysts* arise from the distension of cavities which are not provided with excretory ducts, such as those in the thyreoid.

Implantation cysts are caused by the accidental transference of portions of the epidermis into the underlying connective tissue, as may occur in wounds by needles, awls, forks, or thorns. The implanted epidermis proliferates and forms a small cyst. They are met with chiefly on the palmar aspect of the

[3] Cysts which form in relation to new-growths have been considered with tumours.

fingers, and vary in size from a split pea to a cherry. The treatment consists in removing them by dissection.

Parasitic cysts are produced by the growth within the tissues of cyst-forming parasites, the best known being the tænia echinococcus, which gives rise to the *hydatid cyst*. The liver is by far the most common site of hydatid cysts in the human subject.

With regard to the further life-history of hydatids, the living elements of the cyst may die and degenerate, or the cyst may increase in size until it ruptures. As a result of pyogenic infection the cyst may be converted into an abscess.

The *clinical features* of hydatids vary so much with their situation and size, that they are best discussed with the individual organs. In general it may be said that there is a slow formation of a globular, elastic, fluctuating, painless swelling. Fluctuation is detected when the cyst approaches the surface, and it is then also that percussion may elicit the "hydatid thrill" or fremitus. This thrill is not often obtainable, and in any case is not pathognomonic of hydatids, as it may be elicited in ascites and in other abdominal cysts. Pressure of the cyst upon adjacent structures, and the occurrence of suppuration, are attended with characteristic clinical features.

The *diagnosis* of hydatids will be considered with the individual organs. The disease is more common in certain parts of Australia and in Shetland and Iceland than in countries where the association of dogs in the domestic life of the inhabitants is less intimate. Pfeiler, who has worked at the *serum diagnosis of hydatid disease*, regards the complement deviation method as the most reliable; he believes that a positive reaction may almost be regarded as absolutely diagnostic of an echinococcal lesion.

The *treatment* is to excise the cyst completely, or to inject into it a 1 per cent. solution of formalin. In operating upon hydatids the utmost care must be taken to avoid leakage of the contents of the cyst, as these may readily disseminate the infection.

A *blood cyst* or hæmatoma results from the encapsulation of extravasated blood in the tissues, from hæmorrhage taking place into a preformed cyst, or from the saccular pouching of a varicose vein.

A *lymph cyst* usually results from a contusion in which the skin is forcibly displaced from the subjacent tissues, and lymph vessels are thereby torn across. The cyst is usually situated between the skin and fascia, and contains clear or blood-stained serum. At first it is lax and fluctuates readily, later it becomes larger and more tense. The treatment consists in drawing off the contents through a hollow needle and applying firm pressure. Apart from injury, lymph cysts are met with as the result of the distension of lymph spaces and vessels (*lymphangiectasis*); and in lymphangiomas, of which the best-known example is the cystic hygroma or hydrocele of the neck.

GANGLION

This term is applied to a cyst filled with a clear colourless jelly or colloid material, met with in the vicinity of a joint or tendon sheath.

The commonest variety—the *carpal ganglion*—popularly known as a sprained sinew—is met with as a smooth, rounded, or oval swelling on the dorsal aspect of the carpus, usually towards its radial side (Fig. 60). It is situated over one of the intercarpal or other joints in this region, and may be connected with one or other of the extensor tendons. The skin and fascia are movable over the cyst. The cyst varies in size from a pea to a pigeon's egg, and usually attains its maximum size within a few months and then remains stationary. It becomes tense and prominent when the hand is flexed towards the palm. Its appearance is usually ascribed to some strain of the wrist—for example, in girls learning gymnastics. It may cause no symptoms or it may interfere with the use of the hand, especially in grasping movements and when the hand is dorsiflexed. In girls it may give rise to pain which shoots up the arm. Ganglia are also met with on the dorsum of the metacarpus and on the palmar aspect of the wrist.

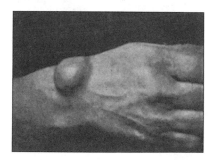

FIG. 60. Carpal Ganglion in a woman æt. 25.

The *tarsal ganglion* is situated on the dorsum of the foot over one or other of the intertarsal joints. It is usually smaller, flatter, and more tense than that met with over the wrist, so that it is sometimes mistaken for a bony tumour. It rarely causes symptoms, unless so situated as to be pressed upon by the boot.

Ganglia in the region of the knee are usually situated over the interval between the femur and tibia, most often on the lateral aspect of the joint in front of the tendon of the biceps (Fig. 61). The swelling, which may attain the size of half a walnut, is tense and hard when the knee is extended, and becomes softer and more prominent when it is flexed. They are met with in young adults who follow laborious occupations or who indulge in athletics, and they cause stiffness, discomfort, and impairment of the use of the limb. A ganglion is sometimes met with on the median aspect of the head of the metatarsal bone of the great toe and may be the cause of considerable suffering; it is indistinguishable from the thickened and enlarged bursa so commonly present in this situation in the condition known as bunion.

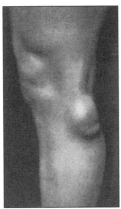

FIG. 61. Ganglion on lateral aspect of Knee in a young woman.

Ganglionic cysts are met with in other situations than those mentioned, but they are so rare as not to require separate description.

Ganglia are to be diagnosed by their situation and physical characters; enlarged bursæ, synovial cysts, and new-growths are the swellings most likely to be mistaken for them. The diagnosis is sometimes only cleared up by withdrawing the clear, jelly-like contents through a hollow needle.

Pathological Anatomy.—The wall of the cyst is composed of fibrous tissue closely adherent to or fused with the surrounding tissues, so that it cannot be shelled out. There is no endothelial lining, and the fibrous tissue of the wall is in immediate contact with the colloid material in the interior, which appears to be derived by a process of degeneration from the surrounding connective tissue. In the region of the knee the ganglion is usually multilocular, and consists of a meshwork of fibrous tissue, the meshes of which are occupied by colloid material.

It is often stated that a ganglion originates from a hernial protrusion of the synovial membrane of a joint or tendon sheath. We have not been able to demonstrate any communication between the cavity of the cyst and that of an adjacent tendon sheath or joint. It is possible, however, that the cyst may originate from a minute portion of synovial membrane being protruded and strangulated so that it becomes disconnected from that to which it originally belonged; it may then degenerate and give rise to colloid material, which accumulates and forms a cyst. Ledderhose and others regard ganglia as entirely new formations in the peri-articular tissues, resulting from colloid degeneration of the fibrous tissue of the capsular ligament, occurring at first in numerous small areas which later coalesce. Ganglia are probably, therefore, of the nature of degeneration cysts arising in the capsule of joints, in tendons, and in their sheaths.

Treatment.—A ganglion can usually be got rid of by a modification of the old-fashioned seton. The skin and cyst wall are transfixed by a stout needle carrying a double thread of silkworm gut; some of the colourless jelly escapes from the punctures; the ends of the thread are tied and cut short, and a dressing is applied. A week later the threads are removed and the minute punctures are sealed with collodion. The action of the threads is to convert the cyst wall into granulation tissue, which undergoes the usual conversion into scar tissue. If the cyst re-forms, it should be removed by open dissection under local anæsthesia. Puncture with a tenotomy knife and scraping the interior, and the injection of irritants, are alternative, but less satisfactory, methods of treatment.

Ganglia in the substance of *tendons* are rare. The diagnosis rests on the observation that the small tumour is cystic, and that it follows the movements of the tendon. The cyst is at first multiple, but the partitions disappear, and the spaces are thrown into one. The tendon is so weakened that it readily ruptures. The best treatment is to resect the affected segment of tendon.

The so-called "compound palmar ganglion" is a tuberculous disease of the tendon sheaths, and is described with diseases of tendon sheaths.

• XI •

INJURIES

Contusions • Wounds: Varieties • Wounds by Firearms and Explosives: Pistol-shot Wounds; Wounds by Sporting Guns; Wounds by Rifle Bullets; Wounds Received in Warfare; Shell Wounds • Embedded Foreign Bodies • Burns and Scalds • Injuries Produced by Electricity: X-ray and Radium; Electrical Burns; Lightning Stroke.

CONTUSIONS

A contusion or bruise is a laceration of the subcutaneous soft tissues, without solution of continuity of the skin. When the integument gives way at the same time, a *contused-wound* results. Bruising occurs when force is applied to a part by means of a blunt object, whether as a direct blow, a crush, or a grazing form of violence. If the force acts at right angles to the part, it tends to produce localised lesions which extend deeply; while, if it acts obliquely, it gives rise to lesions which are more diffuse, but comparatively superficial. It is well to remember that those who suffer from scurvy, or hæmophilia (bleeders), and fat and anæmic females, are liable to be bruised by comparatively trivial injuries.

Clinical Features.—The less severe forms of contusion are associated with *ecchymosis*, numerous minute and discrete punctate hæmorrhages being scattered through the superficial layers of the skin, which is slightly oedematous. The effused blood is soon reabsorbed.

The more severe forms are attended with *extravasation*, the extravasated blood being widely diffused through the cellular tissue of the part, especially where this is loose and lax, as in the region of the orbit, the scrotum and perineum, and on the chest wall. A blue or bluish-black discoloration occurs in patches, varying in size and depth with the degree of force which produced the injury, and in shape with the instrument employed. It is most intense in

205

regions where the skin is naturally thin and pigmented. In parts where the extravasated blood is only separated from the oxygen of the air by a thin layer of epidermis or by a mucous membrane, it retains its bright arterial colour. These points are often well illustrated in cases of black eye, where the blood effused under the conjunctiva is bright red, while that in the eyelids is almost black. In severe contusions associated with great tension of the skin—for example, over the front of the tibia or around the ankle—blisters often form on the surface and constitute a possible avenue of infection. When deeply situated, the blood tends to spread along the lines of least resistance, partly under the influence of gravity, passing under fasciæ, between muscles, along the sheaths of vessels, or in connective-tissue spaces, so that it may only reach the surface after some time, and at a considerable distance from the seat of injury. This fact is sometimes of importance in diagnosis, as, for example, in certain fractures of the base of the skull, where discoloration appears under the conjunctiva or behind the mastoid process some days after the accident.

Blood extravasated deeply in the tissues gives rise to a firm, resistant, doughy swelling, in which there may be elicited on deep palpation a peculiar sensation, not unlike the crepitus of fracture.

It frequently happens that, from the tearing of lymph vessels, serous fluid is extravasated, and a *lymphatic* or *serous cyst* may form.

In all contusions accompanied by extravasation, there is marked swelling of the area involved, as well as pain and tenderness. The temperature may rise to 101° F., or, in the large extravasations that occur in bleeders, even higher—a form of aseptic fever. The degree of shock is variable, but sudden syncope frequently results from severe bruises of the testicle, abdomen, or head, and occasionally marked nervous depression follows these injuries.

Contusion of muscles or nerves may produce partial atrophy and paresis, as is often seen after injuries in the region of the shoulder.

In alcoholic or other debilitated patients, suppuration is liable to ensue in bruised parts, infection taking place from cocci circulating in the blood, or through the overlying skin.

Terminations of Contusions.—The usual termination is a complete return to the normal, some of the extravasated blood being organised, but most of it being reabsorbed. During the process characteristic alterations in the colour of the effused blood take place as a result of changes in the blood pigment. In from twenty-four to forty-eight hours the margins of the blue area become of a violet hue, and as time goes on the discoloured area increases in size, and becomes successively green, yellow, and lemon-coloured at its margins, the central part being the last to change. The rate at which this play of colours proceeds is so variable, and depends on so many circumstances, that no time-limits can be laid down. During the disintegration of the effused blood the adjacent lymph glands may become enlarged, and on dissection may be found to be pigmented. Sometimes the blood persists as a collection of fluid with a newly formed connective-tissue capsule, constituting a *hæmatoma* or *blood cyst*, more often met with in the scalp than in other parts.

The impairment of the blood supply of the skin may lead to the formation of *blisters*, or to *necrosis*. Death of skin is more liable to occur in bleeders, and when the slough separates the blood-clot is exposed and the reparative changes go on extremely slowly. *Suppuration* may occur and lead to the formation of an abscess as a result of direct infection from the skin or through the circulation.

Treatment.—If the patient is seen immediately after the accident, elevation of the part, and firm pressure applied by means of a thick pad of cotton wool and an elastic bandage, are useful in preventing effusion of blood. Ice-bags and evaporating lotions are to be used with caution, as they are liable to lower the vitality of the damaged tissues and lead to necrosis of the skin.

When extravasation has already taken place, massage is the most speedy and efficacious means of dispersing the effused blood. The part should be massaged several times a day, unless the presence of blebs or abrasions of the skin prevents this being done. When this is the case, the use of antiseptic dressings is called for to prevent infection and to promote healing, after which massage is employed.

When the tension caused by the extravasated blood threatens the vitality of the skin, incisions may be made, if asepsis can be assured. The blood from a hæmatoma may be withdrawn by an exploring needle, and the puncture sealed with collodion. Infective complications must be looked for and dealt with on general principles.

WOUNDS

A wound is a solution in the continuity of the skin or mucous membrane and of the underlying tissues, caused by violence.

Three varieties of wounds are described: incised, punctured, and contused and lacerated.

Incised Wounds.—Typical examples of incised wounds are those made by the surgeon in the course of an operation, wounds accidentally inflicted by cutting instruments, and suicidal cut-throat wounds. It should be borne in mind in connection with medico-legal inquiries, that wounds of soft parts that closely overlie a bone, such as the skull, the tibia, or the patella, although, inflicted by a blunt instrument, may have all the appearances of incised wounds.

Clinical Features.—One of the characteristic features of an incised wound is its tendency to gape. This is evident in long skin wounds, and especially when the cut runs across the part, or when it extends deeply enough to divide muscular fibres at right angles to their long axis. The gaping of a wound, further, is more marked when the underlying tissues are in a state of tension—as, for example, in inflamed parts. Incised wounds in the palm of the hand, the sole of the foot, or the scalp, however, have little tendency to gape, because of the close attachment of the skin to the underlying fascia.

Incised wounds, especially in inflamed tissues, tend to bleed profusely; and when a vessel is only partly divided and is therefore unable to contract, it continues to bleed longer than when completely cut across.

The *special risks* of incised wounds are: (1) division of large blood vessels, leading to profuse hæmorrhage; (2) division of nerve-trunks, resulting in motor and sensory disturbances; and (3) division of tendons or muscles, interfering with movement.

Treatment.—If hæmorrhage is still going on, it must be arrested by pressure, torsion, or ligature, as the accumulation of blood in a wound interferes with union. If necessary, the wound should be purified by washing with saline solution or eusol, and the surrounding skin painted with iodine, after which the edges are approximated by sutures. The raw surfaces must be brought into accurate apposition, care being taken that no inversion of the cutaneous surface takes place. In extensive and deep wounds, to ensure more complete closure and to prevent subsequent stretching of the scar, it is advisable to unite the different structures—muscles, fasciæ, and subcutaneous tissue—by separate series of *buried sutures* of catgut or other absorbable material. For the approximation of the skin edges, stitches of horse-hair, fishing-gut, or fine silk are the most appropriate. These *stitches of coaptation* may be interrupted or continuous. In small superficial wounds on exposed parts, stitch marks may be avoided by approximating the edges with strips of gauze fixed in position by collodion, or by subcutaneous sutures of fine catgut. Where the skin is loose, as, for example, in the neck, on the limbs, or in the scrotum, the use of Michel's clips is advantageous in so far as these bring the deep surfaces of the skin into accurate apposition, are introduced with comparatively little pain, and leave only a slight mark if removed within forty-eight hours.

When there is any difficulty in bringing the edges of the wound into apposition, a few interrupted *relaxation stitches* may be introduced wide of the margins, to take the strain off the coaptation stitches. Stout silk, fishing-gut, or silver wire may be employed for this purpose. When the tension is extreme, Lister's button suture may be employed. The tension is relieved and death of skin prevented by scoring it freely with a sharp knife. Relaxation stitches should be removed in four or five days, and stitches of coaptation in from seven to ten days. On the face and neck, wounds heal rapidly, and stitches may be removed in two or three days, thus diminishing the marks they leave.

Drainage.—In wounds in which no cavity has been left, and in which there is no reason to suspect infection, drainage is unnecessary. When, however, the deeper parts of an extensive wound cannot be brought into accurate apposition, and especially when there is any prospect of oozing of blood or serum—as in amputation stumps or after excision of the breast—drainage is indicated. It is a wise precaution also to insert drainage tubes into wounds in fat patients when there is the slightest reason to suspect the presence of infection. Glass or rubber tubes are the best drains; but where it is desirable to leave little mark, a few strands of horse-hair, or a small roll of rubber, form a satisfactory substitute. Except when infection occurs, the drain is removed in from one to four days and the opening closed with a Michel's clip or a suture.

Punctured Wounds.—Punctured wounds are produced by narrow, pointed instruments, and the sharper and smoother the instrument the more does the resulting injury resemble an incised wound; while from more rounded and rougher instruments the edges of the wound are more or less contused or lacerated. The depth of punctured wounds greatly exceeds their width, and the damage to subcutaneous parts is usually greater than that to the skin. When the instrument transfixes a part, the edges of the wound of entrance may be inverted, and those of the exit wound everted. If the instrument is a rough one, these conditions may be reversed by its sudden withdrawal.

Punctured wounds neither gape nor bleed much. Even when a large vessel is implicated, the bleeding usually takes place into the tissues rather than externally.

The *risks* incident to this class of wounds are: (1) the extreme difficulty, especially when a dense fascia has been perforated, of rendering them aseptic, on account of the uncertainty as to their depth, and of the way in which the surface wound closes on the withdrawal of the instrument; (2) different forms of aneurysm may result from the puncture of a large vessel; (3) perforation of a joint, or of a serous cavity, such as the abdomen, thorax, or skull, materially adds to the danger.

Treatment.—The first indication is to purify the whole extent of the wound, and to remove any foreign body or blood-clot that may be in it. It is usually necessary to enlarge the wound, freely dividing injured fasciæ, paring away bruised tissues, and purifying the whole wound-surface. Any blood vessel that is punctured should be cut across and tied; and divided muscles, tendons, or nerves must be sutured. After hæmorrhage has been arrested, iodoform and bismuth paste is rubbed into the raw surface, and the wound closed. If there is any reason to doubt the asepticity of the wound, it is better treated by the open method, and a Bier's bandage should be applied.

Contused and Lacerated Wounds.—These may be considered together, as they so occur in practice. They are produced by crushing, biting, or tearing forms of violence—such as result from machinery accidents, firearms, or the bites of animals. In addition to the irregular wound of the integument, there is always more or less bruising of the parts beneath and around, and the subcutaneous lesions are much wider than appears on the surface.

Wounds of this variety usually gape considerably, especially when there is much laceration of the skin. It is not uncommon to have considerable portions of skin, muscle, or tendon completely torn away.

Hæmorrhage is seldom a prominent feature, as the crushing or tearing of the vessel wall leads to the obliteration of the lumen.

The *special risks* of these wounds are: (1) Sloughing of the bruised tissues, especially when attempts to sterilise the wound have not been successful. (2) Reactionary hæmorrhage after the initial shock has passed off. (3) Secondary hæmorrhage as a result of infective processes ensuing in the wound. (4) Loss of muscle or tendon, interfering with motion. (5) Cicatricial contraction. (6) Gangrene, which may follow occlusion of main vessels, or virulent infective processes. (7) It is not uncommon to have particles of carbon embedded in the tissues after lacerated wounds, leaving unsightly, pigmented scars. This is often seen in coal-miners, and in those injured by firearms, and is to be prevented by removing all gross dirt from the edges of the wound.

Treatment.—In severe wounds of this class implicating the extremities, the most important question that arises is whether or not the limb can be saved. In examining the limb, attention should first be directed to the state of the main blood vessels, in order to determine if the vascular supply of the part beyond the lesion is sufficient to maintain its vitality. Amputation is usually called for if there is complete absence of pulsation in the distal arteries and if the part beyond is cold. If at the same time important nerve-trunks are lacerated, so that the function of the limb would be seriously impaired, it is not worth running the risk of attempting to save it. If, in addition, there is extensive destruction of large muscular masses or of important tendons, or comminution of the bones, amputation is usually imperative. Stripping of large areas of skin is not in itself a reason for removing a limb, as much can be done by skin grafting, but when it is associated with other lesions it favours amputation. In considering these points, it must be borne in mind that the damage to the deeper tissues is always more extensive than appears on the surface, and that in many cases it is only possible to estimate the real extent of the injury by administering an anæsthetic and exploring the wound. In doubtful cases the possibility of rendering the parts aseptic will often decide the question for or against amputation. If thorough purification is accomplished, the success which attends conservative measures is often remarkable. It is permissible to run an amount of risk to save an upper extremity which would be unjustifiable in the case of a lower limb. The age and occupation of the patient must also be taken into account.

It having been decided to try and save the limb, the question is only settled for the moment; it may have to be reconsidered from day to day, or even from hour to hour, according to the progress of the case.

When it is decided to make the attempt to save the limb, the wound must be thoroughly purified. All bruised tissue in which gross dirt has become engrained should be cut away with knife or scissors. The raw surface is then cleansed with eusol, washed with sterilised salt solution followed by methylated spirit, and rubbed all over with "bipp" paste. If the purification is considered satisfactory the wound may be closed, otherwise it is left open, freely drained or packed with gauze, and the limb is immobilised by suitable splints.

WOUNDS BY FIREARMS AND EXPLOSIVES

It is not necessary here to do more than indicate the general characters of wounds produced by modern weapons. For further details the reader is referred to works on military surgery. Experience has shown that the nature and severity of the injuries sustained in warfare vary widely in different campaigns, and even in different fields of the same campaign. Slight variations in the size, shape, and weight of rifle bullets, for example, may profoundly modify the lesions they produce: witness the destructive effect of the pointed bullet compared with that of the conical form previously used. The conditions under which the fighting is carried on also influence the wounds. Those sustained in the open, long-range fighting of the South African campaign of 1899-1902 were very different from those met with in the entrenched warfare in France in 1914-1918. It has been found also that the infective complications are greatly influenced by the terrain in which the fighting takes place. In the dry, sandy, uncultivated veldt of South Africa, bullet wounds seldom became infected, while those sustained in the highly manured fields of Belgium were almost invariably contaminated with putrefactive organisms, and gaseous gangrene and tetanus were common complications. It has been found also that wounds inflicted in naval engagements present different characters from those sustained on land. Many other factors, such as the physical and mental condition of the men, the facilities for affording first aid, and the transport arrangements, also play a part in determining the nature and condition of the wounds that have to be dealt with by military surgeons.

Whatever the nature of the weapon concerned, the wound is of the *punctured, contused, and lacerated* variety. Its severity depends on the size, shape, and velocity of the missile, the range at which the weapon is discharged, and the part of the body struck.

Shock is a prominent feature, but its degree, as well as the time of its onset, varies with the extent and seat of the injury, and with the mental state of the patient when wounded. We have observed pronounced shock in children after being shot even when no serious injury was sustained. At the moment of injury the patient experiences a sensation which is variously described as being like the lash of a whip, a blow with a stick, or an electric shock. There is not much pain at first, but later it may become severe, and is usually associated with intense thirst, especially when much blood has been lost.

In all forms of wounds sustained in warfare, septic infection constitutes the main risk, particularly that resulting from streptococci. The presence of anaërobic organisms introduces the additional danger of gaseous forms of gangrene.

The earlier the wound is disinfected the greater is the possibility of diminishing this risk. If cleansing is carried out within the first six hours the chance of eliminating sepsis is good; with every succeeding six hours it diminishes, until after twenty-four hours it is seldom possible to do more than mitigate sepsis. (J. T. Morrison.)

The presence of a metallic foreign body having been determined and its position localised by means of the X-rays, all devitalised and contaminated tissue is excised, the foreign material, *e.g.*, a missile, fragments of clothing, gravel and blood-clot, removed, the wound purified with antiseptics and closed or drained according to circumstances.

Pistol-shot Wounds.—Wounds inflicted by pistols, revolvers, and small air-guns are of frequent occurrence in civil practice, the weapon being discharged usually by accident, but frequently with suicidal, and sometimes with homicidal intent.

With all calibres and at all ranges, except actual contact, the wound of entrance is smaller than the bullet. If the weapon is discharged within a foot of the body, the skin surrounding the wound is usually stained with powder and burned, and the hair singed. At ranges varying from six inches to thirty feet, grains of powder may be found embedded in the skin or lying loose on the surface, the greater the range the wider being the area of spread. When black powder is used, the embedded grains usually leave a permanent bluish-black tattooing of the skin. When the weapon is placed in contact with the skin, the subcutaneous tissues are lacerated over an area of two or three inches around the opening made by the bullet and smoke and powder-staining and scorching are more marked than at longer ranges.

When the bullet perforates, the exit wound is usually larger and more extensively lacerated than the wound of entrance. Its margins are as a rule everted, and it shows no marks of flame, smoke, or powder. These features are common to all perforations caused by bullets.

Pistol wounds only produce dangerous effects when fired at close range, and when the cavities of the skull, the thorax, or the abdomen are implicated. In the abdomen a lethal injury may readily be caused even by pistols of the "toy" order. These injuries will be described with regional surgery.

Pistol-shot wounds of *joints* and *soft parts* are seldom of serious import apart from the risk of hæmorrhage and of infection.

Treatment.—The treatment of wounds of the soft parts consists in purifying the wounds of entrance and exit and the surrounding skin, and in providing for drainage if this is indicated.

There being no urgency for the removal of the bullet, time should be taken to have it localised by the X-rays, preferably by stereoscopic plates. In some cases it is not necessary to remove the bullet.

Wounds by Sporting Guns.—In the common sporting or scatter gun, with which accidents so commonly occur during the shooting season, the charge of small shot or pellets leave the muzzle of the gun as a solid mass which makes a single ragged wound having much the appearance of that caused by a single bullet. At a distance of from four to five feet from the muzzle the pellets begin to disperse so that there are separate punctures around the main central wound. As the range increases, these outlying punctures make a wider and wider pattern, until at a distance of from eighteen to twenty feet from the muzzle, the scattering is complete, there is no longer any central wound, and each individual pellet makes its own puncture. From these elementary data, it is usually possible, from the features of the wound, to arrive at an approximately accurate conclusion regarding the range at which the gun was discharged, and this may have an important bearing on the question of accident, suicide, or murder.

As regards the effects on the tissues at close range, that is, within a few feet, there is widespread laceration and disruption; if a bone is struck it is shattered, and portions of bone may be displaced or even driven out through the exit wound.

When the charge impinges over one of the large cavities of the body, the shot may scatter widely through the contained viscera, and there is often no exit wound. In the thorax, for example, if a rib is struck, the charge and possibly fragments of bone, will penetrate the pleura, and be dispersed throughout the lung; in the head, the skull may be shattered and the brain torn up; and in the abdomen, the hollow viscera may be perforated in many places and the solid organs lacerated.

On covered parts the clothing, by deflecting the shot, influences the size and shape of the wound; the entrance wound is increased in size and more ragged, and portions of the clothes may be driven into the tissues.

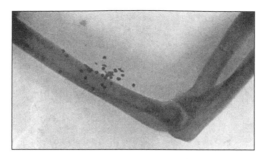

FIG. 62. Radiogram showing Pellets embedded in Arm. (Mr. J. W. Dowden's case.)

A charge of small shot is much more destructive to blood vessels, tendons, and ligaments than a single bullet, which in many cases pushes such structures aside without dividing them. In the abdomen and chest, also, the damage done by a full charge of shot is much more extensive than that inflicted by a single bullet, the deflection of the pellets leading to a greater number of perforations of the intestine and more widespread laceration of solid viscera.

When the charge impinges on one of the extremities at close range, we often have the opportunity of observing that the exit wound is larger, more ragged than that of entrance, and that its edges are everted; the extensive tearing and bruising of all the tissues, including the bones, and the marked tendency to early and progressive septic infection, render amputation compulsory in the majority of such cases.

At a range of from twenty to thirty feet, although the scatter is complete, the pellets are still close together, so that if they encounter the shaft of a long bone, even the femur, they fracture the bone across, often along with some longitudinal splintering.

Individual pellets striking the shafts of long bones become flattened or distorted, and when cancellated bone is struck they become embedded in it (Fig. 62).

The skin, when it is closely peppered with shot, is liable to lose its vitality, and with the addition of a little sepsis, readily necroses and comes away as a slough.

When the shot have diverged so as to strike singly, they seldom do much harm, but fatal damage may be done to the brain or to the aorta, or the eye may be seriously injured by a single pellet.

Small shot fired at longer ranges—over about a hundred and fifty feet—usually go through the skin, but seldom pierce the fascia, and lie embedded in the subcutaneous tissue, from which they can readily be extracted.

The wad of the cartridge behaves erratically: so long as it remains flat it goes off with the rest of the charge, and is often buried in the wound; but if it curls up or turns on its side, it is usually deflected and flies clear of the shot. It may make a separate wound.

Wounds from sporting guns are to be *treated* on the usual lines, the early efforts being directed to the alleviation of shock and the prevention of septic infection. There is rarely any urgency in the removal of pellets from the tissues.

Wounds by Rifle Bullets.—The vast majority of wounds inflicted by rifle bullets are met with in the field during active warfare, and fall to be treated by military surgeons. They occasionally occur accidentally, however, during range practice for example, and may then come under the notice of the civil surgeon.

It is only necessary here to consider the effects of modern small-bore rifle or machine-gun bullets.

The trajectory is practically flat up to 675 yards. In destructive effect there is not much difference between the various high velocity bullets used in different armies; they will kill up to a distance of two miles. The hard covering is employed to enable the bullet to take the grooves in the rifle, and to prevent it stripping as it passes through the barrel. It also increases the penetrating power of the missile, but diminishes its "stopping" power, unless a vital part or a long bone is struck. By removing the covering from the point of the bullet, as is done in the Dum-Dum bullet, or by splitting the end, the bullet is made to expand or "mushroom" when it strikes the body, and its stopping power is thereby greatly increased, the resulting wound being much more severe. These "soft-nosed" expanding bullets are to be distinguished from "explosive" bullets which contain substances which detonate on impact. High velocity bullets are unlikely to lodge in the body unless spent, or pulled up by a sandbag, or metal buckle on a belt, or a book in the pocket, or the core and the case separating—"stripping" of the bullet. Spent shot may merely cause bruising of the surface, or they may pass through the skin and lodge in the subcutaneous tissue, or may even damage some deeper structure such as a nerve trunk.

A blank cartridge fired at close range may cause a severe wound, and, if charged with black powder, may leave a permanent bluish-black pigmentation of the skin.

The lesions of individual tissues—bones, nerves, blood vessels—are considered with these.

Treatment of Gunshot Wounds under War Conditions.—It is only necessary to indicate briefly the method of dealing with gunshot wounds in warfare as practised in the European War.

1. *On the Field.*—Hæmorrhage is arrested in the limbs by an improvised tourniquet; in the head by a pad and bandage; in the thorax or abdomen by packing if necessary, but this should be avoided if possible, as it favours septic infection. If a limb is all but detached it should be completely severed. A full dose of morphin is given hypodermically. The ampoule of iodine carried by the wounded man is broken, and its contents are poured over and around the wound, after which the field dressing is applied. In extensive wounds, the "shell-dressing" carried by the stretcher bearers is preferred. All bandages are applied loosely to allow for subsequent swelling. The fragments of fractured bones are immobilised by some form of emergency splint.

2. *At the Advanced Dressing Station*, after the patient has had a liberal allowance of warm fluid nourishment, such as soup or tea, a full dose of antitetanic serum is injected. The tourniquet is removed and the wound inspected. Urgent amputations are performed. Moribund patients are detained lest they die *en route*.

3. *In the Field Ambulance or Casualty Clearing Station* further measures are employed for the relief of shock, and urgent operations are performed, such as amputation for gangrene, tracheotomy for dyspnoea, or laparotomy for perforated or lacerated intestine. In the majority of cases the main object is to guard against infection; the skin is disinfected over a wide area and surrounded with towels; damaged tissue, especially muscle, is removed with the knife or scissors, and foreign bodies are extracted. Torn blood vessels, and, if possible, nerves and tendons are repaired. The wound is then partly closed, provision being made for free drainage, or some special method of irrigation, such as that of Carrel, is adopted. Sometimes the wound is treated with bismuth, iodoform, and paraffin paste (B.I.P.P.) and sutured.

4. *In the Base Hospital or Hospital Ship* various measures may be called for according to the progress of the wound and the condition of the patient.

Shell Wounds and Wounds produced by Explosions.—It is convenient to consider together the effects of the bursting of shells fired from heavy ordnance and those resulting in the course of blasting operations from the discharge of dynamite or other explosives, or from the bursting of steam boilers or pipes, the breaking of machinery, and similar accidents met with in civil practice.

Wounds inflicted by shell fragments and shrapnel bullets tend to be extensive in area, and show great contusion, laceration, and destruction of the tissues. The missiles frequently lodge and carry portions of the clothing and, it may be, articles from the man's pocket, with them. Shell wounds are attended with a considerable degree of shock. On account of the wide area of contusion which surrounds the actual wound produced by shell fragments, amputation, when called for, should be performed some distance above the torn tissues, as there is considerable risk of sloughing of the flaps.

Wounds produced by dynamite explosions and the bursting of boilers have the same general characters as shell wounds. Fragments of stone, coal, or metal may lodge in the tissues, and favour the occurrence of infective complications.

All such injuries are to be treated on the general principles governing contused and lacerated wounds.

EMBEDDED FOREIGN BODIES

In the course of many operations foreign substances are introduced into the tissues and intentionally left there, for example, suture and ligature materials, steel or aluminium plates, silver wire or ivory pegs used to secure the fixation of bones, or solid paraffin employed to correct deformities. Other substances, such as gauze, drainage tubes, or metal instruments, may be unintentionally left in a wound.

Foreign bodies may also lodge in accidentally inflicted wounds, for example, bullets, needles, splinters of wood, or fragments of clothing. The needles of hypodermic syringes sometimes break and a portion remains embedded in the tissues. As a result of explosions, particles of carbon, in the form of coal-dust or gunpowder, or portions of shale, may lodge in a wound.

The embedded foreign body at first acts as an irritant, and induces a reaction in the tissues in which it lodges, in the form of hyperæmia, local leucocytosis, proliferation of fibroblasts, and the formation of granulation tissue. The subsequent changes depend upon whether or not the wound is infected with pyogenic bacteria. If it is so infected, suppuration ensues, a sinus forms, and persists until the foreign body is either cast out or removed.

If the wound is aseptic, the fate of the foreign body varies with its character. A substance that is absorbable, such as catgut or fine silk, is surrounded and permeated by the phagocytes, which soften and disintegrate it, the debris being gradually absorbed in much the same manner as a fibrinous exudate. Minute bodies that are not capable of being absorbed, such as particles of carbon, or of pigment used in tattooing, are taken up by the phagocytes, and in course of time removed. Larger bodies, such as needles or bullets, which are not capable of being destroyed by the phagocytes, become encapsulated. In the granulation tissue by which they are surrounded large multinuclear giant-cells appear ("*foreign-body giant-cells*") and attach themselves to the foreign body, the fibroblasts proliferate and a capsule of scar tissue is eventually formed around the body. The tissues of the capsule may show evidence of iron pigmentation. Sometimes fluid accumulates around a foreign body within its capsule, constituting a cyst.

Substances like paraffin, strands of silk used to bridge a gap in a tendon, or portions of calcined bone, instead of being encapsulated, are gradually permeated and eventually replaced by new connective tissue.

Embedded bodies may remain in the tissues for an indefinite period without giving rise to inconvenience. At any time, however, they may cause trouble, either as a result of infective complications, or by inducing the formation of a mass of inflammatory tissue around them, which may simulate a gumma, a tuberculous focus, or a sarcoma. This latter condition may give rise to difficulties in diagnosis, particularly if there is no history forthcoming of the entrance of the foreign body. The ignorance of patients regarding the possible lodgment in the tissues of a foreign body—even of considerable size—is remarkable. In such cases the X-rays will reveal the presence of the foreign body if it is sufficiently opaque to cast a shadow. The heavy, lead-containing varieties of glass throw very definite shadows little inferior in sharpness and definition to those of metal; almost all the ordinary forms of commercial glass also may be shown up by the X-rays.

Foreign bodies encapsulated in the peritoneal cavity are specially dangerous, as the proximity of the intestine furnishes a constant possibility of infection.

The question of removal of the foreign body must be decided according to the conditions present in individual cases; in searching for a foreign body in the tissues, unless it has been accurately located, a general anæsthetic is to be preferred.

BURNS AND SCALDS

The distinction between a burn which results from the action of dry heat on the tissues of the body and a scald which results from the action of moist heat, has no clinical significance.

In young and debilitated subjects hot poultices may produce injuries of the nature of burns. In old people with enfeebled circulation mere exposure to a strong fire may cause severe degrees of burning, the clothes covering the part being uninjured. This may also occur about the feet, legs, or knees of persons while intoxicated who have fallen asleep before the fire.

The damage done to the tissues by strong caustics, such as fuming nitric acid, sulphuric acid, caustic potash, nitrate of silver, or arsenical paste, presents pathological and clinical features almost identical with those resulting from heat. Electricity and the Röntgen rays also produce lesions of the nature of burns.

Pathology of Burns.—Much discussion has taken place regarding the explanation of the rapidly fatal issue in extensive superficial burns. On post-mortem examination the lesions found in these cases are: (1) general hyperæmia of all the organs of the abdominal, thoracic, and cerebro-spinal cavities; (2) marked leucocytosis, with destruction of red corpuscles, setting free hæmoglobin which lodges in the epithelial cells of the tubules of the kidneys; (3) minute thrombi and extravasations throughout the tissues of the body; (4) degeneration of the ganglion cells of the solar plexus; (5) oedema and degeneration of the lymphoid tissue throughout the body; (6) cloudy swelling of the liver and kidneys, and softening and enlargement of the spleen. Bardeen suggests that these morbid phenomena correspond so closely to those met with where the presence of a toxin is known to produce them, that in all probability death is similarly due to the action of some poison produced by the action of heat on the skin and on the proteins of the blood.

Clinical Features—Local Phenomena.—The most generally accepted classification of burns is that of Dupuytren, which is based upon the depth of the lesion. Six degrees are thus, recognised: (1) hyperæmia or erythema; (2) vesication; (3) partial destruction of the true skin; (4) total destruction of the true skin; (5) charring of muscles; (6) charring of bones.

It must be observed, however, that burns met with at the bedside always illustrate more than one of these degrees, the deeper forms always being associated with those less deep, and the clinical picture is made up of the combined characters of all. A burn is classified in terms of its most severe portion. It is also to be remarked that the extent and severity of a burn usually prove to be greater than at first sight appears.

Burns of the first degree are associated with erythema of the skin, due to hyperæmia of its blood vessels, and result from scorching by flame, from contact with solids or fluids below 212° F., or from exposure to the sun's rays. They are characterised clinically by acute pain, redness, transitory swelling from oedema, and subsequent desquamation of the surface layers of the epidermis. A special form of pigmentation of the skin is seen on the front of the legs of women from exposure to the heat of the fire.

Burns of Second Degree—Vesication of the Skin.—These are characterised by the occurrence of vesicles or blisters which are scattered over the hyperæmic area, and contain a clear yellowish or brownish fluid. On removing the raised epidermis, the congested and highly sensitive papillæ of the skin are exposed. Unna has found that pyogenic bacteria are invariably present in these blisters. Burns of the second degree leave no scar but frequently a persistent discoloration. In rare instances the burned area becomes the seat of a peculiar overgrowth of fibrous tissue of the nature of keloid (p 401).

Burns of Third Degree—Partial Destruction of the Skin.—The epidermis and papillæ are destroyed in patches, leaving hard, dry, and insensitive sloughs of a yellow or black colour. The pain in these burns is intense, but passes off during the first or second day, to return again, however, when, about the end of a week, the sloughs separate and expose the nerve filaments of the underlying skin. Granulations spring up to fill the gap, and are rapidly covered by epithelium, derived partly from the margins and partly from the remains of skin glands which have not been completely destroyed. These latter appear on the surface of the granulations as small bluish islets which gradually increase in size, become of a greyish-white colour, and ultimately blend with one another and with the edges. The resulting cicatrix may be slightly depressed, but otherwise exhibits little tendency to contract and cause deformity.

Burns of Fourth Degree—Total Destruction of the Skin.—These follow the more prolonged action of any form of intense heat. Large, black, dry eschars are formed, surrounded by a zone of intense congestion. Pain is less severe, and is referred to the parts that have been burned to a less degree. Infection is liable to occur and to lead to wide destruction of the surrounding skin. The amount of granulation tissue necessary to fill the gap is therefore great; and as the epithelial covering can only be derived from the margins—the skin glands being completely destroyed—the healing process is slow. The resulting scars are irregular, deep and puckered, and show a great tendency to contract. Keloid frequently develops in such cicatrices. When situated in the region of the face, neck, or flexures of joints, much deformity and impairment of function may result (Fig. 63).

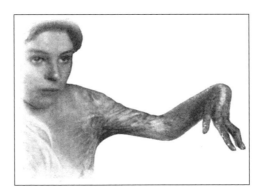

FIG. 63. Cicatricial Contraction following Severe Burn.

In *burns of the fifth degree* the lesion extends through the subcutaneous tissue and involves the muscles; while in those of the *sixth degree* it passes still more deeply and implicates the bones. These burns are comparatively limited in area, as they are usually produced by prolonged contact with hot metal or caustics. Burns of the fifth and sixth degrees are met with in epileptics or intoxicated persons who fall into the fire. Large blood vessels, nerve-trunks, joints, or serous cavities may be implicated.

General Phenomena.—It is customary to divide the clinical history of a severe burn into three periods; but it is to be observed that the features characteristic of the periods have been greatly modified since burns have been treated on the same lines as other wounds.

The first period lasts for from thirty-six to forty-eight hours, during which time the patient remains in a more or less profound state of *shock*, and there is a remarkable absence of pain. When shock is absent or little marked, however, the amount of suffering may be great. When the injury proves fatal during this period, death is due to shock, probably aggravated by the absorption of poisonous substances produced in the burned tissues. In fatal cases there is often evidence of cerebral congestion and oedema.

The *second period* begins when the shock passes off, and lasts till the sloughs separate. The outstanding feature of this period is *toxæmia*, manifested by fever, the temperature rising to 102°, 103°, or 104° F., and congestive or inflammatory conditions of internal organs, giving rise to such clinical complications as bronchitis, broncho-pneumonia, or pleurisy—especially in burns of the thorax; or meningitis and cerebritis, when the neck or head is the seat of the burn. Intestinal catarrh associated with diarrhoea is not uncommon; and ulceration of the duodenum leading to perforation has been met with in a few cases. These phenomena are much more prominent when bacterial infection has taken place, and it seems probable that they are to be attributed chiefly to the infection, as they have become less frequent and less severe since burns have been treated like other breaches of the surface. Albuminuria is a fairly constant symptom in severe burns, and is associated with congestion of the kidneys. In burns implicating the face, neck, mouth, or pharynx, oedema of the glottis is a dangerous complication, entailing as it does the risk of suffocation.

The *third period* begins when the sloughs separate, usually between the seventh and fourteenth days, and lasts till the wound heals, its duration depending upon the size, depth, and asepticity of the raw area. The chief causes of death during this period are toxin absorption in any of its forms; waxy disease of the liver, kidneys, or intestine; less commonly erysipelas, tetanus, or other diseases due to infection by specific organisms. We have seen nothing to substantiate the belief that duodenal ulcers are liable to perforate during the third period.

The *prognosis* in burns depends on (1) the superficial extent, and, to a much less degree, the depth of the injury. When more than one-third of the entire surface of the body is involved, even in a mild degree, the prognosis is grave. (2) The situation of the burn is important. Burns over the serous cavities—abdomen, thorax, or skull—are, other things being equal, much more dangerous than burns of the limbs. The risk of oedema of the glottis in burns about the neck and mouth has already been referred to. (3) Children are more liable to succumb to shock during the early period, but withstand prolonged suppuration better than adults. (4) When the patient survives the shock, the presence or absence of infection is the all-important factor in prognosis.

Treatment.—The *general treatment* consists in combating the shock. When pain is severe, morphin must be injected.

Local Treatment.—The local treatment must be carried out on antiseptic lines, a general anæsthetic being administered, if necessary, to enable the purification to be carried out thoroughly. After carefully removing the clothing, the whole of the burned area is gently, but thoroughly, cleansed with peroxide of hydrogen or warm boracic lotion, followed by sterilised saline solution. As pyogenic bacteria are invariably found in the blisters of burns, these must be opened and the raised epithelium removed.

The dressings subsequently applied should meet the following indications: the relief of pain; the prevention of sepsis; and the promotion of cicatrisation.

An application which satisfactorily fulfils these requirements is *picric acid*. Pads of lint or gauze are lightly wrung out of a solution made up of picric acid, 1½ drams; absolute alcohol, 3 ounces; distilled water, 40 ounces, and applied over the whole of the reddened area. These are covered with antiseptic wool, *without* any waterproof covering, and retained in position by a many-tailed bandage. The dressing should be changed once or twice a week, under the guidance of the temperature chart, any portion of the original dressing which remains perfectly dry being left undisturbed. The value of a general anæsthetic in dressing extensive burns, especially in children, can scarcely be overestimated.

Picric acid yields its best results in superficial burns, and it is useful as *a primary dressing* in all. As soon as the sloughs separate and a granulating surface forms, the ordinary treatment for a healing sore is instituted. Any slough under which pus has collected should be cut away with scissors to permit of free drainage.

An occlusive dressing of melted *paraffin* has also been employed. A useful preparation consists of: Paraffin molle 25 per cent., paraffin durum 67 per cent., olive oil 5 per cent., oil of eucalyptus 2 per cent., and beta-naphthol ¼ per cent. It has a melting point of 48° C. It is also known as *Ambrine* and *Burnol*. After the burned area has been cleansed and thoroughly dried, it is sponged or painted with the melted paraffin, and before solidification takes place a layer of sterilised gauze is applied and covered with a second coating of paraffin. Further coats of paraffin are applied every other day to prevent the gauze sticking to the skin.

An alternative method of treating extensive burns is by immersing the part, or even the whole body when the trunk is affected, in a bath of boracic lotion kept at the body temperature, the lotion being frequently renewed.

If a burn is already infected when first seen, it is to be treated on the same principles as govern the treatment of other infected wounds.

All moist or greasy applications, such as Carron oil, carbolic oil and ointments, and all substances like collodion and dry powders, which retain discharges, entirely fail to meet the indications for the rational treatment of burns, and should be abandoned.

Skin-grafting is of great value in hastening healing after extensive burns, and in preventing cicatricial contraction. The *deformities* which are so liable to develop from contraction of the cicatrices are treated on general principles. In the region of the face, neck, and flexures of joints (Fig. 63), where they are most marked, the contracted bands may be divided and the parts stretched, the raw surface left being covered by Thiersch grafts or by flaps of skin raised from adjacent surfaces or from other parts of the body (Fig. 1).

INJURIES PRODUCED BY ELECTRICITY

Injuries produced by Exposure to X-Rays and Radium.—In the routine treatment of disease by radiations, injury is sometimes done to the tissues, even when the greatest care is exercised as to dosage and frequency of application. Robert Knox describes the following ill-effects.

Acute dermatitis varying in degree from a slight erythema to deep ulceration or even necrosis of skin. When ulcers form they are extremely painful and slow to heal. When hair-bearing areas are affected, epilation may occur without destroying the hair follicles and the hairs are reproduced, but if the reaction is excessive permanent alopecia may result.

Chronic dermatitis, which results from persistence of the acute form, is most intractable and may assume malignant characters. X-ray warts are a late manifestation of chronic dermatitis and may become malignant.

Among the *late manifestations* are neuritis, telangiectasis, and a painful and intractable form of ulceration, any of which may come on months or even years after the cessation of exposure. *Sterility* may be induced in X-ray workers who are imperfectly protected from the effects of the rays.

Electrical burns usually occur in those who are engaged in industrial undertakings where powerful electrical currents are employed.

The lesions—which vary from a slight superficial scorching to complete charring of parts—are most evident at the points of entrance and exit of the current, the intervening tissues apparently escaping injury.

The more superficial degrees of electrical burns differ from those produced by heat in being almost painless, and in healing very slowly, although as a rule they remain dry and aseptic.

The more severe forms are attended with a considerable degree of shock, which is not only more profound, but also lasts much longer than the shock in an ordinary burn of corresponding severity. The parts at the point of entrance of the current are charred to a greater or lesser depth. The eschar is at first dry and crisp, and is surrounded by a zone of pallor. For the first thirty-six to forty-eight hours there is comparatively little suffering, but at the end of that time the parts become exceedingly painful. In a majority of cases, in spite of careful purification, a slow form of moist gangrene sets in, and the slough spreads both in area and in depth, until the muscles and often the large blood vessels and nerves are exposed. A line of demarcation eventually forms, but the sloughs are exceedingly slow to separate, taking from three to five times as long as in an ordinary burn, and during the process of separation there is considerable risk of secondary hæmorrhage from erosion of large vessels.

Treatment.—Electrical burns are treated on the same lines as ordinary burns, by thorough purification and the application of dry dressings, with a view to avoiding the onset of moist gangrene. After granulations have formed, skin-grafting is of value in hastening healing.

Lightning-stroke.—In a large proportion of cases lightning-stroke proves instantly fatal. In non-fatal cases the patient suffers from a profound degree of shock, and there may or may not be any external evidence of injury. In the mildest cases red spots or wheals—closely resembling those of urticaria—may appear on the body, but they usually fade again in the course of twenty-four hours. Sometimes large patches of skin are scorched or stained, the discoloured area showing an arborescent appearance. In other cases the injured skin becomes dry and glazed, resembling parchment. Appearances are occasionally met with corresponding to those of a superficial burn produced by heat. The chief difference from ordinary burns is the extreme slowness with which healing takes place. Localised paralysis of groups of muscles, or even of a whole limb, may follow any degree of lightning-stroke. Treatment is mainly directed towards combating the shock, the surface-lesions being treated on the same lines as ordinary burns.

• XII •

METHODS OF WOUND
TREATMENT

Varieties of Wounds ✦ *Modes of Infection*
Lister's Work ✦ *Means Taken to Prevent Infection of Wounds: Heat;*
Chemical Antiseptics; Disinfection of Hands; Preparation of Skin of
Patient; Instruments; Ligatures; Dressings ✦ *Means Taken to Combat*
Infection: Purification; Open-wound Method.

The surgeon is called upon to treat two distinct classes of wounds: (1) those resulting from injury or disease in which *the skin is already broken*, or in which a communication with a mucous surface exists; and (2) those that he himself makes *through intact skin*, no infected mucous surface being involved.

Infection by bacteria must be assumed to have taken place in all wounds made in any other way than by the knife of the surgeon operating through unbroken skin. On this assumption the modern system of wound treatment is based. Pathogenic bacteria are so widely distributed, that in the ordinary circumstances of everyday life, no matter how trivial a wound may be, or how short a time it may remain exposed, the access of organisms to it is almost certain unless preventive measures are employed.

It cannot be emphasised too strongly that rigid precautions are to be taken to exclude fresh infection, not only in dealing with wounds that are free of organisms, but equally in the management of wounds and other lesions that are already infected. Any laxity in our methods which admits of fresh organisms reaching an infected wound adds materially to the severity of the infective process and consequently to the patient's risk.

There are many ways in which accidental infection may occur. Take, for example, the case of a person who receives a cut on the face by being knocked down in a carriage accident on the street. Organisms may be introduced to such a wound from the shaft or wheel by which he was struck, from the ground on which he lay, from any portion of his clothing that may have come in contact with the wound, or from his own skin. Or, again, the hands of those who render first aid, the water used to bathe the wound, the handkerchief or other extemporised dressing applied to it, may be the means of conveying bacterial infection. Should the wound open on a mucous surface, such as the mouth or nasal cavity, the organisms constantly present in such situations are liable to prove agents of infection.

Even after the patient has come under professional care the risks of his wound becoming infected are not past, because the hands of the doctor, his instruments, dressings, or other appliances may all, unless purified, become the sources of infection.

In the case of an operation carried out through unbroken skin, organisms may be introduced into the wound from the patient's own skin, from the hands of the surgeon or his assistants, through the medium of contaminated instruments, swabs, ligature or suture materials, or other things used in the course of the operation, or from the dressings applied to the wound.

Further, bacteria may gain access to devitalised tissues by way of the bloodstream, being carried hither from some infected area elsewhere in the body.

The Antiseptic System of Surgery.—Those who only know the surgical conditions of to-day can scarcely realise the state of matters which existed before the introduction of the antiseptic system by Joseph Lister in 1867. In those days few wounds escaped the ravages of pyogenic and other bacteria, with the result that suppuration ensued after most operations, and such diseases as erysipelas, pyæmia, and "hospital gangrene" were of everyday occurrence. The mortality after compound fractures, amputations, and many other operations was appalling, and death from blood-poisoning frequently followed even the most trivial operations. An operation was looked upon as a last resource, and the inherent risk from blood-poisoning seemed to have set an impassable barrier to the further progress of surgery. To the genius of Lister we owe it that this barrier was removed. Having satisfied himself that the septic process was due to bacterial infection, he devised a means of preventing the access of organisms to wounds or of counteracting their effects. Carbolic acid was the first antiseptic agent he employed, and by its use in compound fractures he soon obtained results such as had never before been attained. The principle was applied to other conditions with like success, and so profoundly has it affected the whole aspect of surgical pathology, that many of the infective diseases with which surgeons formerly had to deal are now all but unknown. The broad principles upon which Lister founded his system remain unchanged, although the methods employed to put them into practice have been modified.

Means taken to Prevent Infection of Wounds.—The avenues by which infective agents may gain access to surgical wounds are so numerous and so wide, that it requires the greatest care and the most watchful attention on the part of the surgeon to guard them all. It is only by constant practice and patient attention to technical details in the operating room and at the bedside, that the carrying out of surgical manipulations in such a way as to avoid bacterial infection will become an instinctive act and a second nature. It is only possible here to indicate the chief directions in which danger lies, and to describe the means most generally adopted to avoid it.

To prevent infection, it is essential that everything which comes into contact with a wound should be sterilised or disinfected, and to ensure the best results it is necessary that the efficiency of our methods of sterilisation should be periodically tested. The two chief agencies at our disposal are heat and chemical antiseptics.

Sterilisation by Heat.—The most reliable, and at the same time the most convenient and generally applicable, means of sterilisation is by heat. All bacteria and spores are completely destroyed by being subjected for fifteen minutes to *saturated circulating steam* at a temperature of 130° to 145° C. (= 266° to 293° F.). The articles to be sterilised are enclosed in a perforated tin casket, which is placed in a specially constructed steriliser, such as that of Schimmelbusch. This apparatus is so arranged that the steam circulates under a pressure of from two to three atmospheres, and permeates everything contained in it. Objects so sterilised are dry when removed from the steriliser. This method is specially suitable for appliances which are not damaged by steam, such, for example, as gauze swabs, towels, aprons, gloves, and metal instruments; it is essential that the efficiency of the steriliser be tested from time to time by a self-registering thermometer or other means.

The best substitute for circulating steam is *boiling*. The articles are placed in a "fish-kettle steriliser" and boiled for fifteen minutes in a 1 per cent. solution of washing soda.

To prevent contamination of objects that have been sterilised they must on no account be touched by any one whose hands have not been disinfected and protected by sterilised gloves.

Sterilisation by Chemical Agents.—For the purification of the skin of the patient, the hands of the surgeon, and knives and other instruments that are damaged by heat, recourse must be had to chemical agents. These, however, are less reliable than heat, and are open to certain other objections.

Disinfection of the Hands.—It is now generally recognised that one of the most likely sources of wound infection is the hands of the surgeon and his assistants. It is only by carefully studying to avoid all contact with infective matter that the hands can be kept surgically pure, and that this source of wound infection can be reduced to a minimum. The risk of infection from this source has further been greatly reduced by the systematic use of rubber gloves by house-surgeons, dressers, and nurses. The habitual use of gloves has also been adopted by the great majority of surgeons; the minority, who find they are handicapped by wearing gloves as a routine measure, are obliged to do so when operating in infective cases or dressing infected wounds, and in making rectal and vaginal examinations.

The gloves may be sterilised by steam, and are then put on dry, or by boiling, in which case they are put on wet. The gauntlet of the glove should overlap and confine the end of the sleeve of the sterilised overall, and the gloved hands are rinsed in lotion before and at frequent intervals during the operation. The hands are sterilised before putting on the gloves, preferably by a method which dehydrates the skin. Cotton gloves may be worn by the surgeon when tying ligatures, or between operations, and by the anæsthetist during operations on the head, neck, and chest.

The first step in the disinfection of the hands is the mechanical removal of gross surface dirt and loose epithelium by soap, a stream of running water as hot as can be borne, and a loofah or nail-brush, that has been previously sterilised by heat. The nails should be cut down till there is no sulcus between the nail edge and the pulp of the finger in which organisms may lodge. They are next washed for three minutes in methylated spirit to dehydrate the skin, and then for two or three minutes in 70 per cent. sublimate or biniodide alcohol (1 in 1000). Finally, the hands are rubbed with dry sterilised gauze.

Preparation of the Skin of the Patient.—In the purification of the skin of the patient before operation, reliance is to be placed chiefly in the mechanical removal of dirt and grease by the same means as are taken for the cleansing of the surgeon's hands. Hair-covered parts should be shaved. The skin is then dehydrated by washing with methylated spirit, followed by 70 per cent. sublimate or biniodide alcohol (1 in 1000). This is done some hours before the operation, and the part is then covered with pads of dry sterilised gauze or a sterilised towel. Immediately before the operation the skin is again purified in the same way.

The *iodine method* of disinfecting the skin introduced by Grossich is simple, and equally efficient. The day before operation the skin, after being washed with soap and water, is shaved, dehydrated by means of methylated spirit, and then painted with a 5 per cent. solution of iodine in rectified spirit. The painting with iodine is repeated just before the operation commences, and again after it is completed. The final application is omitted in the case of children. In emergency operations the skin is shaved dry and dehydrated with spirit, after which the iodine is applied as described above. The staining of the skin is an advantage, as it enables the operator to recognise the area that has been prepared.

If any acne pustules or infected sinuses are present, they should be destroyed or purified by means of the thermo-cautery or pure carbolic acid, after the patient is anæsthetised.

Appliances used at Operation.—*Instruments* that are not damaged by heat must be boiled in a fish-kettle or other suitable steriliser for fifteen minutes in a 1 per cent. solution of cresol or washing soda. Just before the operation begins they are removed in the tray of the steriliser and placed on a sterilised towel within reach of the surgeon or his assistant. Knives and instruments that are liable to be damaged by heat should be purified by being soaked in pure cresol for a few minutes, or in 1 in 20 carbolic for at least an hour.

Pads of Gauze sterilised by compressed circulating steam have almost entirely superseded marine sponges for operative purposes. To avoid the risk of leaving swabs in the peritoneal cavity, large square pads of gauze, to one corner of which a piece of strong tape about a foot long is securely stitched, should be employed. They should be removed from the caskets in which they are sterilised by means of sterilised forceps, and handed direct to the surgeon. The assistant who attends to the swabs should wear sterilised gloves.

Ligatures and Sutures.—To avoid the risk of implanting infective matter in a wound by means of the materials used for ligatures and sutures, great care must be taken in their preparation.

Catgut.—The following methods of preparing catgut have proved satisfactory: (1) The gut is soaked in juniper oil for at least a month; the juniper oil is then removed by ether and alcohol, and the gut preserved in 1 in 1000 solution of corrosive sublimate in alcohol (Kocher). (2) The gut is placed in a brass receiver and boiled for three-quarters of an hour in a solution consisting of 85 per cent. absolute alcohol, 10 per cent. water, and 5 per cent. carbolic acid, and is then stored in 90 per cent. alcohol. (3) Cladius recommends that the catgut, just as it is bought from the dealers, be loosely rolled on a spool, and then immersed in a solution of—iodine, 1 part; iodide of potassium, 1 part; distilled water, 100 parts. At the end of eight days it is ready for use. Moschcowitz has found that the tensile strength of catgut so prepared is increased if it is kept dry in a sterile vessel, instead of being left indefinitely in the iodine solution. If Salkindsohn's formula is used—tincture of iodine, 1 part; proof spirit, 15 parts—the gut can be kept permanently in the solution without becoming brittle. To avoid contamination from the hands, catgut should be removed from the bottle with aseptic forceps and passed direct to the surgeon. Any portion unused should be thrown away.

Silk is prepared by being soaked for twelve hours in ether, for other twelve in alcohol, and then boiled for ten minutes in 1 in 1000 sublimate solution. It is then wound on spools with purified hands protected by sterilised gloves, and kept in absolute alcohol. Before an operation the silk is again boiled for ten minutes in the same solution, and is used directly from this (Kocher). Linen thread is sterilised in the same way as silk.

Fishing-gut and silver wire, as well as the needles, should be boiled along with the instruments. Horse-hair and fishing-gut may be sterilised by prolonged immersion in 1 in 20 carbolic, or in the iodine solutions employed to sterilise catgut.

The field of operation is surrounded by sterilised towels, clipped to the edges of the wound, and securely fixed in position so that no contamination may take place from the surroundings.

The surgeon and his assistants, including the anæsthetist, wear overalls sterilised by steam. To avoid the risk of infection from dust, scurf, or drops of perspiration falling from the head, the surgeon and his assistants may wear sterilised cotton caps. To obviate the risk of infection taking place by drops of saliva projected from the mouth in talking or coughing in the vicinity of a wound, a simple mask may be worn.

The risk of infection from the *air* is now known to be very small, so long as there is no excess of floating dust. All sweeping, dusting, and disturbing of curtains, blinds, or furniture must therefore be avoided before or during an operation.

It has been shown that the presence of spectators increases the number of organisms in the atmosphere. In teaching clinics, therefore, the risk from air infection is greater than in private practice.

To facilitate primary union, all hæmorrhage should be arrested, and the accumulation of fluid in the wound prevented. When much oozing is antici-pated, a glass or rubber drainage-tube is inserted through a small opening specially made for the purpose. In aseptic wounds the tube may be removed in from twenty-four to forty-eight hours, and where it is important to avoid a scar, the opening should be closed with a Michel's clip; in infected wounds the tube must remain as long as the discharge continues.

The fascia and skin should be brought into accurate apposition by sutures. If any cavity exists in the deeper part of the wound it should be obliterated by buried sutures, or by so adjusting the dressing as to bring its walls into apposition.

If these precautions have been successful, the wound will heal under the original dressing, which need not be interfered with for from seven to ten days, according to the nature of the case.

Dressings.—*Gauze*, sterilised by heat, is almost universally employed for the dressing of wounds. *Double cyanide gauze* may be used in such regions as the neck, axilla, or groin, where complete sterilisation of the skin is difficult to attain, and where it is desirable to leave the dressing undisturbed for ten days or more. *Iodoform* or *bismuth gauze* is of special value for the packing of wounds treated by the open method.

One variety or another of *wool*, rendered absorbent by the extraction of its fat, and sterilised by heat, forms a part of almost every surgical dressing, and various antiseptic agents may be added to it. Of these, corrosive sublimate is the most generally used. Wood-wool dressings are more highly and more uniformly absorbent than cotton wools. As evaporation takes place through wool dressings, the discharge becomes dried, and so forms an unfavourable medium for bacterial growth.

Pads of *sphagnum moss*, sterilised by heat, are highly absorbent, and being economical are used when there is much discharge, and in cases where a leakage of urine has to be soaked up.

Means adopted to combat Infection.—As has already been indicated, the same antiseptic precautions are to be taken in dealing with infected as with aseptic wounds.

In *recent injuries* such as result from railway or machinery accidents, with bruising and crushing of the tissues and grinding of gross dirt into the wounds, the scissors must be freely used to remove the tissues that have been devitalised or impregnated with foreign material. Hair-covered parts should be shaved and the surrounding skin painted with iodine. Crushed and contaminated portions of bone should be chiselled away. Opinions differ as to the benefit derived from washing such wounds with chemical antiseptics, which are liable to devitalise the tissues with which they come in contact, and so render them less able to resist the action of any organisms that may remain in them. All are agreed, however, that free washing with normal salt solution is useful in mechanically cleansing the injured parts. Peroxide of hydrogen sprayed over such wounds is also beneficial in virtue of its oxidising properties. Efficient drainage must be provided, and stitches should be used sparingly, if at all.

The best way in which to treat such wounds is by the *open method*. This consists in packing the wound with iodoform or bismuth gauze, which is left in position as long as it adheres to the raw surface. The packing may be renewed at intervals until the wound is filled by granulations; or, in the course of a few days when it becomes evident that the infection has been overcome, *secondary* sutures may be introduced and the edges drawn together, provision being made at the ends for further packing or for drainage-tubes.

If earth or street dirt has entered the wound, the surface may with advantage be painted over with pure carbolic acid, as virulent organisms, such as those of tetanus or spreading gangrene, are liable to be present. Prophylactic injection of tetanus antitoxin may be indicated.

・ XIII ・

CONSTITUTIONAL EFFECTS OF INJURIES

Syncope ◆ Shock ◆ Collapse
Fat Embolism ◆ Traumatic Asphyxia
Delirium in Surgical Patients: Delirium in General; Delirium Tremens;
Traumatic Delirium

SYNCOPE, SHOCK, AND COLLAPSE

Syncope, shock, and collapse are clinical conditions which, although depending on different causes, bear a superficial resemblance to one another.

Syncope or Fainting.—Syncope is the result of a suddenly produced anæmia of the brain from temporary weakening or arrest of the heart's action. In surgical practice, this condition is usually observed in nervous persons who have been subjected to pain, as in the reduction of a dislocation or the incision of a whitlow; or in those who have rapidly lost a considerable quantity of blood. It may also follow the sudden withdrawal of fluid from a large cavity, as in tapping an abdomen for ascites, or withdrawing fluid from the pleural cavity. Syncope sometimes occurs also during the administration of a general anæsthetic, especially if there is a tendency to sickness and the patient is not completely under. During an operation the onset of syncope is often recognised by the cessation of oozing from the divided vessels before the general symptoms become manifest.

Clinical Features.—When a person is about to faint he feels giddy, has surging sounds in his ears, and haziness of vision; he yawns, becomes pale and sick, and a free flow of saliva takes place into the mouth. The pupils dilate; the pulse becomes small and almost imperceptible; the respirations shallow and hurried; consciousness gradually fades away, and he falls in a heap on the floor.

Sometimes vomiting ensues before the patient completely loses consciousness, and the muscular exertion entailed may ward off the actual faint. This is frequently seen in threatened syncopal attacks during chloroform administration.

Recovery begins in a few seconds, the patient sighing or gasping, or, it may be, vomiting; the strength of the pulse gradually increases, and consciousness slowly returns. In some cases, however, syncope is fatal.

Treatment.—The head should at once be lowered—in imitation of nature's method—to encourage the flow of blood to the brain, the patient, if necessary, being held up by the heels. All tight clothing, especially round the neck or chest, must be loosened. The heart may be stimulated reflexly by dashing cold water over the face or chest, or by rubbing the face vigorously with a rough towel. The application of volatile substances, such as ammonia or smelling-salts, to the nose; the administration by the mouth of sal-volatile, whisky or brandy, and the intra-muscular injection of ether, are the most speedily efficacious remedies. In severe cases the application of hot cloths over the heart, or of the faradic current over the line of the phrenic nerve, just above the clavicle, may be called for.

Surgical Shock.—The condition known as surgical shock may be looked upon as a state of profound exhaustion of the mechanism that exists in the body for the transformation of energy. This mechanism consists of (1) the *brain*, which, through certain special centres, regulates all vital activity; (2) the *adrenal glands*, the secretion of which—adrenalin—acting as a stimulant of the sympathetic system, so controls the tone of the blood vessels as to maintain efficient oxidation of the tissues; and (3) *the liver*, which stores and delivers glycogen as it is required by the muscles, and in addition, deals with the by-products of metabolism.

Crile and his co-workers have shown that in surgical shock histological changes occur in the cells of the brain, the adrenals, and the liver, and that these are identical, whatever be the cause that leads to the exhaustion of the energy-transforming mechanism. These changes vary in degree, and range from slight alterations in the structure of the protoplasm to complete disorganisation of the cell elements.

The influences which contribute to bring about this form of exhaustion that we call shock are varied, and include such emotional states as fear, anxiety, or worry, physical injury and toxic infection, and the effects of these factors are augmented by anything that tends to lower the vitality, such as loss of blood, exposure, insufficient food, loss of sleep or antecedent illness.

Any one or any combination of these influences may cause shock, but the most potent, and the one which most concerns the surgeon, is physical injury, *e.g.*, a severe accident or an operation (*traumatic shock*). This is usually associated with some emotional disturbance, such as fear or anxiety (*emotional shock*), or with hæmorrhage; and may be followed by septic infection (*toxic shock*).

The exaggerated afferent impulses reaching the brain as a result of trauma, inhibit the action of the nuclei in the region of the fourth ventricle and cerebellum which maintain the muscular tone, with the result that the muscular tone is diminished and there is a marked fall in the arterial blood pressure. The capillaries dilate—the blood stagnating in them and giving off its oxygen and transuding its fluid elements into the tissues—with the result that an insufficient quantity of oxygenated blood reaches the heart to enable it to maintain an efficient circulation. As the sarco-lactic acid liberated in the muscles is not oxygenated a condition of acidosis ensues.

The more highly the injured part is endowed with sensory nerves the more marked is the shock; a crush of the hand, for example, is attended with a more intense degree of shock than a correspondingly severe crush of the foot; and injuries of such specially innervated parts as the testis, the urethra, the face, or the spinal cord, are associated with severe degrees, as are also those of parts innervated from the sympathetic system, such as the abdominal or thoracic viscera. It is to be borne in mind that a state of general anæsthesia does not prevent injurious impulses reaching the brain and causing shock during an operation. If the main nerves of the part are "blocked" by injection of a local anæsthetic, however, the central nervous system is protected from these impulses.

While the aged frequently manifest but few signs of shock, they have a correspondingly feeble power of recovery; and while many young children suffer little, even after severe operations, others with much less cause succumb to shock.

When the injured person's mind is absorbed with other matters than his own condition,—as, for example, during the heat of a battle or in the excitement of a railway accident or a conflagration,—even severe injuries may be unattended by pain or shock at the time, although when the period of excitement is over, the severity of the shock is all the greater. The same thing is observed in persons injured while under the influence of alcohol.

Clinical Features.—The patient is in a state of prostration. He is roused from his condition of indifference with difficulty, but answers questions intelligently, if only in a whisper. The face is pale, beads of sweat stand out on the brow, the features are drawn, the eyes sunken, and the cheeks hollow. The lips and ears are pallid; the skin of the body of a greyish colour, cold, and clammy. The pulse is rapid, fluttering, and often all but imperceptible at the wrist; the respiration is irregular, shallow, and sighing; and the temperature may fall to 96° F. or even lower. The mouth is parched, and the patient complains of thirst. There is little sensibility to pain.

Except in very severe cases, shock tends towards recovery within a few hours, the *reaction*, as it is called, being often ushered in by vomiting. The colour improves; the pulse becomes full and bounding; the respiration deeper and more regular; the temperature rises to 100° F. or higher; and the patient begins to take notice of his surroundings. The condition of neurasthenia which sometimes follows an operation may be associated with the degenerative changes in nerve cells described by Crile.

In certain cases the symptoms of traumatic shock blend with those resulting from toxin absorption, and it is difficult to estimate the relative importance of the two factors in the causation of the condition. The conditions formerly known as "delayed shock" and "prostration with excitement" are now generally recognised to be due to toxæmia.

Question of Operating during Shock.—Most authorities agree that operations should only be undertaken during profound shock when they are imperatively demanded for the arrest of hæmorrhage, the prevention of infection of serous cavities, or for the relief of pain which is producing or intensifying the condition.

Prevention of Operation Shock.—In the preparation of a patient for operation, drastic purgation and prolonged fasting must be avoided, and about half an hour before a severe operation a pint of saline solution should be slowly introduced into the rectum; this is repeated, if necessary, during the operation, and at its conclusion. The operating-room must be warm—not less than 70° F.—and the patient should be wrapped in cotton wool and blankets, and surrounded by hot-bottles. All lotions used must be warm (100° F.); and the operation should be completed as speedily and as bloodlessly as possible. The element of fear may to some extent be eliminated by the preliminary administration of such drugs as scopolamin or morphin, and with a view to preventing the passage of exciting afferent impulses, Crile advocates "blocking" of the nerves by the injection of a 1 per cent. solution of novocaine into their substance on the proximal side of the field of operation. To prevent after-pain in abdominal wounds he recommends injecting the edges with quinine and urea hydrochlorate before suturing, the resulting anæsthesia lasting for twenty-four to forty-eight hours. To these preventive measures the term *anoci-association* has been applied. In selecting an anæsthetic, it may be borne in mind that chloroform lowers the blood pressure more than ether does, and that with spinal anæsthesia there is no lowering of the blood pressure.

Treatment.—A patient suffering from shock should be placed in the recumbent position, with the foot of the bed raised to facilitate the return circulation in the large veins, and so to increase the flow of blood to the brain. His bed should be placed near a large fire, and the patient himself surrounded by cotton wool and blankets and hot-bottles. If he has lost much blood, the limbs should be wrapped in cotton wool and firmly bandaged from below upwards, to conserve as much of the circulating blood as possible in the trunk and head. If the shock is moderate in degree, as soon as the patient has been put to bed, about a pint of saline solution should be introduced into the rectum, and 10 to 15 minims of adrenalin chloride (1 in 1000) may with advantage be added to the fluid. The injection should be repeated every two hours until the circulation is sufficiently restored. In severe cases, especially when associated with hæmorrhage, transfusion of whole blood from a compatible donor, is the most efficient means (*Op. Surg.*, p. 37). Cardiac stimulants such as strychnin, digitalin, or strophanthin are contra-indicated in shock, as they merely exhaust the already impaired vaso-motor centre.

Artificial respiration may be useful in tiding a patient over the critical period of shock, especially at the end of a severe operation.

Failing this, the introduction of saline solution at a temperature of about 105° F. into a vein or into the subcutaneous tissue is useful where much blood has been lost (p. 276). Two or three pints may be injected into a vein, or smaller quantities under the skin.

Thirst is best met by giving small quantities of warm water by the mouth, or by the introduction of saline solution into the rectum. Ice only relieves thirst for a short time, and as it is liable to induce flatulence should be avoided, especially in abdominal cases. Dryness of the tongue may be relieved by swabbing the mouth with a mixture of glycerine and lemon juice.

If severe pain calls for the use of morphin, 1/120th grain of atropin should be added, or heroin alone may be given in doses of 1/24th to 1/12th grain.

Collapse is a clinical condition which comes on more insidiously than shock, and which does not attain its maximum degree of severity for several hours. It is met with in the course of severe illnesses, especially such as are associated with the loss of large quantities of fluid from the body—for example, by severe diarrhoea, notably in Asiatic cholera; by persistent vomiting; or by profuse sweating, as in some cases of heat-stroke. Severe degrees of collapse follow sudden and profuse loss of blood.

Collapse often follows upon shock—for example, in intestinal perforations, or after abdominal operations complicated by peritonitis, especially if there is vomiting, as in cases of obstruction high up in the intestine. The symptoms of collapse are aggravated if toxin absorption is superadded to the loss of fluid.

The *clinical features* of this condition are practically the same as those of shock; and it is treated on the same lines.

FAT EMBOLISM.—After various injuries and operations, but especially such as implicate the marrow of long bones—for example, comminuted fractures, osteotomies, resections of joints, or the forcible correction of deformities—fluid fat may enter the circulation in variable quantity. In the vast majority of cases no ill effects follow, but when the quantity is large or when the absorption is long continued certain symptoms ensue, either immediately, or more frequently not for two or three days. These are mostly referable to the lungs and brain.

In the lung the fat collects in the minute blood vessels and produces venous congestion and oedema, and sometimes pneumonia. Dyspnoea, with cyanosis, a persistent cough and frothy or blood-stained sputum, a feeble pulse and low temperature, are the chief symptoms.

When the fat lodges in the capillaries of the brain, the pulse becomes small, rapid, and irregular, delirium followed by coma ensues, and the condition is usually rapidly fatal.

Fat is usually to be detected in the urine, even in mild cases.

The *treatment* consists in tiding the patient over the acute stage of his illness, until the fat is eliminated from the blood vessels.

TRAUMATIC ASPHYXIA OR TRAUMATIC CYANOSIS.—This term has been applied to a condition which results when the thorax is so forcibly compressed that respiration is mechanically arrested for several minutes. It has occurred from being crushed in a struggling crowd, or under a fall of masonry, and in machinery accidents. When the patient is released, the face and the neck as low down as the level of the clavicles present an intense coloration, varying from deep purple to blue-black. The affected area is sharply defined, and on close inspection the appearance is found to be due to the presence of countless minute reddish-blue or black spots, with small areas or streaks of normal skin between them. The punctate nature of the coloration is best recognised towards the periphery of the affected area—at the junction of the brow with the hairy scalp, and where the dark patch meets the normal skin of the chest (Beach and Cobb). Pressure over the skin does not cause the colour to disappear as in ordinary cyanosis. It has been shown by Wright of Boston, that the coloration is due to stasis from mechanical over-distension of the veins and capillaries; actual extravasation into the tissues is exceptional. The sharply defined distribution of the coloration is attributed to the absence of functionating valves in the veins of the head and neck, so that when the increased intra-thoracic pressure is transmitted to these veins they become engorged. Under the conjunctivæ there are extravasations of bright red blood; and sublingual hæmatoma has been observed (Beatson).

The discoloration begins to fade within a few hours, and after the second or third day it disappears, without showing any of the chromatic changes which characterise a bruise. The sub-conjunctival ecchymosis, however, persists for several weeks and disappears like other extravasations. Apart from combating the shock, or dealing with concomitant injuries, no treatment is called for.

DELIRIUM IN SURGICAL PATIENTS

Delirium is a temporary disturbance of mind which occurs in the course of certain diseases, and sometimes after injuries or operations. It may be associated with any of the acute pyogenic infections; with erysipelas, especially when it affects the head or face; or with chronic infective diseases of the urinary organs. In the various forms of meningitis also, and in some cases of injury to the head, it is common; and it is sometimes met with after severe hæmorrhage, and in cases of poisoning by such drugs as iodoform, cocain, or alcohol. Delirium may also, of course, be a symptom of insanity.

Often there is merely incoherent muttering regarding past incidents or occupations, or about absent friends; or the condition may assume the form of excitement, of dementia, or of melancholia; and the symptoms are usually worst at night.

Delirium Tremens is seen in persons addicted to alcohol, who, as the result of accident or operation, are suddenly compelled to lie in bed. Although oftenest met with in habitual drunkards or chronic tipplers, it is by no means uncommon in moderate drinkers, and has even been seen in children.

Clinical Features.—The delirium, which has been aptly described as being of a "busy" character, usually manifests itself within a few days of the patient being laid up. For two or three days he refuses food, is depressed, suspicious, sleepless and restless, demanding to be allowed up. Then he begins to mutter incoherently, to pull off the bedclothes, and to attempt to get out of bed. There is general muscular tremor, most marked in the tongue, the lips, and the hands. The patient imagines that he sees all sorts of horrible beings around him, and is sometimes greatly distressed because of rats, mice, beetles, or snakes, which he fancies are crawling over him. The pulse is soft, rapid, and compressible; the temperature is only moderately raised (100°-101° F.), and as a rule there is profuse sweating. The digestion is markedly impaired, and there is often vomiting. Patients in this condition are peculiarly insensitive to pain, and may even walk about with a fractured leg without apparent discomfort.

In most cases the symptoms begin to pass off in three or four days; the patient sleeps, the hallucinations and tremors cease, and he gradually recovers. In other cases the temperature rises, the pulse becomes rapid, and death results from exhaustion.

The main indication in *treatment* is to secure sleep, and this is done by the administration of bromides, chloral, or paraldehyde, or of one or other of the drugs of which sulphonal, trional, and veronal are examples. Heroin in doses of from 1/24th to 1/12th grain is often of service. Morphin must be used with great caution. In some cases hyoscin (1/200 grain) injected hypodermically is found efficacious when all other means have failed, but this drug must be used with great discrimination. The patient must be encouraged to take plenty of easily digested fluid food, supplemented, if necessary, by nutrient enemata and saline infusions.

In the early stage a brisk mercurial purge is often of value. Alcohol should be withheld, unless failing of the pulse strongly indicates its use, and then it should be given along with the food.

A delirious patient must be constantly watched by a trained attendant or other competent person, lest he get out of bed and do harm to himself or others. Mechanical restraint is often necessary, but must be avoided if possible, as it is apt to increase the excitement and exhaust the patient. On account of the extreme restlessness, there is often great difficulty in carrying out the proper treatment of the primary surgical condition, and considerable modifications in splints and other appliances are often rendered necessary.

A form of delirium, sometimes spoken of as **Traumatic Delirium**, may follow on severe injuries or operations in persons of neurotic temperament, or in those whose nervous system is exhausted by overwork. It is met with apart from alcoholic intemperance. This form of delirium seems to be specially prone to ensue on operations on the face, the thyreoid gland, or the genito-urinary organs. The symptoms appear in from two to five days after the operation, and take the form of restlessness, sleeplessness, low incoherent muttering, and picking at the bedclothes. It is not necessarily attended by fever or by muscular tremors. The patient may show hysterical symptoms. This condition is probably to be regarded as a form of insanity, as it is liable to merge into mania or melancholia.

The *treatment* is carried out on the same lines as that of delirium tremens.

· XIV ·

THE BLOOD VESSELS

*Anatomy • Injuries of Arteries: Varieties
Injuries of Veins: Air Embolism • Repair of Blood Vessels and
Natural Arrest of Hæmorrhage • Hæmorrhage: Varieties; Prevention;
Arrest • Constitutional Effects of Hæmorrhage • Hæmophilia •
Disease of Blood Vessels: Thrombosis; Embolism • Arteritis: Varieties;
Arterio-sclerosis • Thrombo-phlebitis • Phlebitis: Varieties
Varix • Angiomata • Nævus: Varieties; Electrolysis • Cirsoid
Aneurysm • Aneurysm: Varieties; Methods of Treatment • Aneurysms
of Individual Arteries.*

Surgical Anatomy.—An *artery* has three coats: an internal coat—the *tunica intima*—made up of a single layer of endothelial cells lining the lumen; outside of this a layer of delicate connective tissue; and still farther out a dense tissue composed of longitudinally arranged elastic fibres—the internal elastic lamina. The tunica intima is easily ruptured. The middle coat, or *tunica media*, consists of non-striped muscular fibres, arranged for the most part concentrically round the vessel. In this coat also there is a considerable proportion of elastic tissue, especially in the larger vessels. The thickness of the vessel wall depends chiefly on the development of the muscular coat. The external coat, or *tunica externa*, is composed of fibrous tissue, containing, especially in vessels of medium calibre, some yellow elastic fibres in its deeper layers.

In most parts of the body the arteries lie in a sheath of connective tissue, from which fine fibrous processes pass to the tunica externa. The connection, however, is not a close one, and the artery when divided transversely is capable of retracting for a considerable distance within its sheath. In some of the larger arteries the sheath assumes the form of a definite membrane.

The arteries are nourished by small vessels—the *vasa vasorum*—which ramify chiefly in the outer coat. They are also well supplied with nerves, which regulate the size of the lumen by inducing contraction or relaxation of the muscular coat.

The *veins* are constructed on the same general plan as the arteries, the individual coats, however, being thinner. The inner coat is less easily ruptured, and the middle coat contains a smaller proportion of muscular tissue. In one important point veins differ structurally from arteries—namely, in being provided with valves which prevent reflux of the blood. These valves are composed of semilunar folds of the tunica intima strengthened by an addition of connective tissue. Each valve usually consists of two semilunar flaps attached to opposite sides of the vessel wall, each flap having a small sinus on its cardiac side. The distension of these sinuses with blood closes the valve and prevents regurgitation. Valves are absent from the superior and inferior venæ cavæ, the portal vein and its tributaries, the hepatic, renal, uterine, and spermatic veins, and from the veins in the lower part of the rectum. They are ill-developed or absent also in the iliac and common femoral veins—a fact which has an important bearing on the production of varix in the veins of the lower extremity.

The wall of *capillaries* consists of a single layer of endothelial cells.

HÆMORRHAGE

Various terms are employed in relation to hæmorrhage, according to its seat, its origin, the time at which it occurs, and other circumstances.

The term *external hæmorrhage* is employed when the blood escapes on the surface; when the bleeding takes place into the tissues or into a cavity it is spoken of as *internal*. The blood may infiltrate the connective tissue, constituting an *extravasation* of blood; or it may collect in a space or cavity and form a *hæmatoma*.

The coughing up of blood from the lungs is known as *hæmoptysis*; vomiting of blood from the stomach, as *hæmatemesis*; the passage of black-coloured stools due to the presence of blood altered by digestion, as *melæna*; and the passage of bloody urine, as *hæmaturia*.

Hæmorrhage is known as arterial, venous, or capillary, according to the nature of the vessel from which it takes place.

In *arterial* hæmorrhage the blood is bright red in colour, and escapes from the cardiac end of the divided vessel in pulsating jets synchronously with the systole of the heart. In vascular parts—for example the face—both ends of a divided artery bleed freely. The blood flowing from an artery may be dark in colour if the respiration is impeded. When the heart's action is weak and the blood tension low the flow may appear to be continuous and not in jets. The blood from a divided artery at the bottom of a deep wound, escapes on the surface in a steady flow.

Venous bleeding is not pulsatile, but occurs in a continuous stream, which, although both ends of the vessel may bleed, is more copious from the distal end. The blood is dark red under ordinary conditions, but may be purplish, or even black, if the respiration is interfered with. When one of the large veins in the neck is wounded, the effects of respiration produce a rise and fall in the stream which may resemble arterial pulsation.

In *capillary* hæmorrhage, red blood escapes from numerous points on the surface of the wound in a steady ooze. This form of bleeding is serious in those who are the subjects of hæmophilia.

INJURIES OF ARTERIES

The following description of the injuries of arteries refers to the larger, named trunks. The injuries of smaller, unnamed vessels are included in the consideration of wounds and contusions.

Contusion.—An artery may be contused by a blow or crush, or by the oblique impact of a bullet. The bruising of the vessel wall, especially if it is diseased, may result in the formation of a thrombus which occludes the lumen temporarily or even permanently, and in rare cases may lead to gangrene of the limb beyond.

Subcutaneous Rupture.—An artery may be ruptured subcutaneously by a blow or crush, or by a displaced fragment of bone. This injury has been produced also during attempts to reduce dislocations, especially those of old standing at the shoulder. It is most liable to occur when the vessels are diseased. The rupture may be incomplete or complete.

Incomplete Subcutaneous Rupture.—In the majority of cases the rupture is incomplete—the inner and middle coats being torn, while the outer remains intact. The middle coat contracts and retracts, and the internal, because of its elasticity, curls up in the interior of the vessel, forming a valvular obstruction to the blood-flow. In most cases this results in the formation of a thrombus which occludes the vessel. In some cases the blood-pressure gradually distends the injured segment of the vessel wall and leads to the formation of an aneurysm. The pulsation in the vessels beyond the seat of rupture is arrested—for a time at least—owing to the occlusion of the vessel, and the limb becomes cold and powerless. The pulsation seldom returns within five or six weeks of the injury, if indeed it is not permanently arrested, but, as a rule, a collateral circulation is rapidly established, sufficient to nourish the parts beyond. If the pulsation returns within a week of the injury, the presumption is that the occlusion was due to pressure from without—for example, by hæmorrhage into the sheath or the pressure of a fragment of bone.

Complete Subcutaneous Rupture.—When the rupture is complete, all the coats of the vessel are torn and the blood escapes into the surrounding tissues. If the original injury is attended with much shock, the bleeding may not take place until the period of reaction. Rupture of the popliteal artery in association with fracture of the femur, or of the axillary or brachial artery with fracture of the humerus or dislocation of the shoulder, are familiar examples of this injury.

Like incomplete rupture, this lesion is accompanied by loss of pulsation and power, and by coldness of the limb beyond; a tense and excessively painful swelling rapidly appears in the region of the injury, and, where the cellular tissue is loose, may attain a considerable size. The pressure of the effused blood occludes the veins and leads to congestion and oedema of the limb beyond. The interference with the circulation, and the damage to the tissues, may be so great that gangrene ensues.

Treatment.—When an artery has been contused or ruptured, the limb must be placed in the most favourable condition for restoration of the circulation. The skin is disinfected and the limb wrapped in cotton wool to conserve its heat, and elevated to such an extent as to promote the venous return without at the same time interfering with the inflow of blood. A careful watch must be kept on the state of nutrition of the limb, lest gangrene occurs.

If no complications supervene, the swelling subsides, and recovery may be complete in six or eight weeks. If the extravasation is great and the skin threatens to give way, or if the vitality of the limb is seriously endangered, it is advisable to expose the injured vessel, and, after clearing away the clots, to attempt to suture the rent in the artery, or, if torn across, to join the ends after paring the bruised edges. If this is impracticable, a ligature is applied above and below the rupture. If gangrene ensues, amputation must be performed.

These descriptions apply to the larger arteries of the extremities. A good illustration of subcutaneous rupture of the arteries of the head is afforded by the tearing of the middle meningeal artery caused by the application of blunt violence to the skull; and of the arteries of the trunk—caused by the tearing of the renal artery in rupture of the kidney.

Open Wounds of Arteries—Laceration.—Laceration of large arteries is a common complication of machinery and railway accidents. The violence being usually of a tearing, twisting, or crushing nature, such injuries are seldom associated with much hæmorrhage, as torn or crushed vessels quickly become occluded by contraction and retraction of their coats and by the formation of a clot. A whole limb even may be avulsed from the body with comparatively little loss of blood. The risk in such cases is secondary hæmorrhage resulting from pyogenic infection.

The *treatment* is that applicable to all wounds, with, in addition, the ligation of the lacerated vessels.

Punctured wounds of blood vessels may result from stabs, or they may be accidentally inflicted in the course of an operation.

The division of the coats of the vessel being incomplete, the natural hæmostasis that results from curling up of the intima and contraction of the media, fails to take place, and bleeding goes on into the surrounding tissues, and externally. If the sheath of the vessel is not widely damaged, the gradually increasing tension of the extravasated blood retained within it may ultimately arrest the hæmorrhage. A clot then forms between the lips of the wound in the vessel wall and projects for a short distance into the lumen, without, however, materially interfering with the flow through the vessel. The organisation of this clot results in the healing of the wound in the vessel wall.

In other cases the blood escapes beyond the sheath and collects in the surrounding tissues, and a traumatic aneurysm results. Secondary hæmorrhage may occur if the wound becomes infected.

The *treatment* consists in enlarging the external wound to permit of the damaged vessel being ligated above and below the puncture. In some cases it may be possible to suture the opening in the vessel wall. When circumstances prevent these measures being taken, the bleeding may be arrested by making firm pressure over the wound with a pad; but this procedure is liable to be followed by the formation of an aneurysm.

Minute puncture of arteries such as frequently occur in the hypodermic administration of drugs and in the use of exploring needles, are not attended with any escape of blood, chiefly because of the elastic recoil of the arterial wall; a tiny thrombus of platelets and thrombus forms at the point where the intima is punctured.

Incised Wounds.—We here refer only to such incised wounds as partly divide the vessel wall.

Longitudinal wounds show little tendency to gape, and are therefore not attended with much bleeding. They usually heal rapidly, but, like punctured wounds, are liable to be followed by the formation of an aneurysm.

When, however, the incision in the vessel wall is oblique or transverse, the retraction of the muscular coat causes the opening to gape, with the result that there is hæmorrhage, which, even in comparatively small arteries, may be so profuse as to prove dangerous. When the associated wound in the soft parts is valvular the hæmorrhage is arrested and an aneurysm may develop.

When a large arterial trunk, such as the external iliac, the femoral, the common carotid, the brachial, or the popliteal, has been partly divided, for example, in the course of an operation, the opening should be closed with sutures—*arteriorrhaphy*. The circulation being controlled by a tourniquet, or the artery itself occluded by a clamp, fine silk or catgut stitches are passed through the outer and middle coats after the method of Lembert, a fine, round needle being employed. The sheath of the vessel or an adjacent fascia should be stitched over the line of suture in the vessel wall. If infection be excluded, there is little risk of thrombosis or secondary hæmorrhage; and even if thrombosis should develop at the point of suture, the artery is obstructed gradually, and the establishment of a collateral circulation takes place better than after ligation. In the case of smaller trunks, or when suture is impracticable, the artery should be tied above and below the opening, and divided between the ligatures.

Gunshot Wounds of Blood Vessels.—In the majority of cases injuries of large vessels are associated with an external wound; the profusion of the bleeding indicates the size of the damaged vessel, and the colour of the blood and the nature of the flow denote whether an artery or a vein is implicated.

When an artery is wounded a firm *hæmatoma* may form, with an expansile pulsation and a palpable thrill—whether such a hæmatoma remains circumscribed or becomes diffuse depends upon the density or laxity of the tissues around it. In course of time a *traumatic arterial aneurysm* may develop from such a hæmatoma.

When an artery and its companion vein are injured simultaneously an *arterio-venous aneurysm* (p. 310) may develop. This frequently takes place without the formation of a hæmatoma as the arterial blood finds its way into the vein and so does not escape into the tissues. Even if a hæmatoma forms it seldom assumes a great size. In time a swelling is recognised, with a palpable thrill and a systolic bruit, loudest at the level of the communication and accompanied by a continuous venous hum.

If leakage occurs into the tissues, the extravasated blood may occlude the vein by pressure, and the symptoms of arterial aneurysm replace those of the arterio-venous form, the systolic bruit persisting, while the venous hum disappears.

Gangrene may ensue if the blood supply is seriously interfered with, or the signs of *ischæmia* may develop; the muscles lose their elasticity, become hard and paralysed, and anæsthesia of the "glove" or "stocking" type, with other alterations of sensation ensue. Apart from ischæmia, *reflex paralysis* of motion and sensation of a transient kind may follow injury of a large vessel.

Treatment is carried out on the same lines as for similar injuries due to other causes.

INJURIES OF VEINS

Veins are subject to the same forms of injury as arteries, and the results are alike in both, such variations as occur being dependent partly on the difference in their anatomical structure, and partly on the conditions of the circulation through them.

Subcutaneous rupture of veins occur most frequently in association with fractures and in the reduction of dislocations. The veins most commonly ruptured are the popliteal, the axillary, the femoral, and the subclavian. On account of the smaller amount of elastic and muscular tissue in the wall of a vein, the contraction and retraction of its walls are less than in an artery, and so bleeding may continue for a longer period. On the other hand, owing to the lower blood-pressure the outflow goes on more slowly, and the gradually increasing pressure produced by the extravasated blood is usually sufficient to arrest the hæmorrhage before it becomes serious. As an aid in diagnosing the source of the bleeding, it should be remembered that the rupture of a vein does not affect the pulsation in the limb beyond. The risks are practically the same as when an artery is ruptured, excepting that of aneurysm, and the treatment is carried out on the same lines, but it is seldom necessary to operate for the purpose of applying a ligature to the injured vein.

Wounds of veins—punctured and incised—frequently occur in the course of operations; for example, in the removal of tumours or diseased glands from the neck, the axilla, or the groin. They are also met with as a result of accidental stabs and of suicidal or homicidal injuries. The hæmorrhage from a large vein so damaged is usually profuse, but it is more readily controlled by external pressure than that from an artery. When a vein is merely punctured, the bleeding may be arrested by pressure with a pad of gauze, or by a lateral ligature—that is, picking up the margins of the rent in the wall and securing them with a ligature without occluding the lumen. In the large veins, such as the internal jugular, the femoral, or the axillary, it is usually possible to suture the opening in the wall. This does not necessarily result in thrombosis in the vessel, or in obliteration of its lumen.

When an *artery and vein are simultaneously wounded*, the features peculiar to each are present in greater or less degree. In the limbs gangrene may ensue, especially if the wound is infected. Punctured and gun-shot wounds implicating both artery and vein are liable to be followed by the development of arterio-venous aneurysm.

Entrance of Air into Veins—Air Embolism.—This serious, though fortunately rare, accident is apt to occur in the course of operations in the region of the thorax, neck, or axilla, if a large vein is opened and fails to collapse on account of the rigidity of its walls, its incorporation in a dense fascia, or from traction being made upon it. If the wound in a vein is thus held open, the negative pressure during inspiration sucks air into the right side of the heart. This is accompanied by a hissing or gurgling sound, and with the next expiration some frothy blood escapes from the wound. The patient instantly becomes pale, the pupils dilate, respiration becomes laboured, and although the heart may continue to beat forcibly, the peripheral pulse is weak, and may even be imperceptible. On auscultating the heart, a churning sound may be heard. Death may result in a few minutes; or the heart may slowly regain its power and recovery take place.

Prevention.—In operations in the "dangerous area"—as the region of the root of the neck is called in this connection—care must be taken not to cut or divide any vein before it has been secured by forceps, and to apply ligatures securely and at once. Deep wounds in this region should be kept filled with normal salt solution. Immediately a cut is recognised in a vein, a finger should be placed over the vessel on the cardiac side of the wound, and kept there until the opening is secured.

Treatment.—Little can be done after the air has actually entered the vein beyond endeavouring to maintain the heart's action by hypodermic injections of ether or strychnin and the application of mustard or hot cloths over the chest. The head at the same time should be lowered to prevent syncope. Attempts to withdraw the air by suction, and the employment of artificial respiration, have proved futile, and are, by some, considered dangerous. In a desperate case massage of the heart might be tried.

THE NATURAL ARREST OF HÆMORRHAGE AND THE REPAIR OF BLOOD VESSELS

Primary Hæmorrhage.—The term primary hæmorrhage is applied to the bleeding which follows immediately on the wounding of a blood vessel. The natural process by which such hæmorrhage is arrested varies with the character of the wound in the vessel and may be modified by accidental circumstances.

(a) *Repair of completely divided Artery.*—When an artery is *completely* divided, the circular fibres of the muscular coat contract, so that the lumen of the cut ends is diminished, and at the same time each segment retracts within its sheath in virtue of the recoil of the elastic elements in its walls, the tunica intima curls up in the interior of the vessel, and the tunica externa collapses over the cut ends. The blood that escapes from the injured vessel fills the interstices of the tissues, and, coagulating, forms a clot which temporarily arrests the bleeding. That part of the clot which lies between the divided ends of the vessel and in the cellular tissue outside, is known as the *external clot*, while the portion which projects into the lumen of the vessel is known as the *internal clot*, and it usually extends as far as the nearest collateral branch.

255

These processes constitute what is known as the *temporary arrest of hæmorrhage*, which, it will be observed, is effected by the contraction and retraction of the divided artery and by clotting.

The *permanent arrest* takes place by the transformation of the clot into scar tissue. The internal clot plays the most important part in the process; it becomes invaded by leucocytes and proliferating endothelial and connective-tissue cells, and new blood vessels permeate the mass, which is thus converted into granulation tissue. This is ultimately replaced by fibrous tissue, which permanently occludes the end of the vessel. Concurrently and by the same process the external clot is converted into scar tissue.

If a divided artery is *ligated at its cut end*, the tension of the ligature is usually sufficient to rupture the inner and middle coats, which curl up within the lumen, the outer coat alone being held in the grasp of the ligature. An internal clot forms and, becoming organised, permanently occludes the vessel as above described. The ligature and the small portion of vessel beyond it are subsequently absorbed.

In course of time the collateral branches of the vessel above and below the level of section enlarge and their inter-communication becomes more free, so that even when large trunks have been divided the vascular supply of the parts beyond may be completely restored. This is known as the development of the *collateral circulation*.

Imperfect Collateral Circulation.—While the development of the collateral circulation after the ligation or obstruction from other cause of a main arterial trunk may be sufficient to prevent gangrene of the limb, it may be insufficient for its adequate nourishment; it may be cold, bluish in colour, and there may be necrosis of the skin over bony points; this is notably the case in the lower extremity after ligation of the femoral or popliteal artery, when patches of skin may die over the prominence of the heel, the balls of the toes, the projecting base of the fifth metatarsal and the external malleolus.

If, during the period of reaction, the blood-pressure rises considerably, the occluding clot at the divided end of the vessel may be washed away or the ligature displaced, permitting of fresh bleeding taking place—*reactionary* or *intermediary hæmorrhage* (p. 272).

In the event of the wound becoming infected with pyogenic organisms, the occluding blood-clot or the young fibrous tissue may become disintegrated in the suppurative process, and the bleeding start afresh—*secondary hæmorrhage* (p. 273).

(b) If an artery is only *partly cut across*, the divided fibres of the tunica muscularis contract and those of the tunica externa retract, with the result that a more or less circular hole is formed in the wall of the vessel, from which free bleeding takes place, as the conditions are unfavourable for the formation of an occluding clot. Even if a clot does form, when the blood-pressure rises it is readily displaced, leading to reactionary hæmorrhage. Should the wound become infected, secondary hæmorrhage is specially liable to occur. A further risk attends this form of injury, in that the intra-vascular tension may in time lead to gradual stretching of the scar tissue which closes the gap in the vessel wall, with the result that a localised dilatation or diverticulum forms, constituting a *traumatic aneurysm*.

(c) When the injury merely takes the form of a *puncture* or *small incision* a blood-clot forms between the edges, becomes organised, and is converted into cicatricial tissue which seals the aperture. Such wounds may also be followed by reactionary or secondary hæmorrhage, or later by the formation of a traumatic aneurysm.

Conditions which influence the Natural Arrest of Hæmorrhage.—The natural arrest of bleeding is favoured by tearing or crushing of the vessel walls, owing to the contraction and retraction of the coats and the tendency of blood to coagulate when in contact with damaged tissue. Hence the primary hæmorrhage following lacerated wounds is seldom copious. The occurrence of syncope or of profound shock also helps to stop bleeding by reducing the force of the heart's action.

On the other hand, there are conditions which retard the natural arrest. When, for example, a vessel is only partly divided, the contraction and retraction of the muscular coat, instead of diminishing the calibre of the artery, causes the wound in the vessel to gape; by completing the division of the vessel under these circumstances the bleeding can often be arrested. In certain situations, also, the arteries are so intimately connected with their sheaths, that when cut across they were unable to retract and contract—for example, in the scalp, in the penis, and in bones—and copious bleeding may take place from comparatively small vessels. This inability of the vessels to contract and retract is met with also in inflamed and oedematous parts and in scar tissue. Arteries divided in the substance of a muscle also sometimes bleed unduly. Any increase in the force of the heart's action, such as may result from exertion, excitement, or over-stimulation, also interferes with the natural arrest. Lastly, in bleeders, there are conditions which interfere with the natural arrest of hæmorrhage.

Repair of a Vessel ligated in its Continuity.—When a ligature is applied to an artery it should be pulled sufficiently tight to occlude the lumen without causing rupture of its coats. It often happens, however, that the compression causes rupture of the inner and middle coats, so that only the outer coat remains in the grasp of the ligature. While this weakens the wall of the vessel, it has the advantage of hastening coagulation, by bringing the blood into contact with damaged tissue. Whether the inner and middle coats are ruptured or not, blood coagulates both above and below the ligature, the proximal clot being longer and broader than that on the distal side. In small arteries these clots extend as far as the nearest collateral branch, but in the larger trunks their length varies. The permanent occlusion of those portions of the vessel occupied by clot is brought about by the formation of granulation tissue, and its replacement by cicatricial tissue, so that the occluded segment of the vessel is represented by a fibrous cord. In this process the coagulum only plays a passive rôle by forming a scaffolding on which the granulation tissue is built up. The ligature surrounding the vessel, and the elements of the clot, are ultimately absorbed.

Repair of Veins.—The process of repair in veins is the same as that in arteries, but the thrombosed area may become canalised and the circulation through the vessel be re-established.

HÆMORRHAGE IN SURGICAL OPERATIONS

The management of the hæmorrhage which accompanies an operation includes (a) preventive measures, and (b) the arrest of the bleeding.

Prevention of Hæmorrhage.—Whenever possible, hæmorrhage should be controlled by *digital compression* of the main artery supplying the limb rather than by a tourniquet. If efficiently applied compression reduces the immediate loss of blood to a minimum, and the bleeding from small vessels that follows the removal of the tourniquet is avoided. Further, the pressure of a tourniquet has been shown to be a material factor in producing shock.

In selecting a point at which to apply digital compression, it is essential that the vessel should be lying over a bone which will furnish the necessary resistance. The common carotid, for example, is pressed backward and medially against the transverse process (carotid tubercle) of the sixth cervical vertebra; the temporal against the temporal process (zygoma) in front of the ear; and the facial against the mandible at the anterior edge of the masseter.

In the upper extremity, the subclavian is pressed against the first rib by making pressure downwards and backwards in the hollow above the clavicle; the axillary and brachial by pressing against the shaft of the humerus.

In the lower extremity, the femoral is controlled by pressing in a direction backward and slightly upward against the brim of the pelvis, midway between the symphysis pubis and the anterior superior iliac spine.

The abdominal aorta may be compressed against the bodies of the lumbar vertebræ opposite the umbilicus, if the spine is arched well forwards over a pillow or sand-bag, or by the method suggested by Macewen, in which the patient's spine is arched forwards by allowing the lower extremities and pelvis to hang over the end of the table, while the assistant, standing on a stool, applies his closed fist over the abdominal aorta and compresses it against the vertebral column. Momburg recommends an elastic cord wound round the body between the iliac crest and the lower border of the ribs, but this procedure has caused serious damage to the intestine.

When digital compression is not available, the most convenient and certain means of preventing hæmorrhage—say in an amputation—is by the use of some form of *tourniquet*, such as the elastic tube of Esmarch or of Foulis, or an elastic bandage, or the screw tourniquet of Petit. Before applying any of these it is advisable to empty the limb of blood. This is best done after the manner suggested by Lister: the limb is held vertical for three or four minutes; the veins are thus emptied by gravitation, and they collapse, and as a physiological result of this the arteries reflexly contract, so that the quantity of blood entering the limb is reduced to a minimum. With the limb still elevated the tourniquet is firmly applied, a part being selected where the vessel can be pressed directly against a bone, and where there is no risk of exerting injurious pressure on the nerve-trunks. The tourniquet should be applied over several layers of gauze or lint to protect the skin, and the first turn of the tourniquet must be rapidly and tightly applied to arrest completely the arterial flow, otherwise the veins only are obstructed and the limb becomes congested. In the lower extremity the best place to apply a tourniquet is the middle third of the thigh; in the upper extremity, in the middle of the arm. A tourniquet should never be applied tighter or left on longer than is absolutely necessary.

The screw tourniquet of Petit is to be preferred when it is desired to intermit the flow through the main artery as in operations for aneurysm.

When a tourniquet cannot conveniently be applied, or when its presence interferes with the carrying out of the operation—as, for example, in amputations at the hip or shoulder—the hæmorrhage may be controlled by preliminary ligation of the main artery above the seat of operation—for instance, the external iliac or the subclavian. For such contingencies also the steel skewers used by Spence and Wyeth, or a special clamp or forceps, such as that suggested by Lynn Thomas, may be employed. In the case of vessels which it is undesirable to occlude permanently, such as the common carotid, the temporary application of a ligature or clamp is useful.

Arrest of Hæmorrhage.—*Ligature.*—This is the best means of securing the larger vessels. The divided vessel having been caught with forceps as near to its cut end as possible, a ligature of catgut or silk is tied round it. When there is difficulty in applying a ligature securely, for example in a dense tissue like the scalp or periosteum, or in a friable tissue like the thyreoid gland or the mesentery, a stitch should be passed so as to surround the bleeding vessel a short distance from its end, in this way ensuring a better hold and preventing the ligature from slipping.

If the hæmorrhage is from a partly divided vessel, this should be completely cut across to enable its walls to contract and retract, and to facilitate the application of forceps and ligatures.

Torsion.—This method is seldom employed except for comparatively small vessels, but it is applicable to even the largest arteries. In employing torsion, the end of the vessel is caught with forceps, and the terminal portion twisted round several times. The object is to tear the inner and middle coats so that they curl up inside the lumen, while the outer fibrous coat is twisted into a cord which occludes the end of the vessel.

Forci-pressure.—Bleeding from the smallest arteries and from arterioles can usually be arrested by firmly squeezing them for a few minutes with artery forceps. It is usually found that on the removal of the forceps at the end of an operation no further hæmorrhage takes place. By the use of specially strong clamps, such as the angiotribes of Doyen, large trunks may be occluded by pressure.

Cautery.—The actual cautery or Paquelin's thermo-cautery is seldom employed to arrest hæmorrhage, but is frequently useful in preventing it, as, for example, in the removal of piles, or in opening the bowel in colostomy. It is used at a dull-red heat, which sears the divided ends of the vessel and so occludes the lumen. A bright-red or a white heat cuts the vessel across without occluding it. The separation of the slough produced by the charring of the tissues is sometimes attended with secondary bleeding.

Hæmostatics or *Styptics.*—The local application of hæmostatics is seldom to be recommended. In the treatment of epistaxis or bleeding from the nose, of hæmorrhage from the socket of a tooth, and sometimes from ulcerating or granulating surfaces, however, they may be useful. All clots must be removed and the drug applied directly to the bleeding surface. Adrenalin and turpentine are the most useful drugs for this purpose.

Hæmorrhage from bone, for example the skull, may be arrested by means of Horsley's aseptic plastic wax. To stop persistent oozing from soft tissues, Horsley successfully applied a portion of living vascular tissue, such as a fragment of muscle, which readily adheres to the oozing surface and yields elements that cause coagulation of the blood by thrombo-kinetic processes. When examined after two or three days the muscle has been found to be closely adherent and undergoing organisation.

Arrest of Accidental Hæmorrhage.—The most efficient means of temporarily controlling hæmorrhage is by pressure applied with the finger, or with a pad of gauze, directly over the bleeding point. While this is maintained an assistant makes digital pressure, or applies a tourniquet, over the main vessel of the limb on the proximal side of the bleeding point. A useful *emergency tourniquet* may be improvised by folding a large handkerchief *en cravatte*, with a cork or piece of wood in the fold to act as a pad. The handkerchief is applied round the limb, with the pad over the main artery, and the ends knotted on the lateral aspect of the limb. With a strong piece of wood the handkerchief is wound up like a Spanish windlass, until sufficient pressure is exerted to arrest the bleeding.

When hæmorrhage is taking place from a number of small vessels, its arrest may be effected by elevation of the bleeding part, particularly if it is a

limb. By this means the force of the circulation is diminished and the formation of coagula favoured. Similarly, in wounds of the hand or forearm, or of
the foot or leg, bleeding may be arrested by placing a pad in the flexure and
acutely flexing the limb at the elbow or knee respectively.

Reactionary Hæmorrhage.—Reactionary or intermediary hæmorrhage is
really a recurrence of primary bleeding. As the name indicates, it occurs during the period of reaction—that is, within the first twelve hours after an
operation or injury. It may be due to the increase in the blood-pressure that
accompanies reaction displacing clots which have formed in the vessels, or
causing vessels to bleed which did not bleed during the operation; to the
slipping of a ligature; or to the giving way of a grossly damaged portion of
the vessel wall. In the scrotum, the relaxation of the dartos during the first
few hours after operation occasionally leads to reactionary hæmorrhage.

As a rule, reactionary hæmorrhage takes place from small vessels as a
result of the displacement of occluding clots, and in many cases the hæmorrhage stops when the bandages and soaked dressings are removed. If not, it
is usually sufficient to remove the clots and apply firm pressure, and in the
case of a limb to elevate it. Should the hæmorrhage recur, the wound must be
reopened, and ligatures applied to the bleeding vessels. Douching the wound
with hot sterilised water (about 110° F.), and plugging it tightly with gauze,
are often successful in arresting capillary oozing. When the bleeding is more
copious, it is usually due to a ligature having slipped from a large vessel such
as the external jugular vein after operations in the neck, and the wound must
be opened up and the vessel again secured. The internal administration of
heroin or morphin, by keeping the patient quiet, may prove useful in preventing the recurrence of hæmorrhage.

Secondary Hæmorrhage.—The term secondary hæmorrhage refers to
bleeding that is delayed in its onset and is due to pyogenic infection of the
tissues around an artery. The septic process causes softening and erosion of
the wall of the artery so that it gives way under the pressure of the contained
blood. The leakage may occur in drops, or as a rush of blood, according to
the extent of the erosion, the size of the artery concerned, and the relations
of the erosion to the surrounding tissues. When met with as a complication
of a wound there is an interval—usually a week to ten days—between the
receipt of the wound and the first hæmorrhage, this time being required for
the extension of the septic process to the wall of the artery and the conse-

quent erosion of its coats. When secondary hæmorrhage occurs apart from a wound, there is a similar septic process attacking the wall of the artery from the outside; for example in sloughing sore-throat, the separation of a slough may implicate the wall of an artery and be followed by serious and it may be fatal hæmorrhage. The mechanical pressure of a fragment of bone or of a rubber drainage tube upon the vessel may aid the septic process in causing erosion of the artery. In pre-Listerian days, the silk ligature around the artery likewise favoured the changes that lead to secondary hæmorrhage, and the interesting observation was often made, that when the collateral circulation was well established, the leakage occurred on the *distal* side of the ligature. While it may happen that the initial hæmorrhage is rapidly fatal, as for example when the external carotid or one of its branches suddenly gives way, it is quite common to have one, two or more *warning hæmorrhages* before the leakage on a large scale, which is rapidly fatal.

The *appearances of the wound* in cases complicated by secondary hæmorrhage are only characteristic in so far that while obviously infected, there is an absence of all reaction; instead of frankly suppurating, there is little or no discharge and the surrounding cellular tissue and the limb beyond are oedematous and pit on pressure.

The *general symptoms* of septic poisoning in cases of secondary hæmorrhage vary widely in severity: they may be so slight that the general health is scarcely affected and the convalescence from an operation, for example, may be apparently normal except that the wound does not heal satisfactorily. For example, a patient may be recovering from an operation such as the removal of an epithelioma of the mouth, pharynx or larynx and the associated lymph glands in the neck, and be able to be up and going about his room, when, suddenly, without warning and without obvious cause, a rush of blood occurs from the mouth or the incompletely healed wound in the neck, causing death within a few minutes.

On the other hand, the toxæmia may be of a profound type associated with marked pallor and progressive failure of strength, which, of itself, even when the danger from hæmorrhage has been overcome, may have a fatal termination. The *prognosis* therefore in cases of secondary hæmorrhage can never be other than uncertain and unfavourable; the danger from loss of blood *per se* is less when the artery concerned is amenable to control by surgical measures.

Treatment.—The treatment of secondary hæmorrhage includes the use of local measures to arrest the bleeding, the employment of general measures to counteract the accompanying toxæmia, and when the loss of blood has been considerable, the treatment of the bloodless state.

Local Measures to arrest the Hæmorrhage.—The occurrence of even slight hæmorrhages from a septic wound in the vicinity of a large blood vessel is to be taken seriously; it is usually necessary to *open up the wound*, clear out the clots and infected tissues with a sharp spoon, disinfect the walls of the cavity with eusol or hydrogen peroxide, and *pack* it carefully but not too tightly with gauze impregnated with some antiseptic, such as "bipp," so that, if the bleeding does not recur, it may be left undisturbed for several days. The packing should if possible be brought into actual contact with the leaking point in the vessel, and so arranged as to make pressure on the artery above the erosion. The dressings and bandage are then applied, with the limb in the attitude that will diminish the force of the stream through the main artery, for example, flexion at the elbow in hæmorrhage from the deep palmar arch. Other measures for combating the local sepsis, such as the irrigation method of Carrel, may be considered.

If the wound involves one of the extremities, it may be useful; and it imparts confidence to the nurse, and, it may be, to the patient, if a Petit's tourniquet is loosely applied above the wound, which the nurse is instructed to tighten up in the event of bleeding taking place.

Ligation of the Artery.—If the hæmorrhage recurs in spite of packing the wound, or if it is serious from the outset and likely to be critical if repeated, ligation of the artery itself or of the trunk from which it springs, at a selected spot higher up, should be considered. This is most often indicated in wounds of the extremities.

As examples of proximal ligation for secondary hæmorrhage may be cited ligation of the hypogastric artery for hæmorrhage in the buttock, of the common iliac for hæmorrhage in the thigh, of the brachial in the upper arm for hæmorrhage from the deep palmar arch, and of the posterior tibial behind the medial malleolus for hæmorrhage from the sole of the foot.

Amputation is the last resource, and should be decided upon if the hæmorrhage recurs after proximal ligation, or if this has been followed by gangrene of the limb; it should also be considered if the nature of the wound and the virulence of the sepsis would of themselves justify removal of the limb. Every surgeon can recall cases in which a timely amputation has been the means of saving life.

The *counteraction of the toxæmia* and the *treatment of the bloodless state*, are carried out on the usual lines.

Hæmorrhage of Toxic Origin.—Mention must also be made of hæmorrhages which depend upon infective or toxic conditions and in which no gross lesion of the vessels can be discovered. The bleeding occurs as an oozing, which may be comparatively slight and unimportant, or by its persistence may become serious. It takes place into the superficial layers of the skin, from mucous membranes, and into the substance of such organs as the pancreas. Hæmorrhage from the stomach and intestine, attended with a brown or black discoloration of the vomit and of the stools, is one of the best known examples: it is not uncommonly met with in infective conditions originating in the appendix, intestine, gall-bladder, and other abdominal organs. Hæmorrhage from the mucous membrane of the stomach after abdominal operations—apparently also due to toxic causes and not to the operation—gives rise to the so-called *post-operative hæmatemesis.*

Constitutional Effects of Hæmorrhage.—The severity of the symptoms resulting from hæmorrhage depends as much on the rapidity with which the bleeding takes place as on the amount of blood lost. The sudden loss of a large quantity, whether from an open wound or into a serous cavity—for example, after rupture of the liver or spleen—is attended with marked pallor of the surface of the body and coldness of the skin, especially of the face, feet, and hands. The skin is moist with a cold, clammy sweat, and beads of perspiration stand out on the forehead. The pulse becomes feeble, soft, and rapid, and the patient is dull and listless, and complains of extreme thirst. The temperature is usually sub-normal; and the respiration rapid, shallow, and sighing in character. Abnormal visual sensations, in the form of flashes of light or spots before the eyes; and rushing, buzzing, or ringing sounds in the ears, are often complained of.

In extreme cases, phenomena which have been aptly described as those of "air-hunger" ensue. On account of the small quantity of blood circulating through the body, and the diminished hæmoglobin content of the blood, the tissues are imperfectly oxygenated, and the patient becomes extremely restless, gasping for breath, constantly throwing about his arms and baring his chest in the vain attempt to breath more freely. Faintness and giddiness are marked features. The diminished supply of oxygen to the brain and to the muscles produces muscular twitchings, and sometimes convulsions. Finally the pupils dilate, the sphincters relax, and death ensues.

Young children stand the loss of blood badly, but they quickly recover, as the regeneration of blood takes place rapidly. In old people also, and especially when they are fat, the loss of blood is badly borne, and the ill effects last longer. Women, on the whole, stand loss of blood better than men, and in them the blood is more rapidly re-formed. A few hours after a severe hæmorrhage there is usually a leucocytosis of from 15,000 to 30,000.

Treatment of the Bloodless State.—The patient should be placed in a warm, well-ventilated room, and the foot of the bed elevated. Cardiac stimulants, such as strychnin or alcohol, must be judiciously administered, over-stimulation being avoided. The inhalation of oxygen has been found useful in relieving the urgent symptoms of dyspnoea.

The blood may be emptied from the limbs into the vessels of the trunk, where it is more needed, by holding them vertically in the air for a few minutes, and then applying a firm elastic bandage over a layer of cotton wool, from the periphery towards the trunk.

Introduction of Fluids into the Circulation.—The most valuable measure for maintaining the circulation, however, is by transfusion of blood (*Op. Surg.*, p. 37). If this is not immediately available the introduction of from one to three pints of physiological salt solution (a teaspoonful of common salt to a pint of water) into a vein, or a 6 per cent. solution of gum acacia, is a useful expedient. The solution is sterilised by boiling, and cooled to a temperature of about 105° F. The addition of 5 to 10 minims of adrenalin solution (1 in 1000) is advantageous in raising the blood-pressure (*Op. Surg.*, p. 565).

When the intra-venous method is not available, one or two pints of saline solution with adrenalin should be slowly introduced into the rectum, by means of a long rubber tube and a filler. Satisfactory, although less rapidly obtained results follow the introduction of saline solution into the cellular tissue—for example, under the mamma, into the axilla, or under the skin of the back.

If the patient can retain fluids taken by the mouth—such as hot coffee, barley water, or soda water—these should be freely given, unless the injury necessitates operative treatment under a general anæsthetic.

Transfusion of blood is most valuable as *a preliminary to operation* in patients who are bloodless as a result of hæmorrhage from gastric and duodenal ulcers, and in bleeders.

HÆMOPHILIA

The term hæmophilia is applied to an inherited disease which renders the patient liable to serious hæmorrhage from even the most trivial injuries; and the subjects of it are popularly known as "bleeders."

The cause of the disease and its true nature are as yet unknown. There is no proof of any structural defect in the blood vessels, and beyond the fact that there is a diminution in the number of blood-plates, it has not been demonstrated that there is any alteration in the composition of the blood.

The affection is in a marked degree hereditary, all the branches of an affected family being liable to suffer. Its mode of transmission to individuals, moreover, is characteristic: the male members of the stock alone suffer from the affection in its typical form, while the tendency is transmitted through the female line. Thus the daughters of a father who is a bleeder, whilst they do not themselves suffer from the disease, transmit the tendency to their male offspring. The sons, on the other hand, neither suffer themselves nor transmit the disease to their children (Fig. 64). The female members of a hæmophilic stock are often very prolific, and there is usually a predominance of daughters in their families.

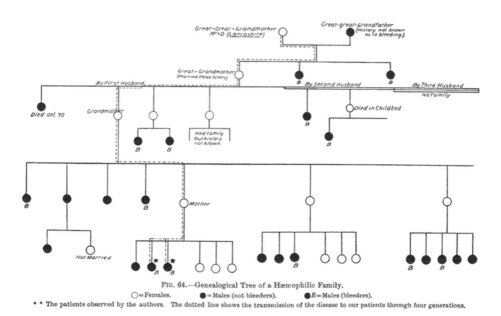

FIG. 64.—Genealogical Tree of a Hæmophilic Family.

○ = Females.　　● = Males (not bleeders).　　●B = Males (bleeders).

* * The patients observed by the authors.　The dotted line shows the transmission of the disease to our patients through four generations.

FIG. 64. Genealogical Tree of a Hæmophilic Family.

The disease is met with in boys who are otherwise healthy, and usually manifests itself during the first few years of life. In rare instances profuse hæmorrhage takes place when the umbilical cord separates. As a rule the first evidence is the occurrence of long-continued and uncontrollable bleeding from a comparatively slight injury, such as the scratch of a pin, the extraction of a tooth, or after the operation of circumcision. The blood oozes slowly from the capillaries; at first it appears normal, but after flowing for some days, or it may be weeks, it becomes pale, thin, and watery, and shows less and less tendency to coagulate.

Female members of hæmophilia families sometimes show a tendency to excessive hæmorrhage, but they seldom manifest the characteristic features met with in the male members.

Sometimes the hæmorrhage takes place apparently spontaneously from the gums, the nasal or the intestinal mucous membrane. In other cases the bleeding occurs into the cellular tissue under the skin or mucous membrane, producing large areas of ecchymosis and discoloration. One of the commonest manifestations of the disease is the occurrence of hæmorrhage into the cavities of the large joints, especially the knee, elbow, or hip. The patient suffers repeatedly from such hæmorrhages, the determining injury being often so slight as to have passed unobserved.

There is evidence that the tendency to bleed is greater at certain times than at others—in some cases showing almost a cyclical character—although nothing is known as to the cause of the variation.

After a severe hæmorrhage into the cellular tissue or into a joint, the patient becomes pale and anæmic, the temperature may rise to 102° or 103° F., the pulse become small and rapid, and hæmic murmurs are sometimes developed over the heart and large arteries. The swelling is tense, fluctuating, and hot, and there is considerable pain and tenderness.

In exceptional cases, blisters form over the seat of the effusion, or the skin may even slough, and the clinical features may therefore come to simulate closely those of an acute suppurative condition. When the skin sloughs, an ulcer is formed with altered blood-clot in its floor like that seen in scurvy, and there is a remarkable absence of any attempt at healing.

The acute symptoms gradually subside, and the blood is slowly absorbed, the discoloration of the skin passing through the same series of changes as occur after an ordinary bruise. The patients seldom manifest the symptoms of the bloodless state, and the blood is rapidly regenerated.

The *diagnosis* is easy if the patient or his friends are aware of the family tendency to hæmorrhage and inform the doctor of it, but they are often sensitive and reticent regarding the fact, and it may only be elicited after close investigation. From the history it is usually easy to exclude scurvy and purpura. Repeated hæmorrhages into a joint may result in appearances which closely simulate those of tuberculous disease. Recent hæmorrhages into the cellular tissue often present clinical features closely resembling those of acute cellulitis or osteomyelitis. A careful examination, however, may reveal ecchymoses on other parts of the body which give a clue to the nature of the condition, and may prevent the disastrous consequences that may follow incision.

These patients usually succumb sooner or later to hæmorrhage, although they often survive several severe attacks. After middle life the tendency to bleed appears to diminish.

Treatment.—As a rule the ordinary means of arresting hæmorrhage are of little avail. From among the numerous means suggested, the following may be mentioned: The application to the bleeding point of gauze soaked in a 1 in 1000 solution of adrenalin; prolonged inhalation of oxygen; freezing the part with a spray of ethyl-chloride; one or more subcutaneous injections of gelatin—5 ounces of a 2½ per cent. solution of white gelatin in normal salt solution being injected at a temperature of about 100° F.; the injection of pituitary extract. The application of a pad of gauze soaked in the blood of a normal person sometimes arrests the bleeding.

To prevent bleeding in hæmophilics, intra-venous or subcutaneous injections of fresh blood serum, taken from the human subject, the sheep, the dog, or the horse, have proved useful. If fresh serum is not available, anti-diphtheritic or anti-tetanic serum or trade preparations, such as hemoplastin, may be employed. We have removed the appendix and amputated through the thigh in hæmophilic subjects without excessive loss of blood after a course of fresh sheep's serum given by the mouth over a period of several weeks.

The chloride and lactate of calcium, and extract of thymus gland have been employed to increase the coagulability of the blood. The patient should drink large quantities of milk, which also increases the coagulability of the blood. Monro has observed remarkable results from the hypodermic injection of emetin hydrochloride in ½-grain doses.

THROMBOSIS AND EMBOLISM

The processes known as thrombosis and embolism are so intimately associated with the diseases of blood vessels that it is convenient to define these terms in the first instance.

Thrombosis.—The term *thrombus* is applied to a clot of blood formed in the interior of the heart or of a blood vessel, and the process by which such a clot forms is known as *thrombosis*. It would appear that slowing or stagnation of the blood-stream, and interference with the integrity of the lining membrane of the vessel wall, are the most important factors determining the formation of the clot. Alterations in the blood itself, such as occur, for example, in certain toxæmias, also favour coagulation. When the thrombus is formed slowly, it consists of white blood cells with a small proportion of fibrin, and, being deposited in successive layers, has a distinctly laminated appearance on section. It is known as a *white thrombus* or laminated clot, and is often met with in the sac of an aneurysm (Fig. 72). When rapidly formed in a vessel in which the blood is almost stagnant—as, for example, in a pouched varicose vein—the blood coagulates *en masse*, and the clot consists of all the elements of the blood, constituting a *red thrombus* (Fig. 66). Sometimes the thrombus is *mixed*—a red thrombus being deposited on a white one, it may be in alternate layers.

When aseptic, a thrombus may become detached and be carried off in the blood-stream as an embolus; it may become organised; or it may degenerate and undergo calcification. Occasionally a small thrombus situated behind a valve in a varicose vein or in the terminal end of a dilated vein—for example in a pile—undergoes calcification, and is then spoken of as a *phlebolith*; it gives a shadow with the X-rays.

When infected with pyogenic bacteria, the thrombus becomes converted into pus and a localised abscess forms; or portions of the thrombus may be carried as emboli in the circulation to distant parts, where they give rise to secondary foci of suppuration—pyæmic abscesses.

Embolism.—The term *embolus* is applied to any body carried along in the circulation and ultimately becoming impacted in a blood vessel. This occurrence is known as *embolism*. The commonest forms of embolus are portions of thrombi or of fibrinous formations on the valves of the heart, the latter being usually infected with micro-organisms.

Embolism plays an important part in determining one form of gangrene, as has already been described. Infective emboli are the direct cause of the secondary abscesses that occur in pyæmia; and they are sometimes responsible for the formation of aneurysm.

Portions of malignant tumours also may form emboli, and their impaction in the vessels may lead to the development of secondary growths in distant parts of the body.

Fat and air embolism have already been referred to.

ARTERITIS

Pyogenic.—Non-suppurative inflammation of the coats of an artery may so soften the wall of the vessel as to lead to aneurysmal dilatation. It is not uncommon in children, and explains the occurrence of aneurysm in young subjects.

When suppuration occurs, the vessel wall becomes disintegrated and gives way, leading to secondary hæmorrhage. If the vessel ruptures into an abscess cavity, dangerous bleeding may occur when the abscess bursts or is opened.

Syphilitic.—The inflammation associated with syphilis results in thickening of the tunica intima, whereby the lumen of the vessel becomes narrowed, or even obliterated—*endarteritis obliterans.* The middle coat usually escapes, but the tunica externa is generally thickened. These changes cause serious interference with the nutrition of the parts supplied by the affected arteries. In large trunks, by diminishing the elasticity of the vessel wall, they are liable to lead to the formation of aneurysm.

Changes in the arterial walls closely resembling those of syphilitic arteritis are sometimes met with in *tuberculous* lesions.

Arterio-sclerosis or **Chronic Arteritis.**—These terms are applied to certain changes which result in narrowing of the lumen and loss of elasticity in the arteries. The condition may affect the whole vascular system or may be confined to particular areas. In the smaller arteries there is more or less uniform thickening of the tunica intima from proliferation of the endothelium and increase in the connective tissue in the elastic lamina—a form of obliterative endarteritis. The narrowing of the vessels may be sufficient to determine gangrene in the extremities. In course of time, particularly in the larger arteries, this new tissue undergoes degeneration, at first of a fatty nature, but progressing in the direction of calcification, and this is followed by the deposit of lime salts in the young connective tissue and the formation of calcareous plates or rings over a considerable area of the vessel wall. To this stage in the process the term *atheromais* applied. The endothelium over these plates often disappears, leaving them exposed to the blood-stream.

Changes of a similar kind sometimes occur in the middle coat, the lime salts being deposited among the muscle fibres in concentric rings.

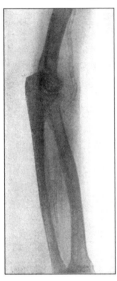

FIG. 65. Radiogram showing Calcareous Degeneration (Atheroma) of Arteries.

The primary cause of arterio-sclerosis is not definitely known, but its almost constant occurrence, to a greater or less degree, in the aged suggests that it is of the nature of a senile degeneration. It is favoured by anything which throws excessive strain on the vessel walls, such as heavy muscular work; by chronic alcoholism and syphilis; or by such general diseases as tend to raise the blood-pressure—for example, chronic Bright's disease or gout. It occurs with greater frequency and with greater severity in men than in women.

Atheromatous degeneration is most common in the large arterial trunks, and the changes are most marked at the arch of the aorta, opposite the flexures of joints, at the mouths of large branches, and at parts where the vessel lies in contact with bone. The presence of diseased patches in the wall of an artery diminishes its elasticity and favours aneurysmal dilatation. Such a vessel also is liable to be ruptured by external violence and so give rise to traumatic aneurysm. Thrombosis is liable to occur when calcareous plates are exposed in the lumen of the vessel by destruction of the endothelium, and this predisposes to embolism. Arterio-sclerosis also interferes with the natural arrest of hæmorrhage, and by rendering the vessels brittle, makes it difficult to secure them by ligature. In advanced cases the accessible arteries—such as the radial, the temporal or the femoral—may be felt as firm, tortuous cords, which are sometimes so hard that they have been aptly compared to "pipe-stems." The pulse is smaller and less compressible than normal, and the vessel moves bodily with each pulsation. It must be borne in mind, however, that the condition of the radial artery may fail to afford a clue to that of the larger arteries. Calcified arteries are readily identified in skiagrams (Fig. 65).

We have met with a chronic form of arterial degeneration in elderly women, affecting especially the great vessels at the root of the neck, in which the artery is remarkably attenuated and dilated, and so friable that the wall readily tears when seized with an artery-forceps, rendering ligation of the vessel in the ordinary way well-nigh impossible. Matas suggests infolding the wall of the vessel with interrupted sutures that do not pierce the intima, and wrapping it round with a strip of peritoneum or omentum.

The most serious form of arterial *thrombosis* is that met with *in the abdominal aorta*, which is attended with violent pains in the lower limbs, rapidly followed by paralysis and arrest of the circulation.

THROMBO-PHLEBITIS AND THROMBOSIS IN VEINS

Thrombosis is more common in veins than in arteries, because slowing of the blood-stream and irritation of the endothelium of the vessel wall are, owing to the conditions of the venous circulation, more readily induced in veins.

Venous thrombosis may occur from purely mechanical causes—as, for example, when the wall of a vein is incised, or the vessel included in a ligature, or when it is bruised or crushed by a fragment of a broken bone or by a bandage too tightly applied. Under these conditions thrombosis is essentially a reparative process, and has already been considered in relation to the repair of blood vessels.

In other cases thrombosis is associated with certain constitutional diseases—gout, for example; the endothelium of the veins undergoing changes—possibly the result of irritation by abnormal constituents in the blood—which favour the formation of thrombi.

Under these various conditions the formation of a thrombus is not necessarily associated with the action of bacteria, although in any of them this additional factor may be present.

The most common cause of venous thrombosis, however, is inflammation of the wall of the vein—phlebitis.

Phlebitis.—Various forms of phlebitis are met with, but for practical purposes they may be divided into two groups—one in which there is a tendency to the formation of a thrombus; the other in which the infective element predominates.

In surgical patients, the *thrombotic form* is almost invariably met with in the lower extremity, and usually occurs in those who are debilitated and anæmic, and who are confined to bed for prolonged periods—for example, during the treatment of fractures of the leg or pelvis, or after such operations as herniotomy, prostatectomy, or appendectomy.

Clinical Features.—The most typical example of this form of phlebitis is that so frequently met with in the great saphena vein, especially when it is varicose. The onset of the attack is indicated by a sudden pain in the lower limb—sometimes below, sometimes above the knee. This initial pain may be associated with shivering or even with a rigor, and the temperature usually rises one or two degrees. There is swelling and tenderness along the line of the affected vein, and the skin over it is a dull-red or purple colour. The swollen vein may be felt as a firm cord, with bead-like enlargements in the position of the valves. The patient experiences a feeling of stiffness and tightness throughout the limb. There is often oedema of the leg and foot, especially when the limb is in the dependent position. The acute symptoms pass off in a few days, but the swelling and tenderness of the vein and the oedema of the limb may last for many weeks.

When the deep veins—iliac, femoral, popliteal—are involved, there is great swelling of the whole limb, which is of a firm almost "wooden" consistence, and of a pale-white colour; the oedema may be so great that it is impossible to feel the affected vein until the swelling has subsided. This is most often seen in puerperal women, and is known as *phlegmasia alba dolens.*

Treatment.—The patient must be placed at absolute rest, with the foot of the bed raised on blocks 10 or 12 inches high, and the limb immobilised by sand-bags or splints. It is necessary to avoid handling the parts, lest the clot be displaced and embolism occur. To avoid frequent movement of the limb, the necessary dressings should be kept in position by means of a many-tailed rather than a roller bandage.

To relieve the pain, warm fomentations or lead and opium lotion should be applied. Later, ichthyol-glycerin, or glycerin and belladonna, may be substituted.

When, at the end of three weeks, the danger of embolism is past, douching and gentle massage may be employed to disperse the oedema; and when the patient gets up he should wear a supporting elastic bandage.

The *infective* form usually begins as a peri-phlebitis arising in connection with some focus of infection in the adjacent tissues. The elements of the vessel wall are destroyed by suppuration, and the thrombus in its lumen becomes infected with pyogenic bacteria and undergoes softening.

Occlusion of the inferior vena cava as a result of infective thrombosis is a well-known condition, the thrombosis extending into the main trunk from some of its tributaries, either from the femoral or iliac veins below or from the hepatic veins above.

Portions of the softened thrombus are liable to become detached and to enter the circulating blood, in which they are carried as emboli. These may lodge in distant parts, and give rise to secondary foci of suppuration—pyæmic abscesses.

Clinical Features.—Infective phlebitis is most frequently met with in the transverse sinus as a sequel to chronic suppuration in the mastoid antrum and middle ear. It also occurs in relation to the peripheral veins, but in these it can seldom be recognised as a separate entity, being merged in the general infective process from which it takes origin. Its occurrence may be inferred, if in the course of a suppurative lesion there is a sudden rise of temperature, with pain, redness, and swelling along the line of a venous trunk, and a rapidly developed oedema of the limb, with pitting of the skin on pressure. In rare cases a localised abscess forms in the vein and points towards the surface.

Treatment.—Attention must be directed towards the condition with which the phlebitis is associated. Ligation of the vein on the cardiac side of the thrombus with a view to preventing embolism is seldom feasible in the peripheral veins, although, as will be pointed out later, the jugular vein is ligated with this object in cases of phlebitis of the transverse sinus.

VARIX—VARICOSE VEINS

The term varix is applied to a condition in which veins are so altered in structure that they remain permanently dilated, and are at the same time lengthened and tortuous. Two types are met with: one in which dilatation of a large superficial vein and its tributaries is the most obvious feature; the other, in which bunches of distended and tortuous vessels develop at one or more points in the course of a vein, a condition to which Virchow applied the term *angioma racemosum venosum.* The two types may occur in combination.

Any vein in the body may become varicose, but the condition is rare except in the veins of the lower extremity, in the veins of the spermatic cord (varicocele), and in the veins of the anal canal (hæmorrhoids).

We are here concerned with varix as it occurs in the veins of the lower extremity.

Etiology.—Considerable difference of opinion exists as to the essential cause of varix. The weight of evidence is in favour of the view that, when dilatation is the predominant element, it results from a congenital deficiency in the number, size, and strength of the valves of the affected veins, and in an inherent weakness in the vessel walls. The *angioma racemosum venosum* is probably also due to a congenital alteration in the structure of the vessels, and is allied to tumours of blood vessels. The view that varix is congenital in origin, as was first suggested by Virchow, is supported by the fact that in a large proportion of cases the condition is hereditary; not only may several members of the same family in succeeding generations suffer from varix, but it is often found that the same vein, or segment of a vein, is involved in all of them. The frequent occurrence of varix in youth is also an indication of its congenital origin.

In the majority of cases it is only when some exciting factor comes into operation that the clinical phenomena associated with varix appear. The most common exciting cause is increased pressure within the veins, and this may be produced in a variety of ways. In certain diseases of the heart, lungs, and liver, for example, the venous pressure may be so raised as to cause a localised dilatation of such veins as are congenitally weak. The direct pressure of a tumour, or of the gravid uterus on the large venous trunks in the pelvis, may so obstruct the flow as to distend the veins of the lower extremity. It is a common experience in women that the signs of varix date from an antecedent pregnancy. The importance of the wearing of tight garters as a factor in the production of varicose veins has been exaggerated, although it must be admitted that this practice is calculated to aggravate the condition when it is once established. It has been proved experimentally that the backward pressure in the veins may be greatly increased by straining, a fact which helps to explain the frequency with which varicosity occurs in the lower limbs of athletes and of those whose occupation involves repeated and violent muscular efforts. There is reason to believe, moreover, that a sudden strain may, by rupturing the valves and so rendering them incompetent, induce varicosity independently of any congenital defect. Prolonged standing or walking, by allowing gravity to act on the column of blood in the veins of the lower limbs, is also an important determining factor in the production of varix.

Thrombosis of the deep veins—in the leg, for example—may induce marked dilatation of the superficial veins, by throwing an increased amount of work upon them. This is to be looked upon rather as a compensatory hypertrophy of the superficial vessels than as a true varix.

Morbid Anatomy.—In the lower extremity the varicosity most commonly affects the vessels of the great saphena system; less frequently those of the small saphena system. Sometimes both systems are involved, and large communicating branches may develop between the two.

The essential lesion is the absence or deficiency of valves, so that they are incompetent and fail to support the column of blood which bears back upon them. Normally the valves in the femoral and iliac veins and in the inferior vena cava are imperfectly developed, so that in the erect posture the great saphena receives a large share of the backward pressure of the column of venous blood.

The whole length of the vein may be affected, but as a rule the disease is confined to one or more segments, which are not only dilated, but are also increased in length, so that they become convoluted. The adjacent loops of the convoluted vein are often bound together by fibrous tissue. All the coats are thickened, chiefly by an increased development of connective tissue, and in some cases changes similar to those of arterio-sclerosis occur. The walls of varicose veins are often exceedingly brittle. In some cases the thickening is uniform, and in others it is irregular, so that here and there thin-walled sacs or pouches project from the side of the vein. These pouches vary in size from a bean to a hen's egg, the larger forms being called *venous cysts*, and being most commonly met with in the region of the

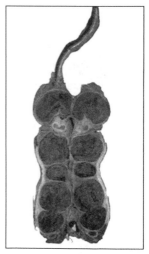

FIG. 66. Thrombosis in Tortuous and Pouched Great Saphena Vein, in longitudinal section.

saphenous opening and of the opening in the popliteal fascia. Such pouches, being exposed to injury, are frequently the seat of thrombosis (Fig. 66).

Clinical Features.—Varix is most frequently met with between puberty and the age of thirty, and the sexes appear to suffer about equally.

The amount of discomfort bears no direct proportion to the extent of the varicosity. It depends rather upon the degree of pressure in the veins, as is shown by the fact that it is relieved by elevation of the limb. When the whole length of the main trunk of the great saphena is implicated, the pressure in the vein is high and the patient suffers a good deal of pain and discomfort. When, on the contrary, the upper part of the saphena and its valves are intact, and only the more distal veins are involved, the pressure is not so high and there is comparatively little suffering. The usual complaint is of a sense of weight and fulness in the limb after standing or walking, sometimes accompanied by actual pain, from which relief is at once obtained by raising the limb. Cramp-like pains in the muscles are often associated with varix of the deep veins.

The dilated and tortuous vein can be readily seen and felt when the patient is examined in the upright posture. In advanced cases, bead-like swellings are sometimes to be detected over the position of the valves, and, on running the fingers along the course of the vessel, a firm ridge, due to periphlebitis, may be detected on each side of the vein. When the limb is oedematous, the outline of the veins is obscured, but they can be identified on palpation as gutter-like tracks. When large veins are implicated, a distinct impulse on coughing may be seen to pass down as far as the knee; and if the vessel is sharply percussed a fluid wave may be detected passing both up and down the vein.

If the patient is placed on a couch and the limb elevated, the veins are emptied, and if pressure is then made over the region of the saphenous opening and the patient allowed to stand up, so long as the great saphena system alone is involved, the veins fill again very slowly from below. If the small saphena system also is involved, and if communicating branches are dilated, the veins fill up from below more rapidly. When the pressure over the saphenous opening is removed, the blood rapidly rushes into the varicose vessels from above; this is known as Trendelenburg's test.

The most marked dilatation usually occurs on the medial side of the limb, between the middle of the thigh and the middle of the calf, the arrangement of the veins showing great variety (Fig. 67).

There are usually one or more bunches of enlarged and tortuous veins in the region of the knee. Frequently a large branch establishes a communication between the systems of the great and small saphenous veins in the region of the popliteal space, or across the front of the upper part of the tibia. The superficial position of this last branch and its proximity to the bone render it liable to injury.

The small veins of the skin of the ankle and foot often show as fine blue streaks arranged in a stellate or arborescent manner, especially in women who have borne children.

Complications.—When the varix is of long standing, the skin in the lower part of the leg sometimes assumes a mahogany-brown or bluish hue, as a result of the *deposit of blood pigment* in the tissues, and this is frequently a precursor of ulceration.

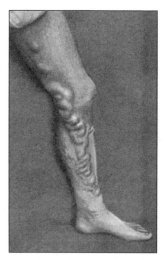

FIG. 67. Extensive Varix of Internal Saphena System on Left Leg, of many years' standing.

Chronic dermatitis (varicose eczema) is often met with in the lower part of the leg, and is due to interference with the nutrition of the skin. The incompetence of the valves allows the pressure in the varicose veins to equal that in the arterioles, so that the capillary circulation is impeded. From the same cause the blood in the deep veins is enabled to enter the superficial veins, where the backward pressure is so great that the blood flows down again, and so a vicious circle is established. The blood therefore loses more and more of its oxygen, and so fails to nourish the tissues.

The *ulcer* of the leg associated with varicose veins has already been described.

Hæmorrhage may take place from a varicose vein as a result of a wound or of ulceration of its wall. Increased intra-venous pressure produced by severe muscular strain may determine rupture of a vein exposed in the floor of an ulcer. If the limb is dependent, the incompetency of the valves permits of rapid and copious bleeding, which may prove fatal, particularly if the patient is intoxicated when the rupture takes place and no means are taken to arrest the hæmorrhage. The bleeding may be arrested at once by elevating the limb, or by applying pressure directly over the bleeding point.

Phlebitis and thrombosis are common sequelæ of varix, and may prove dangerous, either by spreading into the large venous trunks or by giving rise to emboli. The larger the varix the greater is the tendency for a thrombus to spread upwards and to involve the deep veins. Thrombi usually originate in venous cysts or pouches, and at acute bends on the vessel, especially when these are situated in the vicinity of the knee, and are subjected to repeated injuries—for example in riding. Phleboliths sometimes form in such pouches, and may be recognised in a radiogram. In a certain proportion of cases, especially in elderly people, the occurrence of thrombosis leads to cure of the condition by the thrombus becoming organised and obliterating the vein.

Treatment.—At best the treatment of varicose veins is only palliative, as it is obviously impossible to restore to the vessels their normal structure. The patient must avoid wearing anything, such as a garter, which constricts the limb, and any obvious cause of direct pressure on the pelvic veins, such as a tumour, persistent constipation, or an ill-fitting truss, should be removed. Cardiac, renal, or pulmonary causes of venous congestion must also be treated, and the functions of the liver regulated. Severe forms of muscular exertion and prolonged standing or walking are to be avoided, and the patient may with benefit rest the limb in an elevated position for a few hours each day. To support the distended vessels, a closely woven silk or worsted stocking, or a light and porous form of elastic bandage, applied as a puttee, should be worn. These appliances should be put on before the patient leaves his bed in the morning, and should only be removed after he lies down at night. In this way the vessels are never allowed to become dilated. Elastic stockings, and bandages made entirely of india-rubber, are to be avoided. In early and mild cases these measures are usually sufficient to relieve the patient's discomfort.

Operative Treatment.—In aggravated cases, when the patient is suffering pain, when his occupation is interfered with by repeated attacks of phlebitis, or when there are large pouches on the veins, operative treatment is called for. The younger the patient the clearer is the indication to operate. It may be necessary to operate to enable a patient to enter one of the public services, even although no symptoms are present. The presence of an ulcer does not contra-indicate operation; the ulcer should be excised, and the raw surface covered with skin grafts, before dealing with the veins.

The *operation of Trendelenburg* is especially appropriate to cases in which the trunk of the great saphena vein in the thigh is alone involved. It consists in exposing three or four inches of the vein in its upper part, applying a ligature at the upper and lower ends of the exposed portion, and, after tying all tributary branches, resecting this portion of the vein.

The procedure of C. H. Mayo is adapted to cases in which it is desirable to remove longer segments of the veins. It consists in the employment of special instruments known as "ring-enucleators" or "vein-strippers," by means of which long portions of the vein are removed through comparatively small incisions.

An alternative procedure consists in avulsing segments of the vein by means of Babcock's stylet, which consists of a flexible steel rod, 30 inches in length, with acorn-shaped terminals. The instrument is passed along the lumen of the segment to be dealt with, and a ligature applied around the vein above the bulbous end of the stylet enables nearly the whole length of the great saphena vein to be dragged out in one piece. These methods are not suitable when the veins are brittle, when there are pouches or calcareous deposits in their walls, or where there has been periphlebitis binding the coils together.

Mitchell of Belfast advises exposing the varices at numerous points by half-inch incisions, and, after clamping the vein between two pairs of forceps, cutting it across and twisting out the segments of the vein between adjacent incisions. The edges of the incisions are sutured; and the limb is firmly bandaged from below upwards, and kept in an elevated position. We have employed this method with satisfactory results.

The treatment of the complications of varix has already been considered.

ANGIOMA[4]

[4] In the description of angiomas we have followed the teaching of the late John Duncan.

Tumours of blood vessels may be divided, according to the nature of the vessels of which they are composed, into the capillary, the venous, and the arterial angiomas.

CAPILLARY ANGIOMA

The most common form of capillary angioma is the nævus or congenital telangiectasis.

Nævus.—A nævus is a collection of dilated capillaries, the afferent arterioles and the efferent venules of which often share in the dilatation. Little is known regarding the *etiology* of nævi beyond the fact that they are of congenital origin. They often escape notice until the child is some days old, but attention is usually drawn to them within a fortnight of birth. For practical purposes the most useful classification of nævi is into the cutaneous, the subcutaneous, and the mixed forms.

The cutaneous nævus, "mother's mark," or "port-wine stain," consists of an aggregation of dilated capillaries in the substance of the skin. On stretching the skin the vessels can be seen to form a fine network, or to run in leashes parallel to one another. A dilated arteriole or a vein winding about among the capillaries may sometimes be detected. These nævi occur on any part of the body, but they are most frequently met with on the face. They may be multiple, and vary greatly in size, some being no bigger than a pin-head, while others cover large areas of the body. In colour they present every tint from purple to brilliant red; in the majority there is a considerable dash of blue, especially in cold weather.

Unlike the other forms of nævi, the cutaneous variety shows little tendency to disappear, and it is especially persistent when associated with overgrowth of the epidermis and of the hairs—*nævoid mole.*

The *treatment* of the cutaneous nævus is unsatisfactory, owing to the difficulty of removing the nævus without leaving a scar which is even more disfiguring. Very small nævi may be destroyed by a fine pointed Paquelin thermo-cautery, or by escharotics, such as nitric acid. For larger nævi, radium and solidified carbon dioxide ("CO_2 snow") may be used. The extensive port-wine stains so often met with on the face are best left alone.

The *subcutaneous nævus* is comparatively rare. It constitutes a well-defined, localised tumour, which may possess a distinct capsule, especially when it has ceased to grow or is retrogressing. On section, it presents the appearance of a finely reticulated sponge.

Although it may be noticed at, or within a few days of, birth, a subcutaneous nævus is often overlooked, especially when on a covered part of the body, and may not be discovered till the patient is some years old. It forms a rounded, lobulated swelling, seldom of large size and yielding a sensation like that of a sponge; the skin over it is normal, or may exhibit a bluish tinge, especially in cold weather. In some cases the tumour is diminished by pressing the blood out of it, but slowly fills again when the pressure is relaxed, and it swells up when the child struggles or cries. From a cold abscess it is diagnosed by the history and progress of the swelling and by the absence of fluctuation. When situated over one of the hernial openings, it closely simulates a hernia; and when it occurs in the middle line of the face, head, or back, it may be mistaken for such other congenital conditions as meningocele or spina bifida. When other means fail, the use of an exploring needle clears up the diagnosis.

Mixed Nævus.—As its name indicates, the mixed nævus partakes of the characters of the other two varieties; that is, it is a subcutaneous nævus with involvement of the skin.

It is frequently met with on the face and head, but may occur on any part of the body. It also affects parts covered by mucous membrane, such as the cheek, tongue, and soft palate. The swelling is rounded or lobulated, and projects beyond the level of its surroundings. Sometimes the skin is invaded by the nævoid tissue over the whole extent of the tumour, sometimes only over a limited area. Frequently the margin only is of a bright-red colour, while the skin in the centre resembles a cicatrix. The swelling is reduced by steady pressure, and increases in size and becomes tense when the child cries.

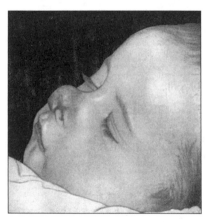

FIG. 68. Mixed Nævus of Nose which was subsequently cured by Electrolysis.

Prognosis.—The rate of growth of the subcutaneous and mixed forms of nævi varies greatly. They sometimes increase rapidly, especially during the first few months of life; after this they usually grow at the same rate as the child, or more slowly. There is a decided tendency to disappearance of these varieties, fully 50 per cent. undergoing natural cure by a process of obliteration, similar to the obliteration of vessels in cicatricial tissue. This usually begins about the period of the first dentition, sometimes at the second dentition, and sometimes at puberty. On the other hand, an increased activity of growth may be shown at these periods. The onset of natural cure is recognised by the tumour becoming firmer and less compressible, and, in the mixed variety, by the colour becoming less bright. Injury, infection, or ulceration of the overlying skin may initiate the curative process.

Towards adult life the spaces in a subcutaneous nævus may become greatly enlarged, leading to the formation of a cavernous angioma.

Treatment.—In view of the frequency with which subcutaneous and mixed nævi disappear spontaneously, interference is only called for when the growth of the tumour is out of proportion to that of the child, or when, from its situation—for example in the vicinity of the eye—any marked increase in its size would render it less amenable to treatment.

The methods of treatment most generally applicable are the use of radium and carbon dioxide snow, igni-puncture, electrolysis, and excision.

For nævi situated on exposed parts, where it is desirable to avoid a scar, the use of *radium* is to be preferred. The tube of radium is applied at intervals to different parts of the nævus, the duration and frequency of the applications varying with the strength of the emanations and the reaction produced. The object aimed at is to induce obliteration of the nævoid tissue by cicatricial contraction without destroying the overlying skin. *Carbon-dioxide snow* may be employed in the same manner, but the results are inferior to those obtained by radium.

Igni-puncture consists in making a number of punctures at different parts of the nævus with a fine-pointed thermo-cautery, with the object of starting at each point a process of cicatrisation which extends throughout the nævoid tissue and so obliterates the vessels.

Electrolysis acts by decomposing the blood and tissues into their constituent elements—oxygen and acids appearing at the positive, hydrogen and bases at the negative electrode. These substances and gases being given off in a nascent condition, at once enter into new combinations with anything in the vicinity with which they have a chemical affinity. In the nævus the practical result of this reaction is that at the positive pole nitric acid, and at the negative pole caustic potash, both in a state of minute subdivision, make their appearance. The effect on the tissues around the positive pole, therefore, is equivalent to that of an acid cauterisation, and on those round the negative pole, to an alkaline cauterisation.

As the process is painful, a general anæsthetic is necessary. The current used should be from 20 to 80 milliampères, gradually increasing from zero, without shock; three to six large Bunsen cells give a sufficient current, and no galvanometer is required. Steel needles, insulated with vulcanite to within an eighth of an inch of their points, are the best. Both poles are introduced into the nævus, the positive being kept fixed at one spot, while the negative is moved about so as to produce a number of different tracks of cauterisation. On no account must either pole be allowed to come in contact with the skin, lest a slough be formed. The duration of the sitting is determined by the effect produced, as indicated by the hardening of the tumour, the average duration being from fifteen to twenty minutes. If pallor of the skin appears, it indicates that the needles are too near the surface, or that the blood supply to the integument is being cut off, and is an indication to stop. To cauterise the track and so prevent bleeding, the needles should be slowly withdrawn while the current is flowing. When the skin is reached the current is turned off. The punctures are covered with collodion. Six or eight weeks should be allowed to elapse before repeating the procedure. From two to eight or ten sittings may be necessary, according to the size and character of the nævus.

Excision is to be preferred for nævi of moderate size situated on covered parts of the body, where a scar is of no importance. Its chief advantages over electrolysis are that a single operation is sufficient, and that the cure is speedy and certain. The operation is attended with much less hæmorrhage than might be expected.

Cavernous Angioma.—This form of angioma consists of a series of large blood spaces which are usually derived from the dilatation of the capillaries of a subcutaneous nævus. The spaces come to communicate freely with one another by the disappearance of adjacent capillary walls. While the most common situation is in the subcutaneous tissue, a cavernous angioma is sometimes met with in internal organs. It may appear at any age from early youth to middle life, and is of slow growth and may become stationary. The swelling is rounded or oval, there is no pulsation or bruit, and the tumour is but slightly compressible. The treatment consists in dissecting it out.

Aneurysm by Anastomosis is the name applied to a vascular tumour in which the arteries, veins, and capillaries are all involved. It is met with chiefly on the upper part of the trunk, the neck, and the scalp. It tends gradually to increase in size, and may, after many years, attain an enormous size. The tumour is ill-defined, and varies in consistence. It is pulsatile, and a systolic bruit or a "thrilling" murmur may be heard over it. The chief risk is hæmorrhage from injury or ulceration.

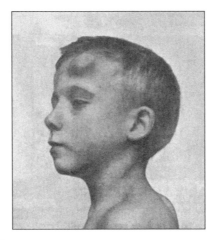

FIG. 69. Cirsoid Aneurysm of Forehead in a boy æt. 10. (Mr. J. W. Dowden's case.)

The *treatment* is conducted on the same lines as for nævus. When electrolysis is employed, it should be directed towards the afferent vessels; and if it fails to arrest the flow through these, it is useless to persist with it. In some cases ligation of the afferent vessels has been successful.

Arterial Angioma or **Cirsoid Aneurysm.**—This is composed of the enlarged branches of an arterial trunk. It originates in the smaller branches of an artery—usually the temporal—and may spread to the main trunk, and may even involve branches of other trunks with which the affected artery anastomoses.

The condition is probably congenital in origin, though its appearance is frequently preceded by an injury. It almost invariably occurs in the scalp, and is usually met with in adolescent young adults.

The affected vessels slowly increase in size, and become tortuous, with narrowings and dilatations here and there. Grooves and gutters are frequently found in the bone underlying the dilated vessels.

There is a constant loud bruit in the tumour, which greatly troubles the patient and may interfere with sleep. There is no tendency either to natural cure or to rupture, but severe and even fatal hæmorrhage may follow a wound of the dilated vessels.

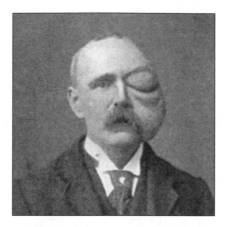

FIG. 70. Cirsoid Aneurysm of Orbit and Face, which developed after a blow on the Orbit with a cricket ball. (From a photograph lent by Sir Montagu Cotterill.)

The condition may be treated by excision or by electrolysis. In excision the hæmorrhage is controlled by an elastic tourniquet applied horizontally round the head, or by ligation of the feeding trunks. In large tumours the bleeding is formidable. In many cases electrolysis is to be preferred, and is performed in the same way as for nævus. The positive pole is placed in the centre of the tumour, while the negative is introduced into the main affluents one after another.

ANEURYSM

An aneurysm is a sac communicating with an artery, and containing fluid or coagulated blood.

Two types are met with—the pathological and the traumatic. It is convenient to describe in this section also certain conditions in which there is an abnormal communication between an artery and a vein—arterio-venous aneurysm.

PATHOLOGICAL ANEURYSM

In this class are included such dilatations as result from weakening of the arterial coats, combined, in most cases, with a loss of elasticity in the walls and increase in the arterial tension due to arterio-sclerosis. In some cases the vessel wall is softened by arteritis—especially the embolic form—so that it yields before the pressure of the blood.

Repeated and sudden raising of the arterial tension, as a result, for example, of violent muscular efforts or of excessive indulgence in alcohol, plays an important part in the causation of aneurysm. These factors probably explain the comparative frequency of aneurysm in those who follow such arduous occupations as soldiers, sailors, dock-labourers, and navvies. In these classes the condition usually manifests itself between the ages of thirty and fifty— that is, when the vessels are beginning to degenerate, although the heart is still vigorous and the men are hard at work. The comparative immunity of women may also be explained by the less severe muscular strain involved by their occupations and recreations.

Syphilis plays an important part in the production of aneurysm, probably by predisposing the patient to arterio-sclerosis and atheroma, and inducing an increase in the vascular tension in the peripheral vessels, from loss of elasticity of the vessel wall and narrowing of the lumen as a result of syphilitic arteritis. It is a striking fact that aneurysm is seldom met with in women who have not suffered from syphilis.

Varieties—Fusiform Aneurysm.—When the *whole circumference* of an artery has been weakened, the tension of the blood causes the walls to dilate uniformly, so that a fusiform or tubular aneurysm results. All the coats of the vessel are stretched and form the sac of the aneurysm, and the affected portion is not only dilated but is also increased in length. This form is chiefly met with in the arch of the aorta, but may occur in any of the main arterial trunks. As the sac of the aneurysm includes all three coats, and as the inner and outer coats are usually thickened by the deposit in them of connective tissue, this variety increases in size slowly and seldom gives rise to urgent symptoms.

As a rule a fusiform aneurysm contains fluid blood, but when the intima is roughened by disease, especially in the form of calcareous plates, shreds of clot may adhere to it.

It has little tendency to natural cure, although this is occasionally effected by the emerging artery becoming occluded by a clot; it has also little tendency to rupture.

Sacculated Aneurysm.—When a *limited area* of the vessel wall is weakened— for example by atheroma or by other form of arteritis—this portion yields before the pressure of the blood, and a sacculated aneurysm results. The internal and middle coats being already damaged, or, it may be, destroyed, by the primary disease, the stress falls on the external coat, which in the majority of cases constitutes the sac. To withstand the pressure the external coat becomes thickened, and as the aneurysm increases in size it forms adhesions to surrounding tissues, so that fasciæ, tendons, nerves, and other structures may be found matted together in its wall. The wall is further strengthened by the deposit on its inner aspect of blood-clot, which may eventually become organised.

The contents of the sac consist of fluid blood and a varying amount of clot which is deposited in concentric layers on the inner aspect of the sac, where it forms a pale, striated, firm mass, which constitutes a laminated clot. Near the blood-current the clot is soft, red, and friable (Fig. 72). The laminated clot not only strengthens the sac, enabling it to resist the blood-pressure and so prevent rupture, but, if it increases sufficiently to fill the cavity, may bring about cure. The principle upon which all methods of treatment are based is to imitate nature in producing such a clot.

Sacculated aneurysm, as compared with the fusiform variety, tends to rupture and also to cure by the formation of laminated clot; natural cure is sometimes all but complete when extension and rupture occur and cause death.

An aneurysm is said to be *diffused* when the sac ruptures and the blood escapes into the cellular tissue.

Clinical Features of Aneurysm.—Surgically, the sacculated is by far the most important variety. The outstanding feature is the existence in the line of an artery of a globular swelling, which pulsates. The pulsation is of an expansile character, which is detected by observing that when both hands are placed over the swelling they are separated with each beat of the heart. If the main artery be compressed on the cardiac side of the swelling, the pulsation is arrested and the tumour becomes smaller and less tense, and it may be still further reduced in size by gentle pressure being made over it so as to empty it of fluid blood. On allowing the blood again to flow through the artery, the pulsation returns at once, but several beats are required before the sac regains its former size. In most cases a distinct thrill is felt on placing the hand over the swelling, and a blowing, systolic murmur may be heard with the stethoscope. It is to be borne in mind that occasionally, when the interchange of blood between an aneurysm and the artery from which it arises is small, pulsation and bruit may be slight or even absent. This is also the case when the sac contains a considerable quantity of clot. When it becomes filled with clot—*consolidated aneurysm*—these signs disappear, and the clinical features are those of a solid tumour lying in contact with an artery, and transmitting its pulsation.

A comparison of the pulse in the artery beyond the seat of the aneurysm with that in the corresponding artery on the healthy side, shows that on the affected side the wave is smaller in volume, and delayed in time. A pulse tracing shows that the normal impulse and dicrotic waves are lost, and that the force and rapidity of the tidal wave are diminished.

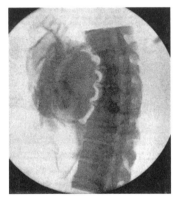

FIG. 71. Radiogram of Aneurysm of Aorta, showing laminated clot and erosion of bodies of vertebræ. The intervertebral discs are intact.

An aneurysm exerts pressure on the surrounding structures, which are usually thickened and adherent to it and to one another. Adjacent veins may be so compressed that congestion and oedema of the parts beyond are produced. Pain, disturbances of sensation, and muscular paralyses may result from pressure on nerves. Such bones as the sternum and vertebræ undergo erosion and are absorbed by the gradually increasing pressure of the aneurysm. Cartilage, on the other hand, being elastic, yields before the pressure, so that the intervertebral discs or the costal cartilages may escape while the adjacent bones are destroyed (Fig. 71). The skin over the tumour becomes thinned and stretched, until finally a slough forms, and when it separates hæmorrhage takes place.

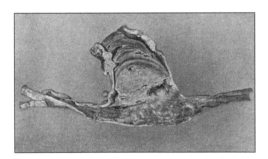

FIG. 72. Sacculated Aneurysm of Abdominal Aorta nearly filled with laminated clot. Note greater density of clot towards periphery.

In the progress of an aneurysm towards rupture, timely clotting may avert death for the moment, but while extension in one direction has been arrested there is apt to be extension in another, with imminence of rupture, or it may be again postponed.

Differential Diagnosis.—The diagnosis is to be made from other pulsatile swellings. Pulsation is sometimes transmitted from a large artery to a tumour, a mass of enlarged lymph glands, or an inflammatory swelling which lies in its vicinity, but the pulsation is not expansile—a most important point in differential diagnosis. Such swellings may, by appropriate manipulation, be moved from the artery and the pulsation ceases, and compression of the artery on the cardiac side of the swelling, although it arrests the pulsation, does not produce any diminution in the size or tension of the swelling, and when the pressure is removed the pulsation is restored immediately.

Fluid swellings overlying an artery, such as cysts, abscesses, or enlarged bursæ, may closely simulate aneurysm. An apparent expansion may accompany the pulsation, but careful examination usually enables this to be distinguished from the true expansion of an aneurysm. Compression of the artery makes no difference in the size or tension of the swelling.

Vascular tumours, such as sarcoma and goitre, may yield an expansile pulsation and a soft, whiffling bruit, but they differ from an aneurysm in that they are not diminished in size by compression of the main artery, nor can they be emptied by pressure.

The exaggerated pulsation sometimes observed in the abdominal aorta, the "pulsating aorta" seen in women, should not be mistaken for aneurysm.

Prognosis.—When *natural cure* occurs it is usually brought about by the formation of laminated clot, which gradually increases in amount till it fills the sac. Sometimes a portion of the clot in the sac is separated and becomes impacted as an embolus in the artery beyond, leading to thrombosis which first occludes the artery and then extends into the sac.

The progress of natural cure is indicated by the aneurysm becoming smaller, firmer, less expansile, and less compressible; the murmur and thrill diminish and the pressure effects become less marked. When the cure is complete the expansile pulsation is lost, and there remains a firm swelling attached to the vessel (*consolidated aneurysm*). While these changes are taking place the collateral arteries become enlarged, and an anastomotic circulation is established.

An aneurysm may prove *fatal* by exerting pressure on important structures, by causing syncope, by rupture, or from the occurrence of suppuration. *Pressure* symptoms are usually most serious from aneurysms situated in the neck, thorax, or skull. Sudden fatal *syncope* is not infrequent in cases of aneurysm of the thoracic aorta.

Rupture may take place through the skin, on a mucous or serous surface, or into the cellular tissue. The first hæmorrhage is often slight and stops naturally, but it soon recurs, and is so profuse, especially when the blood escapes externally, that it rapidly proves fatal. When the bleeding takes place into the cellular tissue, the aneurysm is said to become *diffused*, and the extravasated blood spreads widely through the tissues, exerting great pressure on the surrounding structures.

The *clinical features* associated with rupture are sudden and severe pain in the part, and the patient becomes pale, cold, and faint. If a comparatively small escape of blood takes place into the tissues, the sudden alteration in the size, shape, and tension of the aneurysm, together with loss of pulsation, may be the only local signs. When the bleeding is profuse, however, the parts beyond the aneurysm become greatly swollen, livid, and cold, and the pulse beyond is completely lost. The arrest of the blood supply may result in gangrene. Sometimes the pressure of the extravasated blood causes the skin to slough and, later, give way, and fatal hæmorrhage results.

The *treatment* is carried out on the same lines as for a ruptured artery (p. 261), it being remembered, however, that the artery is diseased and does not lend itself to reconstructive procedures.

Suppuration may occur in the vicinity of an aneurysm, and the aneurysm may burst into the abscess which forms, so that when the latter points the pus is mixed with broken-down blood-clot, and finally free hæmorrhage takes place. It has more than once happened that a surgeon has incised such an abscess without having recognised its association with aneurysm, with tragic results.

Treatment.—In treating an aneurysm, the indications are to imitate Nature's method of cure by means of laminated clot.

Constitutional treatment consists in taking measures to reduce the arterial tension and to diminish the force of the heart's action. The patient must be kept in bed. A dry and non-stimulating diet is indicated, the quantity being gradually reduced till it is just sufficient to maintain nutrition. Saline purges are employed to reduce the vascular tension. The benefit derived from potassium iodide administered in full doses, as first recommended by George W. Balfour, probably depends on its depressing action on the heart and its therapeutic benefit in syphilis. Pain or restlessness may call for the use of opiates, of which heroin is the most efficient.

Local Treatment.—When constitutional treatment fails, local measures must be adopted, and many methods are available.

Endo-aneurysmorrhaphy.—The operation devised by Rudolf Matas in 1888 aims at closing the opening between the sac and its feeding artery, and in addition, folding the wall of the sac in such a way as to leave no vacant space. If there is marked disease of the vessel, Matas' operation is not possible and recourse is then had to ligation of the artery just above the sac.

Extirpation of the Sac—The Old Operation.—The procedure which goes by this name consists in exposing the aneurysm, incising the sac, clearing out the clots, and ligating the artery above and below the sac. This method is suitable to sacculated aneurysm of the limbs, so long as they are circumscribed and free from complications. It has been successfully practised also in aneurysm of the subclavian, carotid, and external iliac arteries. It is not applicable to cases in which there is such a degree of atheroma as would interfere with the successful ligation of the artery. The continuity of the artery may be restored by grafting into the gap left after excision of the sac a segment of the great saphena vein.

Ligation of the Artery.—The object of tying the artery is to diminish or to arrest the flow of blood through the aneurysm so that the blood coagulates both in the sac and in the feeding artery. The ligature may be applied on the cardiac side of the aneurysm—proximal ligation, or to the artery beyond—distal ligation.

Proximal Ligation.—The ligature may be applied immediately above the sac (Anel, 1710) or at a distance above (John Hunter, 1785). The *Hunterian operation* ensures that the ligature is applied to a part of the artery that is presumably healthy and where relations are undisturbed by the proximity of the sac; the best example is the ligation of the superficial femoral artery in Scarpa's triangle or in Hunter's canal for popliteal aneurysm; it is on record that Syme performed this operation with cure of the aneurysm on thirty-nine occasions.

It is to be noted that the Hunterian ligature does not aim at *arresting* the flow of blood through the sac, but is designed so to diminish its volume and force as to favour the deposition within the sac of laminated clot. The development of the collateral circulation which follows upon ligation of the artery at a distance above the sac may be attended with just that amount of return stream which favours the deposit of laminated clot, and consequently the cure of the aneurysm; the return stream may, however, be so forcible as to prevent coagulation of the blood in the sac, or only to allow of the formation of a red thrombus which may in its turn be dispersed so that pulsation in the sac recurs. This does not necessarily imply failure to cure, as the recurrent pulsation may only be temporary; the formation of laminated clot may ultimately take place and lead to consolidation of the aneurysm.

The least desirable result of the Hunterian ligature is met with in cases where, owing to widespread arterial disease, the collateral circulation does not develop and gangrene of the limb supervenes.

Anel's ligature is only practised as part of the operation which deals with the sac directly.

Distal Ligation.—The tying of the artery beyond the sac, or of its two branches where it bifurcates (Brasdor, 1760, and Wardrop, 1825), may arrest or only diminish the flow of blood through the sac. It is less successful than the proximal ligature, and is therefore restricted to aneurysms so situated as not to be amenable to other methods; for example, in aneurysm of the common carotid near its origin, the artery may be ligated near its bifurcation, or in aneurysm of the innominate artery, the carotid and subclavian arteries are tied at the seat of election.

Compression.—Digital compression of the feeding artery has been given up except as a preparation for operations on the sac with a view to favouring the development of a collateral circulation.

Macewen's acupuncture or "needling" consists in passing one or more fine, highly tempered steel needles through the tissues overlying the aneurysm, and through its outer wall. The needles are made to touch the opposite wall of the sac, and the pulsation of the aneurysm imparts a movement to them which causes them to scarify the inner surface of the sac. White thrombus forms on the rough surface produced, and leads to further coagulation. The needles may be left in position for some hours, being shifted from time to time, the projecting ends being surrounded with sterile gauze.

The *Moore-Corradi method* consists in introducing through the wall of the aneurysm a hollow insulated needle, through the lumen of which from 10 to 20 feet of highly drawn silver or other wire is passed into the sac, where it coils up into an open meshwork (Fig. 73). The positive pole of a galvanic battery is attached to the wire, and the negative pole placed over the patient's back. A current, varying in strength from 20 to 70 milliampères, is allowed to flow for about an hour. The hollow needle is then withdrawn, but the wire is left *in situ*. The results are somewhat similar to those obtained by needling, but the clot formed on the large coil of wire is more extensive.

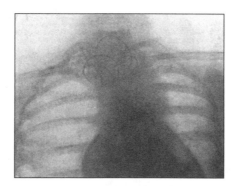

FIG. 73. Radiogram of Innominate Aneurysm after treatment by the Moore-Corradi method. Two feet of finely drawn silver wire were introduced. The patient, a woman, æt. 47, lived for ten months after operation, free from pain (cf. Fig. 75).

Colt's method of wiring has been mainly used in the treatment of abdominal aneurysm; gilt wire in the form of a wisp is introduced through the cannula and expands into an umbrella shape.

Subcutaneous Injections of Gelatin.—Three or four ounces of a 2 per cent. solution of white gelatin in sterilised water, at a temperature of about 100° F., are injected into the subcutaneous tissue of the abdomen every two, three, or four days. In the course of a fortnight or three weeks improvement may begin. The clot which forms is liable to soften and be absorbed, but a repetition of the injection has in several cases established a permanent cure.

Amputation of the limb is indicated in cases complicated by suppuration, by secondary hæmorrhage after excision or ligation, or by gangrene. Amputation at the shoulder was performed by Fergusson in a case of subclavian aneurysm, as a means of arresting the blood-flow through the sac.

TRAUMATIC ANEURYSM

The essential feature of a traumatic aneurysm is that it is produced by some form of injury which divides all the coats of the artery. The walls of the injured vessel are presumably healthy, but they form no part of the sac of the aneurysm. The sac consists of the condensed and thickened tissues around the artery.

The injury to the artery may be a subcutaneous one such as a tear by a fragment of bone: much more commonly it is a punctured wound from a stab or from a bullet.

The aneurysm usually forms soon after the injury is inflicted; the blood slowly escapes into the surrounding tissues, gradually displacing and condensing them, until they form a sac enclosing the effused blood.

Less frequently a traumatic aneurysm forms some considerable time after the injury, from gradual stretching of the fibrous cicatrix by which the wound in the wall of the artery has been closed. The gradual stretching of this cicatrix results in condensation of the surrounding structures which form the sac, on the inner aspect of which laminated clot is deposited.

A traumatic aneurysm is almost always sacculated, and, so long as it remains circumscribed, has the same characters as a pathological sacculated aneurysm, with the addition that there is a scar in the overlying skin. A traumatic aneurysm is liable to become diffuse—a change which, although attended with considerable risk of gangrene, has sometimes been the means of bringing about a cure.

The treatment is governed by the same principles as apply to the pathological varieties, but as the walls of the artery are not diseased, operative measures dealing with the sac and the adjacent segment of the affected artery are to be preferred.

ARTERIO-VENOUS ANEURYSM

An abnormal communication between an artery and a vein constitutes an arterio-venous aneurysm. Two varieties are recognised—one in which the communication is direct—*aneurysmal varix*; the other in which the vein communicates with the artery through the medium of a sac—*varicose aneurysm*.

Either variety may result from pathological causes, but in the majority of cases they are traumatic in origin, being due to such injuries as stabs, punctured wounds, and gun-shot injuries which involve both artery and vein. In former times the most common situation was at the bend of the elbow, the brachial artery being accidentally punctured in blood-letting from the median basilic vein. Arterio-venous aneurysm is a frequent result of injuries by modern high-velocity bullets—for example, in the neck or groin.

In *aneurysmal varix* the higher blood pressure in the artery forces arterial blood into the vein, which near the point of communication with the artery tends to become dilated, and to form a thick-walled sac, beyond which the vessel and its tributaries are distended and tortuous. The clinical features resemble those associated with varicose veins, but the entrance of arterial blood into the dilated veins causes them to pulsate, and produces in them a vibratory thrill and a loud murmur. In those at the groin, the distension of the veins may be so great that they look like sinuses running through the muscles, a feature that must be taken into account in any operation.

As the condition tends to remain stationary, the support of an elastic bandage is all that is required; but when the condition progresses and causes serious inconvenience, it may be necessary to cut down and expose the communication between the artery and vein, and, after separating the vessels, to close the opening in each by suture; this may be difficult or impossible if the parts are matted from former suppuration. If it is impossible thus to obliterate the communication, the artery should be ligated above and below the point of communication; although the risk of gangrene is considerable unless means are taken to develop the collateral circulation beforehand (Makins).

Varicose aneurysm usually develops in relation to a traumatic aneurysm, the sac becoming adherent to an adjacent vein, and ultimately opening into it. In this way a communication between the artery and the vein is established, and the clinical features are those of a combination of aneurysm and aneurysmal varix.

As there is little tendency to spontaneous cure, and as the aneurysm is liable to increase in size and finally to rupture, operative treatment is usually called for. This is carried out on the same lines as for aneurysmal varix, and at the same time incising the sac, turning out the clots, and ligating any branches which open into the sac. If it can be avoided, the vein should not be ligated.

ANEURYSMS OF INDIVIDUAL ARTERIES

Thoracic Aneurysm.—All varieties of aneurysm occur in the aorta, the fusiform being the most common, although a sacculated aneurysm frequently springs from a fusiform dilatation.

The *clinical features* depend chiefly on the direction in which the aneurysm enlarges, and are not always well marked even when the sac is of considerable size. They consist in a pulsatile swelling—sometimes in the supra-sternal notch, but usually towards the right side of the sternum—with an increased area of dulness on percussion. With the X-rays a dark shadow is seen corresponding to the sac. Pain is usually a prominent symptom, and is largely referable to the pressure of the aneurysm on the vertebræ or the sternum, causing erosion of these bones. Pressure on the thoracic veins and on the air-passage causes cyanosis and dyspnoea. When the oesophagus is pressed upon, the patient may have difficulty in swallowing. The left recurrent nerve may be stretched or pressed upon as it hooks round the arch of the aorta, and hoarseness of the voice and a characteristic "brassy" cough may result from paralysis of the muscles of the larynx which it supplies. The vagus, the phrenic, and the spinal nerves may also be pressed upon. When the aneurysm is on the transverse part of the arch, the trachea is pulled down with each beat of the heart—a clinical phenomena known as the "tracheal tug." Aneurysm of the descending aorta may, after eroding the bodies of the vertebræ (Fig. 71) and posterior portions of the ribs, form a swelling in the back to the left of the spine.

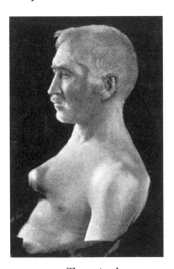

FIG. 74. Thoracic Aneurysm, threatening to rupture externally, but prevented from doing so by Macewen's needling. The needles were left in for forty-eight hours.

Inasmuch as obliteration of the sac and the feeding artery is out of the question, surgical treatment is confined to causing coagulation of the blood in an extension or pouching of the sac, which, making its way through the parietes of the chest, threatens to rupture externally. This may be achieved by Macewen's needles or by the introduction of wire into the sac. We have had cases under observation in which the treatment referred to has been followed by such an amount of improvement that the patient has been able to resume a laborious occupation for one or more years. Christopher Heath found that improvement followed ligation of the left common carotid in aneurysm of the transverse part of the aortic arch.

Abdominal Aneurysm.—Aneurysm is much less frequent in the abdominal than in the thoracic aorta. While any of the large branches in the abdomen may be affected, the most common seats are in the aorta itself, just above the origin of the coeliac artery and at the bifurcation.

The *clinical features* vary with the site of the aneurysm and with its rapidity and direction of growth. A smooth, rounded swelling, which exhibits expansile pulsation, forms, usually towards the left of the middle line. It may extend upwards under cover of the ribs, downwards towards the pelvis, or backward towards the loin. On palpation a systolic thrill may be detected, but the presence of a murmur is neither constant nor characteristic. Pain is usually present; it may be neuralgic in character, or may simulate renal colic. When the aneurysm presses on the vertebræ and erodes them, the symptoms simulate those of spinal caries, particularly if, as sometimes happens, symptoms of compression paraplegia ensue. In its growth the swelling may press upon and displace the adjacent viscera, and so interfere with their functions.

The *diagnosis* has to be made from solid or cystic tumours overlying the artery; from a "pulsating aorta"; and from spinal caries; much help is obtained by the use of the X-rays.

The condition usually proves fatal, either by the aneurysm bursting into the peritoneal cavity, or by slow leakage into the retro-peritoneal tissue.

The Moore-Corradi method has been successfully employed, access to the sac having been obtained by opening the abdomen. Ligation of the aorta has so far been unsuccessful, but in one case operated upon by Keen the patient survived forty-eight days.

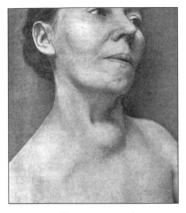

FIG. 75. Innominate Aneurysm in a woman, æt. 47, eight months after treatment by Moore-Corradi method (cf. Fig. 73).

Innominate aneurysm may be of the fusiform or of the sacculated variety, and is frequently associated with pouching of the aorta. It usually grows upwards and laterally, projecting above the sternum and right clavicle, which may be eroded or displaced (Fig. 75). Symptoms of pressure on the structures in the neck, similar to those produced by aortic aneurysm, occur. The pulses in the right upper extremity and in the right carotid and its branches are diminished and delayed. Pressure on the right brachial plexus causes shooting pain down the arm and muscular paresis on that side. Vaso-motor disturbances and contraction of the pupil on the right side may result from pressure on the sympathetic. Death may take place from rupture, or from pressure on the air-passage.

The available methods of treatment are ligation of the right common carotid and third part of the right subclavian (Wardrop's operation), of which a number of successful cases have been recorded. Those most suitable for ligation are cases in which the aneurysm is circumscribed and globular (Sheen). If ligation is found to be impracticable, the Moore-Corradi method or Macewen's needling may be tried.

Carotid Aneurysms.—Aneurysm of the *common carotid* is more frequent on the right than on the left side, and is usually situated either at the root of the neck or near the bifurcation. It is the aneurysm most frequently met with in women. From its position the swelling is liable to press on the vagus, recurrent and sympathetic nerves, on the air-passage, and on the oesophagus, giving rise to symptoms referable to such pressure. There may be cerebral symptoms from interference with the blood supply of the brain.

Aneurysm near the origin has to be diagnosed from subclavian, innominate, and aortic aneurysm, and from other swellings—solid or fluid—met with in the neck. It is often difficult to determine with precision the trunk from which an aneurysm at the root of the neck originates, and not infrequently more than one vessel shares in the dilatation. A careful consideration of the position in which the swelling first appeared, of the direction in which it has progressed, of its pressure effects, and of the condition of the pulses beyond, may help in distinguishing between aortic, innominate, carotid, and subclavian aneurysms. Skiagraphy is also of assistance in recognising the vessel involved.

Tumours of the thyroid, enlarged lymph glands, and fatty and sarcomatous tumours can usually be distinguished from aneurysm by the history of the swelling and by physical examination. Cystic tumours and abscesses in the neck are sometimes more difficult to differentiate on account of the apparently expansile character of the pulsation transmitted to them. The fact that compression of the vessel does not affect the size and tension of these fluid swellings is useful in distinguishing them from aneurysm.

Treatment.—Digital compression of the vessel against the transverse process of the sixth cervical vertebra—the "carotid tubercle"—has been successfully employed in the treatment of aneurysm near the bifurcation. Proximal ligation in the case of high aneurysms, or distal ligation in those situated at the root of the neck, is more certain. Extirpation of the sac is probably the best method of treatment, especially in those of traumatic origin. These operations are attended with considerable risk of hemiplegia from interference with the blood supply of the brain.

The *external carotid* and the cervical portion of the *internal carotid* are seldom the primary seat of aneurysm, although they are liable to be implicated by the upward spread of an aneurysm at the bifurcation of the common trunk. In addition to the ordinary signs of aneurysm, the clinical manifestations are chiefly referable to pressure on the pharynx and larynx, and on the hypoglossal nerve. Aneurysm of the internal carotid is of special importance on account of the way in which it bulges into the pharynx in the region of the tonsil, in some cases closely simulating a tonsillar abscess. Cases are on record in which such an aneurysm has been mistaken for an abscess and incised, with disastrous results.

Aneurysmal varix may occur in the neck as a result of stabs or bullet wounds. The communication is usually between the common carotid artery and the internal jugular vein. The resulting interference with the cerebral circulation causes headache, giddiness, and other brain symptoms, and a persistent loud murmur is usually a source of annoyance to the patient and may be sufficient indication for operative treatment.

Intracranial aneurysm involves the internal carotid and its branches, or the basilar artery, and appears to be more frequently associated with syphilis and with valvular disease of the heart than are external aneurysms. It gives rise to symptoms similar to those of other intracranial tumours, and there is sometimes a loud murmur. It usually proves fatal by rupture, and intracranial hæmorrhage. The treatment is to ligate the common carotid or the vertebral artery in the neck, according to the seat of the aneurysm.

Orbital Aneurysm.—The term pulsating exophthalmos is employed to embrace a number of pathological conditions, including aneurysm, in which the chief symptoms are pulsation in the orbit and protrusion of the eyeball. There may be, in addition, congestion and oedema of the eyelids, and a distinct thrill and murmur, which can be controlled by compression of the common carotid in the neck. Varying degrees of ocular paralysis and of interference with vision may also be present.

These symptoms are due, in the majority of cases, to an aneurysmal varix of the internal carotid artery and cavernous sinus, which is often traumatic in origin, being produced either by fracture of the base of the skull or by a punctured wound of the orbit. In other cases they are due to aneurysm of the ophthalmic artery, to thrombosis of the cavernous sinus, and, in rare instances, to cirsoid aneurysm.

If compression of the common carotid is found to arrest the pulsation, ligation of this vessel is indicated.

Subclavian Aneurysm.—Subclavian aneurysm is usually met with in men who follow occupations involving constant use of the shoulder—for example, dock-porters and coal-heavers. It is more common on the right side.

The aneurysm usually springs from the third part of the artery, and appears as a tense, rounded, pulsatile swelling just above the clavicle and to the outer side of the sterno-mastoid muscle. It occasionally extends towards the thorax, where it may become adherent to the pleura. The radial pulse on the same side is small and delayed. Congestion and oedema of the arm, with pain, numbness, and muscular weakness, may result from pressure on the veins and nerves as they pass under the clavicle; and pressure on the phrenic nerve may induce hiccough. The aneurysm is of slow growth, and occasionally undergoes spontaneous cure.

The conditions most likely to be mistaken for it are a soft, rapidly growing sarcoma, and a normal artery raised on a cervical rib.

On account of the relations of the artery and of its branches, treatment is attended with greater difficulty and danger in subclavian than in almost any other form of external aneurysm. The available operative measures are proximal ligation of the innominate, and distal ligation. In some cases it has been found necessary to combine distal ligation with amputation at the shoulder-joint, to prevent the collateral circulation maintaining the flow through the aneurysm. Matas' operation has been successfully performed by Hogarth Pringle.

Axillary Aneurysm.—This is usually met with in the right arm of labouring men and sailors, and not infrequently follows an injury in the region of the shoulder. The vessel may be damaged by the head of a dislocated humerus or in attempts to reduce the dislocation, by the fragments of a fractured bone, or by a stab or cut. Sometimes the vein also is injured and an arterio-venous aneurysm established.

Owing to the laxity of the tissues, it increases rapidly, and it may soon attain a large size, filling up the axilla, and displacing the clavicle upwards. This renders compression of the third part of the subclavian difficult or impossible. It may extend beneath the clavicle into the neck, or, extending inwards may form adhesions to the chest wall, and, after eroding the ribs, to the pleura.

The usual symptoms of aneurysm are present, and the pressure effects on the veins and nerves are similar to those produced by an aneurysm of the subclavian. Intra-thoracic complications, such as pleurisy or pneumonia, are not infrequent when there are adhesions to the chest wall and pleura. Rupture may take place externally, into the shoulder-joint, or into the pleura.

Extirpation of the sac is the operation of choice, but, if this is impracticable, ligation of the third part of the subclavian may be had recourse to.

Brachial aneurysm usually occurs at the bend of the elbow, is of traumatic origin, and is best treated by excision of the sac.

Aneurysmal varix, which was frequently met with in this situation in the days of the barber-surgeons,—usually as a result of the artery having been accidentally wounded while performing venesection of the median basilic vein,—may be treated, according to the amount of discomfort it causes, by a supporting bandage, or by ligation of the artery above and below the point of communication.

Aneurysms of the vessels of the **forearm and hand** call for no special mention; they are almost invariably traumatic, and are treated by excision of the sac.

Inguinal Aneurysm (*Aneurysm of the Iliac and Femoral Arteries*).—Aneurysms appearing in the region of Poupart's ligament may have their origin in the external or common iliac arteries or in the upper part of the femoral. On account of the tension of the fascia lata, they tend to spread upwards towards the abdomen, and, to a less extent, downwards into the thigh. Sometimes a constriction occurs across the sac at the level of Poupart's ligament.

The pressure exerted on the nerves and veins of the lower extremity causes pain, congestion, and oedema of the limb. Rupture may take place externally, or into the cellular tissue of the iliac fossa.

These aneurysms have to be diagnosed from pulsating sarcoma growing from the pelvic bones, and from an abscess or a mass of enlarged lymph glands overlying the artery and transmitting its pulsation.

The method of treatment that has met with most success is ligation of the common or external iliac, reached either by reflecting the peritoneum from off the iliac fossa (extra-peritoneal operation), or by going through the peritoneal cavity (trans-peritoneal operation).

Gluteal Aneurysm.—An aneurysm in the buttock may arise from the superior or from the inferior gluteal artery, but by the time it forms a salient swelling it is seldom possible to recognise by external examination in which vessel it takes origin. The special symptoms to which it gives rise are pain down the limb from pressure on the sciatic nerve, and interference with the movements at the hip.

Ligation of the hypogastric (internal iliac) by the trans-peritoneal route is the most satisfactory method of treatment. Extirpation of the sac is difficult and dangerous, especially when the aneurysm has spread into the pelvis.

Femoral Aneurysm.—Aneurysm of the femoral artery beyond the origin of the profunda branch is usually traumatic in origin, and is more common in Scarpa's triangle than in Hunter's canal. Any of the methods already described is available for their treatment—the choice lying between Matas' operation and ligation of the external iliac.

Aneurysm of the *profunda femoris* is distinguished from that of the main trunk by the fact that the pulses beyond are, in the former, unaffected, and by the normal artery being felt pulsating over or alongside the sac.

In *aneurysmal varix*, a not infrequent result of a bullet wound or a stab, the communication with the vein may involve the main trunk of the femoral artery. Should operative interference become necessary as a result of progressive increase in size of the tumour, or progressive distension of the veins of the limb, an attempt should be made to separate the vessels concerned and to close the opening in each by suture. If this is impracticable, the artery is tied above and below the communication; gangrene of the limb may supervene, and we have observed a case in which the gangrene extended up to the junction of the middle and lower thirds of the thigh, and in which recovery followed upon amputation of the thigh.

Popliteal Aneurysm.—This is the most common surgical aneurysm, and is not infrequently met with in both limbs. It is generally due to disease of the artery, and repeated slight strains, which are so liable to occur at the knee, play an important part in its formation. In former times it was common in post-boys, from the repeated flexion and extension of the knee in riding.

The aneurysm is usually of the sacculated variety, and may spring from the front or from the back of the vessel. It may exert pressure on the bones and ligaments of the joint, and it has been known to rupture into the articulation. The pain, stiffness, and effusion into the joint which accompany these changes often lead to an erroneous diagnosis of joint disease. The sac may press upon the popliteal artery or vein and their branches, causing congestion and oedema of the leg, and lead to gangrene. Pressure on the tibial and common peroneal nerves gives rise to severe pain, muscular cramp, and weakness of the leg.

The differential diagnosis is to be made from abscess, bursal cyst, enlarged glands, and sarcoma, especially pulsating sarcoma of one of the bones entering into the knee joint.

The choice of operation lies between ligation of the femoral artery in Hunter's canal, and Matas' operation of aneurysmo-arteriorrhaphy. The success which attends the Hunterian operation is evidenced by the fact that Syme performed it thirty-seven times without a single failure. If it fails, the old operation should be considered, but it is a more serious operation, and one which is more liable to be followed by gangrene of the limb. Experience shows that ligation of the vein, or even the removal of a portion of it, is not necessarily followed by gangrene. The risk of gangrene is diminished by a course of digital compression of the femoral artery, before operating on the aneurysm.

Aneurysmal varix is sometimes met with in the region of the popliteal space. It is characterised by the usual symptoms, and is treated by palliative measures, or by ligation of the artery above and below the point of communication.

Aneurysm in the **leg and foot** is rare. It is almost always traumatic, and is treated by excision of the sac.

⋆ XV ⋆

THE LYMPH VESSELS
AND GLANDS

Anatomy and Physiology
Injuries of Lymph Vessels
Wounds of Thoracic Duct
Diseases of Lymph Vessels ⋆ *Lymphangitis: Varieties*
Lymphangiectasis ⋆ *Filarial Disease*
Lymphangioma ⋆ *Diseases of Lymph Glands*
Lymphadenitis: Septic; Tuberculous; Syphilitic
Lymphadenoma ⋆ *Leucocythæmia* ⋆ *Tumours*

Surgical Anatomy and Physiology.—Lymph is essentially blood plasma, which has passed through the walls of capillaries. After bathing and nourishing the tissues, it is collected by lymph vessels, which return it to the blood stream by way of the thoracic duct. These lymph vessels take origin in the lymph spaces of the tissues and in the walls of serous cavities, and they usually run alongside blood vessels—*perivascular lymph vessels.* They have a structure similar to that of veins, but are more abundantly provided with valves. Along the course of the lymph trunks are the *lymph glands*, which possess a definite capsule and are composed of a reticulated connective tissue, the spaces of which are packed with leucocytes. The glands act as filters, arresting not only inert substances, such as blood pigment circulating in the lymph, but also living elements, such as cancer cells or bacteria. As it passes through a gland the lymph is brought into intimate contact with the leucocytes, and in bacterial infections there is always a struggle between the organisms and the leucocytes, so that the glands may be looked upon as an important line of defence, retarding or preventing the passage of bacteria and their products into the general circulation. The infective agent, moreover, in order to reach the blood stream, must usually overcome the resistance of several glands.

307

Lymph glands are, for the most part, arranged in groups or chains, such as those in the axilla, neck, and groin. In any given situation they vary in number and size in different individuals, and fresh glands may be formed on comparatively slight stimulus, and disappear when the stimulus is withdrawn. The best-known example of this is the increase in the number of glands in the axilla which takes place during lactation; when this function ceases, many of the glands become involuted and are transformed into fat, and in the event of a subsequent lactation they are again developed. After glands have been removed by operation, new ones may be formed.

The following are the more important groups of glands, and the areas drained by them in the head and neck and in the extremities.

Head and Neck.—*The anterior auricular (parotid and pre-auricular) glands* lie beneath the parotid fascia in front of the ear, and some are partly embedded in the substance of the parotid gland; they drain the parts about the temple, cheek, eyelids, and auricle, and are frequently the seat of tuberculous disease. *The occipital gland*, situated over the origin of the trapezius from the superior curved line, drains the top and back of the head; it is rarely infected. *The posterior auricular (mastoid) glands* lie over the mastoid process, and drain the side of the head and auricle. These three groups pour their lymph into the superficial cervical glands. *The submaxillary*—two to six in number—lie along the lower order of the mandible from the symphysis to the angle, the posterior ones (paramandibular) being closely connected with the submaxillary salivary gland. They receive lymph from the face, lips, floor of the mouth, gums, teeth, anterior part of tongue, and the alæ nasi, and from the pre-auricular glands. The lymph passes from them into the deeper cervical glands. They are frequently infected with tubercle, with epithelioma which has spread to them from the mouth, and also with pyogenic organisms. *The submental glands* lie in or close to the median line between the anterior bellies of the digastric muscles, and receive lymph from the lips. It is rare for them to be the seat of tubercle, but in epithelioma of the lower lip and floor of the mouth they are infected at an early stage of the disease. *The supra-hyoid gland* lies a little farther back, immediately above the hyoid bone, and receives lymph from the tongue. *The superficial cervical (external jugular) glands*, when present, lie along the external jugular vein, and receives lymph from the occipital and auricular glands and from the auricle. *The sterno-mastoid glands*—glandulæ concatinatæ—form a chain along the posterior edge of the sterno-mastoid muscle, some of them lying beneath the muscle. They are commonly enlarged in secondary syphilis. *The superior deep cervical (internal jugular) glands*—from six to twenty in number—form a continuous chain along the internal jugular vein, beneath the sterno-mastoid muscle. They drain the various groups of glands which lie nearer the surface, also the interior of the skull, the larynx, trachea, thyreoid, and lower part of the pharynx, and pour their lymph into the main trunks at the root of the neck. Belonging to this group is one large gland (the tonsillar gland) which lies behind the posterior belly of the digastric, and rests in the angle between the internal jugular and common facial veins. It is commonly enlarged in affections of the tonsil and posterior part of the tongue. In the same group are three or four glands which lie entirely under cover of the upper end of the sterno-mastoid muscle, and surround the accessory nerve before it perforates the muscle. The deep cervical glands are commonly infected by tubercle and also by epithelioma secondary to disease in the tongue or throat. *The inferior deep cervical (supra-clavicular) glands* lie in the posterior triangle, above the clavicle. They receive lymph from the lowest cervical glands, from the upper part of the chest wall, and from the highest axillary glands. They are frequently infected in cancer of the breast; those on the left side also in cancer of the stomach. The removal of diseased supra-clavicular glands is not to be lightly undertaken, as difficulties are liable to ensue in connection with the thoracic duct, the pleura, or the junction of the subclavian and internal jugular veins. *The retro-pharyngeal glands* lie on each side of the median line upon the rectus capitis anticus major muscle and in front of the pre-vertebral layer of the cervical fascia. They receive part of the lymph from the posterior wall of the pharynx, the interior of the nose and its accessory cavities, the auditory (Eustachian) tube, and the tympanum. When they are infected with pyogenic organisms or with tubercle bacilli, they may lead to the formation of one form of retro-pharyngeal abscess.

Upper Extremity.—*The epi-trochlear and cubital glands* vary in number, that most commonly present lying about an inch and a half above the medial epi-condyle, and other and smaller glands may lie along the medial (internal) bicipital groove or at the bend of the elbow. They drain the ulnar side of the hand and forearm, and pour their lymph into the axillary group. The epi-trochlear gland is sometimes enlarged in syphilis. *The axillary glands* are arranged in groups: a central group lies embedded in the axillary fascia and fat, and is often related to an opening in it; a posterior or subscapular group lies along the line of the subscapular vessels; anterior or pectoral groups lie behind the pectoralis minor, along the medial side of the axillary vein, and an inter-pectoral group, between the two pectoral muscles. The axillary glands receive lymph from the arm, mamma, and side of the chest, and pass it on into the lowest cervical glands and the main lymph trunk. They are frequently the seat of pyogenic, tuberculous, and cancerous infection, and their complete removal is an essential part of the operation for cancer of the breast.

Lower Extremity.—*The popliteal glands* include one superficial gland at the termination of the small saphenous vein, and several deeper ones in relation to the popliteal vessels. They receive lymph from the toes and foot, and transmit it to the inguinal glands. *The femoral glands* lie vertically along the upper part of the great saphenous vein, and receive lymph from the leg and foot; from them the lymph passes to the deep inguinal and external iliac glands. The femoral glands often participate in pyogenic infections entering through the skin of the toes and sole of the foot. *The superficial inguinal glands* lie along the inguinal (Poupart's) ligament, and receive lymph from the external genitals, anus, perineum, buttock, and anterior abdominal wall. The lymph passes on to the deep inguinal and external iliac glands. The superficial glands through their relations to the genitals are frequently the subject of venereal infection, and also of epithelioma when this disease affects the genitals or anus; they are rarely the seat of tuberculosis. *The deep inguinal glands* lie on the medial side of the femoral vein, and sometimes within the femoral canal. They receive lymph from the deep lymphatics of the lower limb, and some of the efferent vessels from the femoral and superficial inguinal glands. The lymph then passes on through the femoral canal to the external iliac glands. The extension of malignant disease, whether cancer or sarcoma, can often be traced along these deeper lymphatics into the pelvis, and as the obstruction to the flow of lymph increases there is a corresponding increase in the swollen dropsical condition of the lower limb on the same side.

The glands of the *thorax* and *abdomen* will be considered with the surgery of these regions.

INJURIES OF LYMPH VESSELS

Lymph vessels are divided in all wounds, and the lymph that escapes from them is added to any discharge that may be present. In injuries of larger trunks the lymph may escape in considerable quantity as a colourless, watery fluid—*lymphorrhagia*; and the opening through which it escapes is known as a *lymphatic fistula*. This has been observed chiefly after extensive operation for the removal of malignant glands in the groin where there already exists a considerable degree of obstruction to the lymph stream, and in such cases the lymph, including that which has accumulated in the vessels of the limb, may escape in such abundance as to soak through large dressings and delay healing. Ultimately new lymph channels are formed, so that at the end of from four to six weeks the discharge of lymph ceases and the wound heals.

Lymphatic Oedema.—When the lymphatic return from a limb has been seriously interfered with,—as, for example, when the axillary contents has been completely cleared out in operating for cancer of the breast,—a condition of lymphatic oedema may result, the arm becoming swollen, tight, and heavy.

Various degrees of the conditions are met with; in the severe forms, there is pain, as well as incapacity of the limb. As in ordinary oedema, the condition is relieved by elevation of the limb, but not nearly to the same degree; in time the tissues become so hard and tense as scarcely to pit on pressure; this is in part due to the formation of new connective tissue and hypertrophy of the skin; in advanced cases there is a gradual transition into one form of elephantiasis.

Handley has devised a method of treatment—*lymphangioplasty*—the object of which is to drain the lymph by embedding a number of silk threads in the subcutaneous cellular tissue.

Wounds of the Thoracic Duct.—The thoracic duct usually opens at the angle formed by the junction of the left internal jugular and subclavian veins, but it may open into either of these vessels by one or by several channels, or the duct may be double throughout its course. There is a smaller duct on the right side—the right lymphatic duct. The duct or ducts may be displaced by a tumour or a mass of enlarged glands, and may be accidentally wounded in dissections at the root of the neck; jets of milky fluid—chyle—may at once escape from it. The jets are rhythmical and coincide with expiration. The injury may, however, not be observed at the time of operation, but later through the dressings being soaked with chyle—*chylorrhoea*. If the wound involves the only existing main duct and all the chyle escapes, the patient suffers from intense thirst, emaciation, and weakness, and may die of inanition; but if, as is usually the case, only one of several collateral channels is implicated, the loss of chyle may be of little moment, as the discharge usually ceases. If the wound heals so that the chyle is prevented from escaping, a fluctuating swelling may form beneath the scar; in course of time it gradually disappears.

An attempt should be made to close the wound in the duct by means of a fine suture; failing this, the duct must be occluded by a ligature as if it were a bleeding artery. The tissues are then stitched over it and the skin wound accurately closed, so as to obtain primary union, firm pressure being applied by dressings and an elastic webbing bandage. Even if the main duct is obliterated, a collateral circulation is usually established. A wound of the right lymphatic duct is of less importance.

Subcutaneous rupture of the thoracic duct may result from a crush of the thorax. The chyle escapes and accumulates in the cellular tissue of the posterior mediastinum, behind the peritoneum, in the pleural cavity (*chylo-thorax*), or in the peritoneal cavity (*chylous ascites*). There are physical signs of fluid in one or other of these situations, but, as a rule, the nature of the lesion is only recognised when chyle is withdrawn by the exploring needle.

DISEASES OF LYMPH VESSELS

Lymphangitis.—Inflammation of peripheral lymph vessels usually results from some primary source of pyogenic infection in the skin. This may be a wound or a purulent blister, and the streptococcus pyogenes is the organism most frequently present. *Septic* lymphangitis is commonly met with in those who, from the nature of their occupation, handle infective material. A *gono-coccal* form has been observed in those suffering from gonorrhoea.

The inflammation affects chiefly the walls of the vessels, and is attended with clotting of the lymph. There is also some degree of inflammation of the surrounding cellular tissue—*peri-lymphangitis*. One or more abscesses may form along the course of the vessels, or a spreading cellulitis may supervene.

The *clinical features* resemble those of other pyogenic infections, and there are wavy red lines running from the source of infection towards the nearest lymph glands. These correspond to the inflamed vessels, and are the seat of burning pain and tenderness. The associated glands are enlarged and painful. In severe cases the symptoms merge into those of septicæmia. When the deep lymph vessels alone are involved, the superficial red lines are absent, but the limb becomes greatly swollen and pits on pressure.

In cases of extensive lymphangitis, especially when there are repeated attacks, the vessels are obliterated by the formation of new connective tissue and a persistent solid oedema results, culminating in one form of elephantiasis.

Treatment.—The primary source of infection is dealt with on the usual lines. If the lymphangitis affects an extremity, Bier's elastic bandage is applied, and if suppuration occurs, the pus is let out through one or more small incisions; in other parts of the body Klapp's suction bells are employed. An autogenous vaccine may be prepared and injected. When the condition has subsided, the limb is massaged and evenly bandaged to promote the disappearance of oedema.

Tuberculous Lymphangitis.—Although lymph vessels play an important rôle in the spread of tuberculosis, the clinical recognition of the disease in them is exceptional. The infection spreads upwards along the superficial lymphatics, which become nodularly thickened; at one or more points, larger, peri-lymphangitic nodules may form and break down into abscesses and ulcers; the nearest group of glands become infected at an early stage. When the disease is widely distributed throughout the lymphatics of the limb, it becomes swollen and hard—a condition illustrated by lupus elephantiasis.

Syphilitic lymphangitis is observed in cases of primary syphilis, in which the vessels of the dorsum of the penis can be felt as indurated cords.

In addition to acting as channels for the conveyance of bacterial infection, *lymph vessels frequently convey the cells of malignant tumours*, and especially cancer, from the seat of the primary disease to the nearest lymph glands, and they may themselves become the seat of cancerous growth forming nodular cords. The permeation of cancer by way of the lymphatics, described by Sampson Handley, has already been referred to.

Lymphangiectasis is a dilated or varicose condition of lymph vessels. It is met with as a congenital affection in the tongue and lips, or it may be acquired as the result of any condition which is attended with extensive obliteration or blocking of the main lymph trunks. An interesting type of lymphangiectasis is that which results from the presence of the *filaria Bancrofti* in the vessels, and is observed chiefly in the groin, spermatic cord, and scrotum of persons who have lived in the tropics.

Filarial disease in the lymphatics of the groin appears as a soft, doughy swelling, varying in size from a walnut to a cocoa-nut; it may partly disappear on pressure and when the patient lies down.

The patient gives a history of feverish attacks of the nature of lymphangitis during which the swelling becomes painful and tender. These attacks may show a remarkable periodicity, and each may be followed by an increase in the size of the swelling, which may extend along the inguinal canal into the abdomen, or down the spermatic cord into the scrotum. On dissection, the swelling is found to be made up of dilated, tortuous, and thickened lymph vessels in which the parent worm is sometimes found, and of greatly enlarged lymph glands which have undergone fibrosis, with giant-cell formation and eosinophile aggregations. The fluid in the dilated vessels is either clear or turbid, in the latter case resembling chyle. The affection is frequently bilateral, and may be associated with lymph scrotum, with elephantiasis, and with chyluria.

The *diagnosis* is to be made from such other swellings in the groin as hernia, lipoma, or cystic pouching of the great saphenous vein. It is confirmed by finding the recently dead or dying worms in the inflamed lymph glands.

Treatment.—When the disease is limited to the groin or scrotum, excision may bring about a permanent cure, but it may result in the formation of lymphatic sinuses and only afford temporary relief.

Lymphangioma.—A lymphangioma is a swelling composed of a series of cavities and channels filled with lymph and freely communicating with one another. The cavities result either from the new formation of lymph spaces or vessels, or from the dilatation of those which already exist; their walls are composed of fibro-areolar tissue lined by endothelium and strengthened by non-striped muscle. They are rarely provided with a definite capsule, and frequently send prolongations of their substance between and into muscles and other structures in their vicinity. They are of congenital origin and usually make their appearance at or shortly after birth. When the tumour is made up of a meshwork of caverns and channels, it is called a *cavernous lymphangioma*; when it is composed of one or more cysts, it is called a *cystic lymphangioma*. It is probable that the cysts are derived from the caverns by breaking down and absorption of the intervening septa, as transition forms between the cavernous and cystic varieties are sometimes met with.

The *cavernous lymphangioma* appears as an ill-defined, soft swelling, presenting many of the characters of a subcutaneous hæmangioma, but it is not capable of being emptied by pressure, it does not become tense when the blood pressure is raised, as in crying, and if the tumour is punctured, it yields lymph instead of blood. It also resembles a lipoma, especially the congenital variety which grows from the periosteum, and the differential diagnosis between these is rarely completed until the swelling is punctured or explored by operation. If treatment is called for, it is carried out on the same lines as for hæmangioma, by means of electrolysis, igni-puncture, or excision. Complete excision is rarely possible because of the want of definition and encapsulation, but it is not necessary for cure, as the parts that remain undergo cicatrisation.

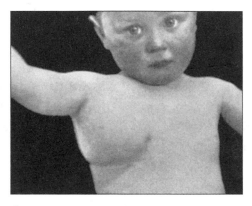

FIG. 76. Congenital Cystic Tumour or Hygroma of Axilla. (From a photograph lent by Dr. Lediard.)

The *cystic lymphangioma, lymphatic cyst*, or *congenital cystic hygroma* is most often met with in the neck—*hydrocele of the neck*; it is situated beneath the deep fascia, and projects either in front of or behind the sterno-mastoid muscle. It may attain a large size, the overlying skin and cyst wall may be so thin as to be translucent, and it has been known to cause serious impairment of respiration through pressing on the trachea. In the axilla also the cystic tumour may attain a considerable size (Fig. 76); less frequent situations are the groin, and the floor of the mouth, where it constitutes one form of ranula.

The nature of these swellings is to be recognised by their situation, by their having existed from infancy, and, if necessary, by drawing off some of the contents of the cyst through a fine needle. They are usually remarkably indolent, persisting often for a long term of years without change, and, like the hæmangioma, they sometimes undergo spontaneous cicatrisation and cure. Sometimes the cystic tumour becomes infected and forms an abscess— another, although less desirable, method of cure. Those situated in the neck are most liable to suppurate, probably because of pyogenic organisms being brought to them by the lymphatics taking origin in the scalp, ear, or throat.

If operative interference is called for, the cysts may be tapped and injected with iodine, or excised; the operation for removal may entail a considerable dissection amongst the deeper structures at the root of the neck, and should not be lightly undertaken; parts left behind may be induced to cicatrise by inserting a tube of radium and leaving it for a few days.

Lymphangiomas are met with in the abdomen in the form of *omental cysts*.

DISEASES OF LYMPH GLANDS

Lymphadenitis.—Inflammation of lymph glands results from the advent of an irritant, usually bacterial or toxic, brought to the glands by the afferent lymph vessels. These vessels may share in the inflammation and be the seat of lymphangitis, or they may show no evidence of the passage of the noxa. It is exceptional for the irritant to reach the gland through the blood-stream.

A strain or other form of trauma is sometimes blamed for the onset of lymphadenitis, especially in the glands of the groin (bubo), but it is usually possible to discover some source of pyogenic infection which is responsible for the mischief, or to obtain a history of some antecedent infection such as gonorrhoea. It is possible for gonococci to lie latent in the inguinal glands for long periods, and only give rise to lymphadenitis if the glands be subsequently subjected to injury. The glands most frequently affected are those in the neck, axilla, and groin.

The characters of the lymphadenitis vary with the nature of the irritant. Sometimes it is mild and evanescent, as in the glandular enlargement in the neck which attends tonsillitis and other forms of sore throat. Sometimes it is more persistent, as in the enlargement that is associated with adenoids, hypertrophied tonsils, carious teeth, eczema of the scalp, and otorrhoea; and it is possible that this indolent enlargement predisposes to tuberculous infection. A similar enlargement is met with in the axilla in cases of chronic interstitial mastitis, and in the groin as a result of chronic irritation about the external genitals, such as balanitis.

Sometimes the lymphadenitis is of an acute character, and the tendency is towards the formation of an abscess. This is illustrated in the axillary glands as a result of infected wounds of the fingers; in the femoral glands in infected wounds or purulent blisters on the foot; in the inguinal glands in gonorrhoea and soft sore; and in the cervical glands in the severer forms of sore throat associated with diphtheria and scarlet fever. The most acute suppurations result from infection with streptococci.

Superficial glands, when inflamed and suppurating, become enlarged, tender, fixed, and matted to one another. In the glands of the groin the suppurative process is often remarkably sluggish; purulent foci form in the interior of individual glands, and some time may elapse before the pus erupts through their respective capsules. In the deeply placed cervical glands, especially in cases of streptococcal throat infections, the suppuration rapidly involves the surrounding cellular tissue, and the clinical features are those of an acute cellulitis and deeply seated abscess. When this is incised the necrosed glands may be found lying in the pus, and on bacteriological examination are found to be swarming with streptococci. In suppuration of the axillary glands the abscess may be quite superficial, or it may be deeply placed beneath the strong fascia and pectoral muscles, according to the group of glands involved.

The *diagnosis* of septic lymphadenitis is usually easy. The indolent enlargements are not always to be distinguished, however, from commencing tuberculous disease, except by the use of the tuberculin test, and by the fact that they usually disappear on removing the peripheral source of irritation.

Treatment.—The first indication is to discover and deal with the source of infection, and in the indolent forms of lymphadenitis this will usually be followed by recovery. In the acute forms following on pyogenic infection, the best results are obtained from the hyperæmic treatment carried out by means of suction bells. If suppuration is not thereby prevented, or if it has already taken place, each separate collection of pus is punctured with a narrow-bladed knife and the use of the suction bell is persevered with. If there is a large periglandular abscess, as is often the case, in the neck and axilla, the opening may require to be made by Hilton's method, and it may be necessary to insert a drainage-tube.

Tuberculous Disease of Glands.—This is a disease of great frequency and importance. The tubercle bacilli usually gain access to the gland through the afferent lymph vessels, which convey them from some lesion of the surface within the area drained by them. Tuberculous infection may supervene in glands that are already enlarged as a result of chronic septic irritation. While any of the glands in the body may be affected, the disease is most often met with in the cervical groups which derive their lymph from the mouth, nose, throat, and ear.

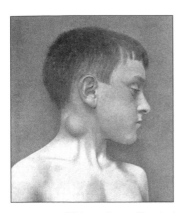

FIG. 77. Tuberculous Cervical Gland with abscess formation in subcutaneous cellular tissue, in a boy æt. 10.

The appearance of the glands on section varies with the stage of the disease. In the early stages the gland is enlarged, it may be to many times its natural size, is normal in appearance and consistence, and as there is no peri-adenitis it is easily shelled out from its surroundings. On microscopical examination, however, there is evidence of infection in the shape of bacilli and of characteristic giant and epithelioid cells. At a later stage, the gland tissue is studded with minute yellow foci which tend to enlarge and in time to become confluent, so that the whole gland is ultimately converted into a caseous mass. This caseous material is surrounded by the thickened capsule which, as a result of peri-adenitis, tends to become adherent to and fused with surrounding structures, and particularly with layers of fascia and with the walls of veins. The caseated tissue often remains unchanged for long periods; it may become calcified, but more frequently it breaks down and liquefies.

Tuberculous disease in the cervical glands is a common accompaniment or sequel of adenoids, enlarged tonsils, carious teeth, pharyngitis, middle-ear disease, and conjunctivitis. These lesions afford the bacilli a chance of entry into the lymph vessels, in which they are carried to the glands, where they give rise to disease.

The enlargement may affect only one gland, usually below the angle of the mandible, and remain confined to it, the gland reaching the size of a hazel-nut, and being ovoid, firm, and painless. More commonly the disease affects several glands, on one or on both sides of the neck. When the disease commences in the pre-auricular or submaxillary glands, it tends to spread to those along the carotid sheath: when the posterior auricular and occipital glands are first involved, the spread is to those along the posterior border of the sterno-mastoid. In many cases all the chains in front of, beneath, and behind this muscle are involved, the enlarged glands extending from the mastoid to the clavicle. They are at first discrete and movable, and may even vary in size from time to time; but with the addition of peri-adenitis they become fixed and matted together, forming lobulated or nodular masses

(Fig. 78). They become adherent not only to one another, but also to the structures in their vicinity,—and notably to the internal jugular vein,—a point of importance in regard to their removal by operation.

At any stage the disease may be arrested and the glands remain for long periods without further change. It is possible that the tuberculous tissue may undergo cicatrisation. More commonly suppuration ensues, and a cold abscess forms, but if there is a mixed infection, the pyogenic factor being usually derived from the throat, it may take on active features.

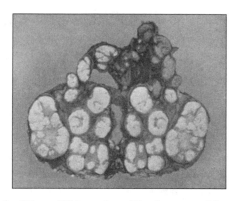

FIG. 78. Mass of Tuberculous Glands removed from Axilla (cf. Fig. 79).

The transition from the solid to the liquefied stage is attended with pain and tenderness in the gland, which at the same time becomes fixed and globular, and finally fluctuation can be elicited.

If left to itself, the softened tubercle erupts through the capsule of the gland and infects the cellular tissue. The cervical fascia is perforated and a cold abscess, often much larger than the gland from which it took origin, forms between the fascia and the overlying skin. The further stages—reddening, undermining of skin and external rupture, with the formation of ulcers and sinuses—have been described with tuberculous abscess. The ulcers and sinuses persist indefinitely, or they heal and then break out again; sometimes the skin becomes infected, and a condition like lupus spreads over a considerable area. Spontaneous healing finally takes place after the caseous tubercle has been extruded; the resulting scars are extremely unsightly, being puckered or bridled, or hypertrophied like keloid.

While the disease is most common in childhood and youth, it may be met with even in advanced life; and although often associated with impaired health and unhealthy surroundings, it may affect those who are apparently robust and are in affluent circumstances.

Diagnosis.—The chief importance lies in differentiating tuberculous disease from lympho-sarcoma and from lymphadenoma, and this is usually possible from the history and from the nature of the enlargement. Signs of liquefaction and suppuration support the diagnosis of tubercle. If any doubt remains, one of the glands should be removed and submitted to microscopical examination. Other forms of sarcoma, and the enlargement of an accessory thyreoid, are less likely to be confused with tuberculous glands. Calcified tuberculous glands give definite shadows with the X-rays.

Enlargement of the cervical glands from secondary cancer may simulate tuberculosis, but is differentiated by its association with cancer in the mouth or throat, and by the characteristic, stone-like induration of epithelioma.

The cold abscess which results from tuberculous glands is to be distinguished from that due to disease in the cervical spine, retro-pharyngeal abscess, as well as from congenital and other cystic swellings in the neck.

Prognosis.—Next to lupus, glandular disease is of all tuberculous lesions the least dangerous to life; but while it is the rule to recover from tuberculous disease of glands with or without an operation, it is unfortunately quite common for such persons to become the subjects of tuberculosis in other parts of the body at any subsequent period of life.

Treatment.—There is considerable difference of opinion regarding the treatment of glandular tuberculosis. Some authorities, impressed with the undoubted possibility of natural cure, are satisfied with promoting this by measures directed towards improving the general health, by the prolonged administration of tuberculin, and by repeated exposures to the X-rays and to sunlight. Others again, influenced by the risk of extension of the disease and by the destruction of tissue and disfigurement caused by breaking down of the tuberculous tissue and mixed infection, advocate the removal of the glands by operation.

The conditions vary widely in different cases, and the treatment should be adapted to the individual requirements. If the disease remains confined to the glands originally infected and there are no signs of breaking down, "expectant measures" may be persevered with.

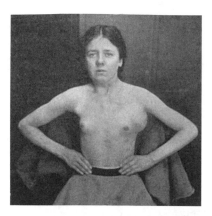

FIG. 79. Tuberculous Axillary Glands (cf. Fig. 78)

If, on the other hand, the disease exhibits aggressive tendencies, the question of operation should be considered. The undesirable results of the breaking down and liquefaction of the diseased gland may be avoided by the timely withdrawal of the fluid contents through a hollow needle.

The excision of tuberculous glands is often a difficult operation, because of the number and deep situation of the glands to be removed, and of the adhesions to surrounding structures. The skin incision must be sufficiently extensive to give access to the whole of the affected area, and to avoid disfigurement should, whenever possible, be made in the line of the natural creases of the skin. In exposing the glands the common facial and other venous trunks may require to be clamped and tied. Care must be taken not to injure the important nerves, particularly the accessory, the vagus, and the phrenic. The inframaxillary branches of the facial, the hypoglossal and its descending branches, and the motor branches of the deep cervical plexus, are also liable to be injured. The dissection is rendered easier and is attended with less risk of injury to the nerves, if the patient is placed in the sitting posture so as to empty the veins, and, instead of a knife, the conical scissors of Mayo are employed. When the glands are extensively affected on both sides of the neck, it is advisable to allow an interval to elapse rather than to operate on both sides at one sitting. (*Op. Surg.*, p. 189.)

If the tonsils are enlarged they should not be removed at the same time, as, by so doing, there is a risk of pyogenic infection from the throat being carried to the wound in the neck, but they should be removed, after an interval, to prevent relapse of disease in the glands.

When the skin is broken and caseous tuberculous tissue is exposed, healing is promoted by cutting away diseased skin, removing the granulation tissue with the spoon, scraping sinuses, and packing the cavity with iodoform worsted and treating it by the open method and secondary suture if necessary. Exposure to the sunshine on the seashore and to the X-rays is often beneficial in these cases.

Tuberculous disease in the axillary glands may be a result of extension from those in the neck, from the mamma, ribs, or sternum, or more rarely from the upper extremity. We have seen it from an infected wound of a finger. In some cases no source of infection is discoverable. The individual glands attain a considerable size, and they fuse together to form a large tumour which fills up the axillary space. The disease progresses more rapidly than it does in the cervical glands, and almost always goes on to suppuration with the formation of sinuses. Conservative measures need not be considered, as the only satisfactory treatment is excision, and that without delay.

Tuberculous disease in the glands of the groin is comparatively rare. We have chiefly observed it in the femoral glands as a result of inoculation tubercle on the toes or sole of the foot. The affected glands nearly always break down and suppurate, and after destroying the overlying skin give rise to fungating ulcers. The treatment consists in excising the glands and the affected skin. The dissection may be attended with troublesome hæmorrhage from the numerous veins that converge towards the femoral trunk.

Tuberculous disease in the *mesenteric* and *bronchial glands* is described with the surgery of regions.

Syphilitic Disease of Glands.—Enlargement of lymph glands is a prominent feature of acquired syphilis, especially in the form of the indolent or bullet-bubo which accompanies the primary lesion, and the general enlargement of glands that occurs in secondary syphilis. Gummatous disease in glands is extremely rare; the affected gland rapidly enlarges to the size of a walnut, and may then persist for a long period without further change; if it breaks down, the overlying skin is destroyed and the caseated tissue of the gumma exposed.

Lymphadenoma.—*Hodgkin's Disease* (Pseudo-leukæmia of German authors).—This is a rare disease, the origin of which is as yet unknown, but analogy would suggest that it is due to infection with a slowly growing micro-organism. It is chiefly met with in young subjects, and is characterised by a painless enlargement of a particular group of glands, most commonly those in the cervical region (Fig. 80).

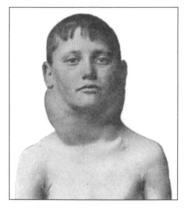

The glands are usually larger than in tuberculosis, and they remain longer discrete and movable; they are firm in consistence, and on section present a granular appearance due to overgrowth of the connective-tissue framework. In time the glandular masses may form enormous projecting tumours, the swelling being added to by lymphatic oedema of the overlying cellular tissue and skin.

The enlargement spreads along the chain of glands to those above the clavicle, to those in the axilla, and to those of the opposite side (Fig. 81). Later, the glands in the groin

FIG. 80. Chronic Hodgkin's Disease in a boy æt. 11.

become enlarged, and it is probable that the infection has spread from the neck along the mediastinal, bronchial, retro-peritoneal, and mesenteric glands, and has branched off to the iliac and inguinal groups.

Two clinical types are recognised, one in which the disease progresses slowly and remains confined to the cervical glands for two or more years; the other, in which the disease is more rapidly disseminated and causes death in from twelve to eighteen months.

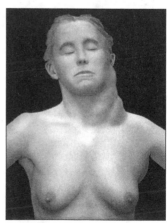

In the acute form, the health suffers, there is fever, and the glands may vary in size with variations in the temperature; the blood presents the characters met with in secondary anæmia. The spleen, liver, testes, and mammæ may be enlarged; the glandular swellings press on important structures, such as the trachea, oesophagus, or great veins, and symptoms referable to such pressure manifest themselves.

Diagnosis.—Considerable difficulty attends the diagnosis of lymphadenoma at an early stage. The negative results of tuberculin tests may assist in the differentiation from tuberculous

FIG. 81. Lymphadenoma (Hodgkin's Disease) affecting left side of neck and left axilla, in a woman æt. 44. Three years' duration.

disease, but the more certain means of excising one of the suspected glands and submitting it to microscopical examination should be had recourse to. The sections show proliferation of endothelial cells, the formation of numerous giant cells quite unlike those of tuberculosis and a progressive fibrosis. Lympho-sarcoma can usually be differentiated by the rapid assumption of the local features of malignant disease, and in a gland removed for examination, a predominance of small round cells with scanty protoplasm. The enlargement associated with leucocythæmia is differentiated by the characteristic changes in the blood.

Treatment.—In the acute form of lymphadenoma, treatment is of little avail. Arsenic may be given in full doses either by the mouth or by subcutaneous injection; the intravenous administration of neo-salvarsan may be tried. Exposure to the X-rays and to radium has been more successful than any other form of treatment. Excision of glands, although sometimes beneficial, seldom arrests the progress of the disease. The ease and rapidity with which large masses of glands may be shelled out is in remarkable contrast to what is observed in tuberculous disease. Surgical interference may give relief when important structures are being pressed upon—tracheotomy, for example, may be required where life is threatened by asphyxia.

Leucocythæmia.—This is a disease of the blood and of the blood-forming organs, in which there is a great increase in the number, and an alteration of the character, of the leucocytes present in the blood. It may simulate lymphadenoma, because, in certain forms of the disease, the lymph glands, especially those in the neck, axilla, and groin, are greatly enlarged.

TUMOURS OF LYMPH GLANDS

Primary Tumours.—*Lympho-sarcoma*, which may be regarded as a sarcoma starting in a lymph gland, appears in the neck, axilla, or groin as a rapidly growing tumour consisting of one enlarged gland with numerous satellites. As the tumour increases in size, the sarcomatous tissue erupts through the capsule of the gland, and infiltrates the surrounding tissues, whereby it becomes fixed to these and to the skin.

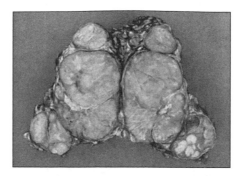

FIG. 82. Lympho-Sarcoma removed from Groin. It will be observed that there is one large central parent tumour surrounded by satellites.

The prognosis is grave in the extreme, and the only hope is in early excision, followed by the use of radium and X-rays. We have observed a case of lympho-sarcoma above the clavicle, in which excision of all that was removable, followed by the insertion of a tube of radium for ten days, was followed by a disappearance of the disease over a period which extended to nearly five years, when death resulted from a tumour in the mediastinum. In a second case in which the growth was in the groin, the patient, a young man, remained well for over two years and was then lost sight of.

Secondary Tumours.—Next to tuberculosis, *secondary cancer* is the most common disease of lymph glands. In the neck it is met with in association with epithelioma of the lip, tongue, or fauces. The glands form tumours of variable size, and are often larger than the primary growth, the characters of which they reproduce. The glands are at first movable, but soon become fixed both to each other and to their surroundings; when fixed to the mandible they form a swelling of bone-like hardness; in time they soften, liquefy, and burst through the skin, forming foul, fungating ulcers. A similar condition is met with in the groin from epithelioma of the penis, scrotum, or vulva. In cancer of the breast, the infection of the axillary glands is an important complication.

In *pigmented* or *melanotic cancers* of the skin, the glands are early infected and increase rapidly, so that, when the primary growth is still of small size—as, for example, on the sole of the foot—the femoral glands may already constitute large pigmented tumours.

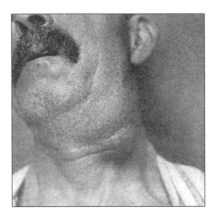

FIG. 83. Cancerous Glands in Neck secondary to Epithelioma of Lip. (Mr. G. L. Chiene's case.)

The implication of the glands in other forms of cancer will be considered with regional surgery.

Secondary sarcoma is seldom met with in the lymph glands except when the primary growth is a lympho-sarcoma and is situated in the tonsil, thyreoid, or testicle.

◆ XVI ◆

THE NERVES

Anatomy ◆ *Injuries of Nerves: Changes in Nerves after Division;*
Repair and its Modifications; Clinical Features; Primary and
Secondary Suture ◆ *Subcutaneous Injuries of Nerves* ◆ *Diseases:*
Neuritis; Tumours
Surgery of the Individual Nerves: Brachial Neuralgia; Sciatica;
Trigeminal Neuralgia

Anatomy.—A nerve-trunk is made up of a variable number of bundles of nerve fibres surrounded and supported by a framework of connective tissue. The nerve fibres are chiefly of the medullated type, and they run without interruption from a nerve cell or *neuron* in the brain or spinal medulla to their peripheral terminations in muscle, skin, and secretory glands.

Each nerve fibre consists of a number of nerve fibrils collected into a central bundle—the axis cylinder—which is surrounded by an envelope, the neurolemma or sheath of Schwann. Between the neurolemma and the axis cylinder is the medullated sheath, composed of a fatty substance known as myelin. This medullated sheath is interrupted at the nodes of Ranvier, and in each internode is a nucleus lying between the myelin and the neurolemma. The axis cylinder is the essential conducting structure of the nerve, while the neurolemma and the myelin act as insulating agents. The axis cylinder depends for its nutrition on the central neuron with which it is connected, and from which it originally developed, and it degenerates if it is separated from its neuron.

The connective-tissue framework of a nerve-trunk consists of the *perineurium*, or general sheath, which surrounds all the bundles; the *epineurium*, surrounding individual groups of bundles; and the *endoneurium*, a delicate connective tissue separating the individual nerve fibres. The blood vessels and lymphatics run in these connective-tissue sheaths.

According to Head and his co-workers, Sherren and Rivers, the afferent fibres in the peripheral nerves can be divided into three systems:—

1. Those which subserve *deep sensibility* and conduct the impulses produced by pressure as well as those which enable the patient to recognise the position of a joint on passive movement (joint-sensation), and the kinæsthetic sense, which recognises that active contraction of the muscle is taking place (active muscle-sensation). The fibres of this system run with the motor nerves, and pass to muscles, tendons, and joints. Even division of both the ulnar and the median nerves above the wrist produces little loss of deep sensibility, unless the tendons are also cut through. The failure to recognise this form of sensibility has been largely responsible for the conflicting statements as to the sensory phenomena following operations for the repair of divided nerves.

2. Those which subserve *protopathic* sensibility—that is, are capable of responding to painful cutaneous stimuli and to the extremes of heat and cold. These also endow the hairs with sensibility to pain. They are the first to regenerate after division.

3. Those which subserve *epicritic* sensibility, the most highly specialised, capable of appreciating light touch, *e.g.* with a wisp of cotton wool, as a well-localised sensation, and the finer grades of temperature, called cool and warm (72°-104° F.), and of discriminating as separate the points of a pair of compasses 2 cms. apart. These are the last to regenerate.

A nerve also exerts a trophic influence on the tissues in which it is distributed.

The researches of Stoffel on the minute anatomy of the larger nerves, and the disposition in them of the bundles of nerve fibres supplying different groups of muscles, have opened up what promises to be a fruitful field of clinical investigation and therapeutics. He has shown that in the larger nerve-trunks the nerve bundles for special groups of muscles are not, as was formerly supposed, arranged irregularly and fortuitously, but that on the contrary the nerve fibres to a particular group of muscles have a typical and practically constant position within the nerve.

In the large nerve-trunks of the limbs he has worked out the exact position of the bundles for the various groups of muscles, so that in a cross section of a particular nerve the component bundles can be labelled as confidently and accurately as can be the cortical areas in the brain. In the living subject, by using a fine needle-like electrode and a very weak galvanic current, he has been able to differentiate the nerve bundles for the various groups of muscles. In several cases of spastic paralysis he succeeded in picking out in the nerve-trunk of the affected limb the nerve bundles supplying the spastic muscles, and, by resecting portions of them, in relieving the spasm. In a case of spastic contracture of the pronator muscles of the forearm, for example, an incision is made along the line of the median nerve above the bend of the elbow. At the lateral side of the median nerve, where it lies in contact with the biceps muscle, is situated a well-defined and easily isolated bundle of fibres which supplies the pronator teres, the flexor carpi radialis, and the palmaris longus muscles. On incising the sheath of the nerve this bundle can be readily dissected up and its identity confirmed by stimulating it with a very weak galvanic current. An inch or more of the bundle is then resected.

INJURIES OF NERVES

Nerves are liable to be cut or torn across, bruised, compressed, stretched, or torn away from their connections with the spinal medulla.

Complete Division of a Mixed Nerve.—Complete division is a common result of accidental wounds, especially above the wrist, where the ulnar, median, and radial nerves are frequently cut across, and in gun-shot injuries.

Changes in Structure and Function.—The mere interruption of the continuity of a nerve results in degeneration of its fibres, the myelin being broken up into droplets and absorbed, while the axis cylinders swell up, disintegrate, and finally disappear. Both the conducting and the insulating elements are thus lost. The degeneration in the central end of the divided nerve is usually limited to the immediate proximity of the lesion, and does not even involve all the nerve fibres. In the distal end, it extends throughout the entire peripheral distribution of the nerve, and appears to be due to the cutting off of the fibres from their trophic nerve cells in the spinal medulla. Immediate suturing of the ends does not affect the degeneration of the distal segment. The peripheral end undergoes complete degeneration in from six weeks to two months.

The physiological effects of complete division are that the muscles supplied by the nerve are immediately paralysed, the area to which it furnishes the sole cutaneous supply becomes insensitive, and the other structures, including tendons, bones, and joints, lose sensation, and begin to atrophy from loss of the trophic influence.

Nerves divided in Amputation.—In the case of nerves divided in an amputation, there is an active, although necessarily abortive, attempt at regeneration, which results in the formation of bulbous swellings at the cut ends of the nerves. When there has been suppuration, and especially if the nerves have been cut so as to be exposed in the wound, these bulbous swellings may attain an abnormal size, and are then known as "amputation" or "stump neuromas" (Fig. 84).

When the nerves in a stump have not been cut sufficiently short, they may become involved in the cicatrix, and it may be necessary, on account of pain, to free them from their adhesions, and to resect enough of the terminal portions to prevent them again becoming adherent. When this is difficult, a portion may be resected from each of the nerve-trunks at a higher level; and if this fails to give relief, a fresh amputation may be performed. When there is agonising pain dependent upon an ascending neuritis, it may be necessary to resect the corresponding posterior nerve roots within the vertebral canal.

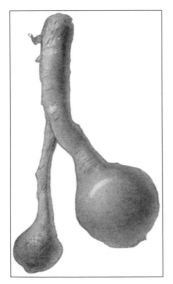

FIG. 84. Stump Neuromas of Sciatic Nerve, excised forty years after the original amputation by Mr. A. G. Miller.

Other Injuries of Nerves.—*Contusion* of a nerve-trunk is attended with extravasation of blood into the connective-tissue sheaths, and is followed by degeneration of the contused nerve fibres. Function is usually restored, the conducting paths being re-established by the formation of new nerve fibres.

When a nerve is *torn across* or badly *crushed*—as, for example, by a fractured bone—the changes are similar to those in a divided nerve, and the ultimate result depends on the amount of separation between the ends and the possibility of the young axis cylinders bridging the gap.

Involvement of Nerves in Scar Tissue.—Pressure or traction may be exerted upon a nerve by contracting scar tissue, or a process of neuritis or perineuritis may be induced.

When terminal filaments are involved in a scar, it is best to dissect out the scar, and along with it the ends of the nerves pressed upon. When a nerve-trunk, such as the sciatic, is involved in cicatricial tissue, the nerve must be exposed and freed from its surroundings (*neurolysis*), and then stretched so as to tear any adhesions that may be present above or below the part exposed. It may be advisable to displace the liberated nerve from its original position so as to minimise the risk of its incorporation in the scar of the original wound or in that resulting from the operation—for example, the radial nerve may be buried in the substance of the triceps, or it may be surrounded by a segment of vein or portion of fat-bearing fascia.

Injuries of nerves resulting from **gun-shot wounds** include: (1) those in which the nerve is directly damaged by the bullet, and (2) those in which the nerve-trunk is involved secondarily either by scar tissue in its vicinity or by callus following fracture of an adjacent bone. The primary injuries include contusion, partial or complete division, and perforation of the nerve-trunk. One of the most constant symptoms is the early occurrence of severe neuralgic pain, and this is usually associated with marked hyperæsthesia.

Regeneration.—*Process of Repair when the Ends are in Contact.*—*If the wound is aseptic*, and the ends of the divided nerve are sutured or remain in contact, they become united, and the conducting paths are re-established by a regeneration of nerve fibres. There is a difference of opinion as to the method of regeneration. The Wallerian doctrine is that the axis cylinders in the central end grow downwards, and enter the nerve sheaths of the distal portion, and continue growing until they reach the peripheral terminations in muscle and skin, and in course of time acquire a myelin sheath; the cells of the neurolemma multiply and form long chains in both ends of the nerve, and are believed to provide for the nourishment and support of the actively lengthening axis cylinders. Another view is that the formation of new axis cylinders is not confined to the central end, but that it goes on also in the peripheral segment, in which, however, the new axis cylinders do not attain maturity until continuity with the central end has been re-established.

If the wound becomes infected and suppuration occurs, the young nerve fibres are destroyed and efficient regeneration is prevented; the formation of scar tissue also may constitute a permanent obstacle to new nerve fibres bridging the gap.

When the ends are not in contact, reunion of the divided nerve fibres does not take place whether the wound is infected or not. At the proximal end there forms a bulbous swelling, which becomes adherent to the scar tissue. It consists of branching axis cylinders running in all directions, these having failed to reach the distal end because of the extent of the gap. The peripheral end is completely degenerated, and is represented by a fibrous cord, the cut end of which is often slightly swollen or bulbous, and is also incorporated with the scar tissue of the wound.

Clinical Features.—The symptoms resulting from division and non-union of a nerve-trunk necessarily vary with the functions of the affected nerve. The following description refers to a mixed sensori-motor trunk, such as the median or radial (musculo-spiral) nerve.

Sensory Phenomena.—Superficial touch is tested by means of a wisp of cotton wool stroked gently across the skin; the capacity of discriminating two points as separate, by a pair of blunt-pointed compasses; the sensation of pressure, by means of a pencil or other blunt object; of pain, by pricking or scratching with a needle; and of sensibility to heat and cold, by test-tubes containing water at different temperatures. While these tests are being carried out, the patient's eyes are screened off.

After division of a nerve containing sensory fibres, there is an area of absolute cutaneous insensibility to touch (anæsthesia), to pain (analgesia), and to all degrees of temperature—*loss of protopathic sensibility*; surrounded by an area in which there is loss of sensation to light touch, inability to recognise minor differences of temperature (72°-104° F.), and to appreciate as separate impressions the contact of the two points of a compass—*loss of epicritic sensibility* (Head and Sherren) (Figs. 91, 92).

Motor Phenomena.—There is immediate and complete loss of voluntary power in the muscles supplied by the divided nerve. The muscles rapidly waste, and within from three to five days, they cease to react to the faradic current. When tested with the galvanic current, it is found that a stronger current must be used to call forth contraction than in a healthy muscle, and the contraction appears first at the closing of the circuit when the anode is used as the testing electrode. The loss of excitability to the interrupted current, and the specific alteration in the type of contraction with the constant current, is known as the *reaction of degeneration*. After a few weeks all electric excitability is lost. The paralysed muscles undergo fatty degeneration, which attains its maximum three or four months after the division of the nerve. Further changes may take place, and result in the transformation of the muscle into fibrous tissue, which by undergoing shortening may cause deformity known as *paralytic contracture*.

Vaso-motor Phenomena.—In the majority of cases there is an initial rise in the temperature of the part (2° to 3° F.), with redness and increased vascularity. This is followed by a fall in the local temperature, which may amount to 8° or 10° F., the parts becoming pale and cold. Sometimes the hyperæmia resulting from vaso-motor paralysis is more persistent, and is associated with swelling of the parts from oedema—the so-called *angio-neurotic oedema*. The vascularity varies with external influences, and in cold weather the parts present a bluish appearance.

Trophic Phenomena.—Owing to the disappearance of the subcutaneous fat, the skin is smooth and thin, and may be abnormally dry. The hair is harsh, dry, and easily shed. The nails become brittle and furrowed, or thick and curved, and the ends of the fingers become club-shaped. Skin eruptions, especially in the form of blisters, occur, or there may be actual ulcers of the skin, especially in winter. In aggravated cases the tips of the fingers disappear from progressive ulceration, and in the sole of the foot a perforating ulcer may develop. Arthropathies are occasionally met with, the joints becoming the seat of a painless effusion or hydrops, which is followed by fibrous thickening of the capsular and other ligaments, and terminates in stiffness and fibrous ankylosis. In this way the fingers are seriously crippled and deformed.

Treatment of Divided Nerves.—The treatment consists in approximating the divided ends of the nerve and placing them under the most favourable conditions for repair, and this should be done at the earliest possible opportunity. (*Op. Surg.*, pp. 45, 46.)

Primary Suture.—The reunion of a recently divided nerve is spoken of as primary suture, and for its success asepsis is essential. As the suturing of the ends of the nerve is extremely painful, an anæsthetic is required.

When the wound is healed and while waiting for the restoration of function, measures are employed to maintain the nutrition of the damaged nerve and of the parts supplied by it. The limb is exercised, massaged, and douched, and protected from cold and other injurious influences. The nutrition of the paralysed muscles is further improved by electricity. The galvanic current is employed, using at first a mild current of not more than 5 milliampères for about ten minutes, the current being made to flow downwards in the course of the nerve, with the positive electrode applied to the spine, and the negative over the affected nerve near its termination. It is an advantage to have a metronome in the circuit whereby the current is opened and closed automatically at intervals, so as to cause contraction of the muscles.

The results of primary suture, when it has been performed under favourable conditions, are usually satisfactory. In a series of cases investigated by Head and Sherren, the period between the operation and the first return of sensation averaged 65 days. According to Purves Stewart protopathic sensation commences to appear in about six weeks and is completely restored in six months; electric sensation and motor power reappear together in about six months, and restoration is complete in a year. When sensation returns, the area of insensibility to pain steadily diminishes and disappears; sensibility to extremes of temperature appears soon after; and last of all, after a considerable interval, there is simultaneous return of appreciation of light touch, moderate degrees of temperature, and the points of a compass.

A clinical means of estimating how regeneration in a divided nerve is progressing has been described by Tinel. He found that a tingling sensation, similar to that experienced in the foot, when it is recovering from the "sleeping" condition induced by prolonged pressure on the sciatic nerve from sitting on a hard bench, can be elicited on percussing over *growing* axis cylinders. Tapping over the proximal end of a *newly divided nerve, e.g.* the common peroneal behind the head of the fibula, produces no tingling, but when in about three weeks axis cylinders begin to grow in the proximal end-bulb, local tingling is induced by tapping there. The downward growth of the axis cylinders can be traced by tapping over the distal segment of the nerve, the tingling sensation being elicited as far down as the young axis cylinders have reached. When the regeneration of the axis cylinders is complete, tapping no longer causes tingling. It usually takes about one hundred days for this stage to be reached.

Tinel's sign is present before voluntary movement, muscular tone, or the normal electrical reactions reappear.

In cases of complete nerve paralysis that have not been operated upon, the tingling test is helpful in determining whether or not regeneration is taking place. Its detection may prevent an unnecessary operation being performed.

Primary suture should not be attempted so long as the wound shows signs of infection, as it is almost certain to end in failure. The ends should be sutured, however, as soon as the wound is aseptic or has healed.

Secondary Suture.—The term secondary suture is applied to the operation of stitching the ends of the divided nerve after the wound has healed.

Results of Secondary Suture.—When secondary suture has been performed under favourable conditions, the prognosis is good, but a longer time is required for restoration of function than after primary suture. Purves Stewart says protopathic sensation is sometimes observed much earlier than in primary suture, because partial regeneration of axis cylinders in the peripheral segment has already taken place. Sensation is recovered first, but it seldom returns before three or four months. There then follows an improvement or disappearance of any trophic disturbances that may be present. Recovery of motion may be deferred for long periods—rather because of the changes in the muscles than from want of conductivity in the nerve—and if the muscles have undergone complete degeneration, it may never take place at all. While waiting for recovery, every effort should be made to maintain the nutrition of the damaged nerve, and of the parts which it supplies.

When suture is found to be impossible, recourse must be had to other methods, known as nerve bridging and nerve implantation.

Incomplete Division of a Mixed Nerve.—The effects of partial division of a mixed nerve vary according to the destination of the nerve bundles that have been interrupted. Within their area of distribution the paralysis is as complete as if the whole trunk had been cut across. The uninjured nerve-bundles continue to transmit impulses with the result that there is a *dissociated paralysis* within the distribution of the affected nerve, some muscles continuing to act and to respond normally to electric stimulation, while others behave as if the whole nerve-trunk had been severed.

In addition to vasomotor and trophic changes, there is often severe pain of a burning kind (*causalgia* or *thermalgia*) which comes on about a fortnight after the injury and causes intense and continuous suffering which may last for months. Paroxysms of pain may be excited by the slightest touch or by heat, and the patient usually learns for himself that the constant application of cold wet cloths allays the pain. The thermalgic area sweats profusely.

335

Operative treatment is indicated where there is no sign of improvement within three months, when recovery is arrested before complete restoration of function is attained, or when thermalgic pain is excessive.

Subcutaneous Injuries of Nerves.—Several varieties of subcutaneous injuries of nerves are met with. One of the best known is the compression paralysis of the nerves of the upper arm which results from sleeping with the arm resting on the back of a chair or the edge of a table—the so-called "drunkard's palsy"; and from the pressure of a crutch in the axilla—"crutch paralysis." In some of these injuries, notably "drunkard's palsy," the disability appears to be due not to damage of the nerve, but to overstretching of the extensors of the wrist and fingers (Jones). A similar form of paralysis is sometimes met with from the pressure of a tourniquet, from tight bandages or splints, from the pressure exerted by a dislocated bone or by excessive callus, and from hyperextension of the arm during anæsthesia.

In all these forms there is impaired sensation, rarely amounting to anæsthesia, marked muscular wasting, and diminution or loss of voluntary motor power, while—and this is a point of great importance—the normal electrical reactions are preserved. There may also develop trophic changes such as blisters, superficial ulcers, and clubbing of the tips of the fingers. The prognosis is usually favourable, as recovery is the rule within from one to three months. If, however, neuritis supervenes, the electrical reactions are altered, the muscles degenerate, and recovery may be retarded or may fail to take place.

Injuries which act abruptly or instantaneously are illustrated in the crushing of a nerve by the sudden displacement of a sharp-edged fragment of bone, as may occur in comminuted fractures of the humerus. The symptoms include perversion or loss of sensation, motor paralysis, and atrophy of muscles, which show the reaction of degeneration from the eighth day onwards. The presence of the reaction of degeneration influences both the prognosis and the treatment, for it implies a lesion which is probably incapable of spontaneous recovery, and which can only be remedied by operation.

The *treatment* varies with the cause and nature of the lesion. When, for example, a displaced bone or a mass of callus is pressing upon the nerve, steps must be taken to relieve the pressure, by operation if necessary. When there is reason to believe that the nerve is severely crushed or torn across, it should be exposed by incision, and, after removal of the damaged ends, should be united by sutures. When it is impossible to make a definite diagnosis as to the state of the nerve, it is better to expose it by operation, and thus learn the exact state of affairs without delay; in the event of the nerve being torn, the ends should be united by sutures.

Dislocation of Nerves.—This injury, which resembles the dislocation of tendons from their grooves, is seldom met with except in the ulnar nerve at the elbow, and is described with injuries of that nerve.

DISEASES OF NERVES

Traumatic Neuritis.—This consists in an overgrowth of the connective-tissue framework of a nerve, which causes irritation and pressure upon the nerve fibres, sometimes resulting in their degeneration. It may originate in connection with a wound in the vicinity of a nerve, as, for example, when the brachial nerves are involved in scar tissue subsequent to an operation for clearing out the axilla for cancer; or in contusion and compression of a nerve—for example, by the pressure of the head of the humerus in a dislocation of the shoulder. Some weeks or months after the injury, the patient complains of increasing hyperæsthesia and of neuralgic pains in the course of the nerve. The nerve is very sensitive to pressure, and, if superficial, may be felt to be swollen. The associated muscles are wasted and weak, and are subject to twitchings. There are also trophic disturbances. It is rare to have complete sensory and motor paralysis. The disease is commonest in the nerves of the upper extremity, and the hand may become crippled and useless.

Treatment.—Any constitutional condition which predisposes to neuritis, such as gout, diabetes, or syphilis, must receive appropriate treatment. The symptoms may be relieved by rest and by soothing applications, such as belladonna, ichthyol, or menthol, by the use of hot-air and electric baths, and in obstinate cases by blistering or by the application of Corrigan's button. When such treatment fails the nerve may be stretched, or, in the case of a purely sensory trunk, a portion may be excised. Local causes, such as involvement of the nerve in a scar or in adhesions, may afford indications for operative treatment.

Multiple Peripheral Neuritis.—Although this disease mainly comes under the cognizance of the physician, it may be attended with phenomena which call for surgical interference. In this country it is commonly due to alcoholism, but it may result from diabetes or from chronic poisoning with lead or arsenic, or from bacterial infections and intoxications such as occur in diphtheria, gonorrhoea, syphilis, leprosy, typhoid, influenza, beri-beri, and many other diseases.

It is, as a rule, widely distributed throughout the peripheral nerves, but the distribution frequently varies with the cause—the alcoholic form, for example, mainly affecting the legs, the diphtheritic form the soft palate and pharynx, and that associated with lead poisoning the forearms. The essential lesion is a degeneration of the conducting fibres of the affected nerves, and the prominent symptoms are the result of this. In alcoholic neuritis there is great tenderness of the muscles. When the legs are affected the patient may be unable to walk, and the toes may droop and the heel be drawn up, resulting in one variety of pes equino-varus. Pressure sores and perforating ulcer of the foot are the most important trophic phenomena.

Apart from the medical *treatment*, measures must be taken to prevent deformity, especially when the legs are affected. The bedclothes are supported by a cage, and the foot maintained at right angles to the leg by sand-bags or splints. When the disease is subsiding, the nutrition of the damaged nerves and muscles should be maintained by massage, baths, passive movements, and the use of the galvanic current. When deformity has been allowed to take place, operative measures may be required for its correction.

NEUROMA[5]

Neuroma is a clinical term applied to all tumours, irrespective of their structure, which have their seat in nerves.

A tumour composed of newly formed nerve tissue is spoken of as a **true neuroma**; when ganglionic cells are present in addition to nerve fibres, the name *ganglionic neuroma* is applied. These tumours are rare, and are chiefly met with in the main cords or abdominal plexuses of the sympathetic system of children or young adults. They are quite insensitive, and their removal is only called for if they cause pain or show signs of malignancy.

A **false neuroma** is an overgrowth of the sheath of a nerve. This overgrowth may result in the formation of a circumscribed tumour, or may take the form of a diffuse fibromatosis.

[5] We have followed the classification adopted by Alexis Thomson in his work *On Neuroma, and Neuro-fibromatosis* (Edinburgh: 1900).

The circumscribed or solitary tumour grows from the sheath of a nerve which is otherwise healthy, and it may be innocent or malignant.

The innocent form is usually fibrous or myxomatous, and is definitely encapsulated. It may become cystic as a result of hæmorrhage or of myxomatous degeneration. It grows very slowly, is usually elliptical in shape, and the solid form is rarely larger than a hazel-nut. The nerve fibres may be spread out all round the tumour, or may run only on one side of it. When subcutaneous and related to the smaller unnamed cutaneous nerves, it is known as a *painful subcutaneous nodule* or *tubercle*. It is chiefly met with about the ankle, and most often in women. It is remarkably sensitive, even gentle handling causing intense pain, which usually radiates to the periphery of the nerve affected. When related to a deeper, named nerve-trunk, it is known as a *trunk-neuroma*. It is usually less sensitive than the "subcutaneous nodule," and rarely gives rise to motor symptoms unless it involves the nerve roots where they pass through bony canals.

A trunk-neuroma is recognised clinically by its position in the line of a nerve, by the fact that it is movable in the transverse axis of the nerve but not in its long axis, and by being unduly painful and sensitive.

Treatment.—If the tumour causes suffering it should be removed, preferably by shelling it out from the investing nerve sheath or capsule. In the subcutaneous nodule the nerve is rarely recognisable, and is usually sacrificed. When removal of the tumour is incomplete, a tube of radium should be inserted into the cavity, to prevent recurrence of the tumour in a malignant form.

The malignant neuroma is a sarcoma growing from the sheath of a nerve. It has the same characters and clinical features as the innocent variety, only it grows more rapidly, and by destroying the nerve fibres causes motor symptoms—jerkings followed by paralysis. The sarcoma tends to spread along the lymph spaces in the long axis of the nerve, as well as to implicate the surrounding

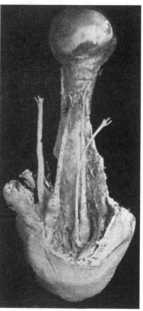

FIG. 85. Amputation Stump of Upper Arm, showing bulbous thickening of the ends of the nerves, embedded in scar tissue at the apex of the stamp.

tissues, and it is liable to give rise to secondary growths. The malignant neuroma is met with chiefly in the sciatic and other large nerves of the limbs.

The *treatment* is conducted on the same lines as sarcoma in other situations; the insertion of a tube of radium after removal of the tumour diminishes the tendency to recurrence; a portion of the nerve-trunk being sacrificed,
means must be taken to bridge the gap. In inoperable cases it may be possible
to relieve pain by excising a portion of the nerve above the tumour, or, when
this is impracticable, by resecting the posterior nerve roots and their ganglia
within the vertebral canal.

The so-called *amputation neuroma* has already been referred to (p. 344).

Diffuse or Generalised Neuro-Fibromatosis—Recklinghausen's Disease.—These
terms are now used to include what were formerly known as "multiple neu-
romata," as well as certain other overgrowths related to nerves. The essential
lesion is an overgrowth of the endoneural connective tissue throughout the
nerves of both the cerebro-spinal and sympathetic systems. The nerves are
diffusely and unequally thickened, so that small twigs may become enlarged
to the size of the median, while at irregular intervals along their course the
connective-tissue overgrowth is exaggerated so as to form tumour-like swellings similar to the trunk-neuroma already described. The tumours, which
vary greatly in size and number—as many as a thousand have been counted
in one case—are enclosed in a capsule derived from the perineurium. The
fibromatosis may also affect the cranial nerves, the ganglia on the posterior
nerve roots, the nerves within the vertebral canal, and the sympathetic nerves
and ganglia, as well as the continuations of the motor nerves within the
muscles. The nerve fibres, although mechanically displaced and dissociated
by the overgrown endoneurium, undergo no structural change except when
compressed in passing through a bony canal.

The disease probably originates before birth, although it may not make
its appearance till adolescence or even till adult life. It is sometimes met with
in several members of one family. It is recognised clinically by the presence
of multiple tumours in the course of the nerves, and sometimes by palpable
enlargement of the superficial nerve-trunks (Fig. 86). The tumours resemble
the solitary trunk-neuroma, are usually quite insensitive, and many of them
are unknown to the patient. As a result of injury or other exciting cause,
however, one or other tumour may increase in size and become extremely
sensitive; the pain is then agonising; it is increased by handling, and interferes

with sleep. In these conditions, a malignant transformation of the fibroma into sarcoma is to be suspected. Motor disturbances are exceptional, unless in the case of tumours within the vertebral canal, which press on the spinal medulla and cause paraplegia.

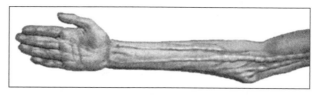

FIG. 86. Diffuse enlargement of Nerves in generalised Neuro-fibromatosis. (After R. W. Smith.)

Neuro-fibromatosis is frequently accompanied by *pigmentation of the skin* in the form of brown spots or patches scattered over the trunk.

The disease is often stationary for long periods. In progressive cases the patient becomes exhausted, and usually dies of some intercurrent affection, particularly phthisis. The treatment is restricted to relieving symptoms and complications; removal of one of the tumours is to be strongly deprecated.

In a considerable proportion of cases one of the multiple tumours takes on the characters of a malignant growth ("secondary malignant neuroma," Garrè). This malignant transformation may follow upon injury, or on an unsuccessful attempt to remove the tumour. The features are those of a rapidly growing sarcoma involving a nerve-trunk, with agonising pain and muscular cramps, followed by paralysis from destruction of the nerve fibres. The removal of the tumour is usually followed by recurrence, so that high amputation is the only treatment to be recommended. Metastasis to internal organs is exceptional.

There are other types of neuro-fibromatosis which require brief mention.

The plexiform neuroma (Fig. 87) is a fibromatosis confined to the distribution of one or more contiguous nerves or of a plexus of nerves, and it may occur either by itself or along with multiple

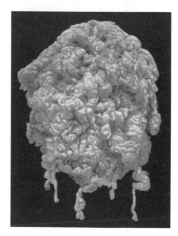

FIG. 87. Plexiform Neuroma of small Sciatic Nerve, from a girl æt. 16. (Mr. Annandale's case.)

tumours of the nerve-trunks and with pigmentation of the skin. The clinical features are those of an ill-defined swelling composed of a number of tortuous, convoluted cords, lying in a loose areolar tissue and freely movable on one another. It is rarely the seat of pain or tenderness. It most often appears in the early years of life, sometimes in relation to a pigmented or hairy mole. It is of slow growth, may remain stationary for long periods, and has little or no tendency to become malignant. It is usually subcutaneous, and is frequently situated on the head or neck in the distribution of the trigeminal or superficial cervical nerves. There is no necessity for its removal, but this may be indicated because of disfigurement, especially on the face or scalp or because its bulk interferes with function. When involving the ophthalmic division of the trigeminus, for example, it may cause enlargement of the upper lid and proptosis, with danger to the function of the globe. The results of excision are usually satisfactory, even if the removal is not complete.

The cutaneous neuro-fibroma or *molluscum fibrosum* has been shown by Recklinghausen to be a soft fibroma related to the terminal filaments of one of the cutaneous nerves (Fig. 88). The disease appears in the form of multiple, soft, projecting tumours, scattered all over the body, except the palms of the hands and soles of the feet. The tumours are of all sizes, some being no larger than a pin's head, whilst many are as big as a filbert and a few even larger. Many are sessile and others are distinctly pedunculated, but all are covered with skin. They are mobile, soft to the touch, and of the consistence of firm fat. In exceptional cases one of the skin tumours may attain an enormous size and cause a hideous deformity, hanging down by its own weight in lobulated or folded masses (pachy-dermatocele). The treatment consists in removing the larger swellings. In some cases molluscum fibrosum is associated with pigmentation of the skin and with multiple tumours of the nerve-trunks. The small multiple tumours rarely call for interference.

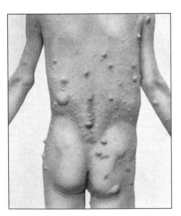

FIG. 88. Multiple Neuro-fibromas of Skin (Molluscum fibrosum, or Recklinghausen's disease).

Elephantiasis neuromatosa is the name applied by Virchow to a condition in which a limb is swollen and misshapen as a result of the extension of a neuro-fibromatosis to the skin and subcutaneous cellular tissue of the extremity as a whole (Fig. 89). It usually begins in early life without apparent cause, and it may be associated with multiple tumours of the nerve-trunks. The inconvenience caused by the bulk and weight of the limb may justify its removal.

SURGERY OF THE INDIVIDUAL NERVES[6]

The Brachial Plexus.—Lesions of the brachial plexus may be divided into those above the clavicle and those below that bone.

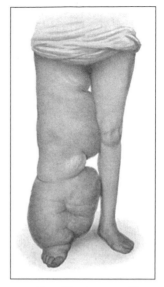

FIG. 89. Elephantiasis Neuromatosa in a woman æt. 28

In the **supra-clavicular injuries**, the violence applied to the head or shoulder causes over-stretching of the anterior branches (primary divisions) of the cervical nerves, the fifth, or the fifth and sixth being those most liable to suffer. Sometimes the traction is exerted upon the plexus from below, as when a man in falling from a height endeavours to save himself by clutching at some projection, and the lesion then mainly affects the first dorsal nerve. There is tearing of the nerve sheaths, with hæmorrhage, but in severe cases partial or complete severance of nerve fibres may occur and these give way at different levels. During the healing process an excess of fibrous tissue is formed, which may interfere with regeneration.

Post-anæsthetic paralysis occurs in patients in whom, during the course of an operation, the arm is abducted and rotated laterally or extended above the head, causing over-stretching of the plexus, especially of the fifth, or fifth and sixth, anterior branches.

A *cervical rib* may damage the plexus by direct pressure, the part usually affected being the medial cord, which is made up of fibres from the eighth cervical and first dorsal nerves.

When a lesion of the plexus complicates a *fracture of the clavicle*, the nerve injury is due, not to pressure on or laceration of the nerves by fragments of

[6]We desire here to acknowledge our indebtedness to Mr. James Sherren's work on *Injuries of Nerves and their Treatment.*

343

bone, but to the violence causing the fracture, and this is usually applied to the point of the shoulder.

Penetrating *wounds*, apart from those met with in military practice, are rare.

In the **infra-clavicular injuries**, the lesion most often results from the pressure of the dislocated head of the humerus; occasionally from attempts made to reduce the dislocation by the heel-in-the-axilla method, or from fracture of the upper end of the humerus or of the neck of the scapula. The whole plexus may suffer, but more frequently the medial cord is alone implicated.

Clinical Features.—Three types of lesion result from indirect violence: the whole plexus; the upper-arm type; and the lower-arm type.

When the whole plexus is involved, sensibility is lost over the entire forearm and hand and over the lateral surface of the arm in its distal two-thirds. All the muscles of the arm, forearm, and hand are paralysed, and, as a rule, also the pectorals and spinati, but the rhomboids and serratus anterior escape. There is paralysis of the sympathetic fibres to the eye and orbit, with narrowing of the palpebral fissure, recession of the globe, and the pupil is slow to dilate when shaded from the light.

The *upper-arm type*—Erb-Duchenne paralysis—is that most frequently met with, and it is due to a lesion of the fifth anterior branch, or, it may be, also of the sixth. The position of the upper limb is typical: the arm and forearm hang close to the side, with the forearm extended and pronated; the deltoid, spinati, biceps, brachialis, and supinators are paralysed, and in some cases the radial extensors of the wrist and the pronator teres are also affected. The patient is unable to supinate the forearm or to abduct the arm, and in most cases to flex the forearm. He may, however, regain some power of flexing the forearm when it is fully pronated, the extensors of the wrist becoming feeble flexors of the elbow. There is, as a rule, no loss of sensibility, but complaint may be made of tickling and of pins-and-needles over the lateral aspect of the arm. The abnormal position of the limb may persist although the muscles regain the power of voluntary movement, and as the condition frequently follows a fall on the shoulder, great care is necessary in diagnosis, as the condition is apt to be attributed to an injury to the axillary (circumflex) nerve.

The *lower-arm type* of paralysis, associated with the name of Klumpke, is usually due to over-stretching of the plexus, and especially affects the anterior branch of the first dorsal nerve. In typical cases all the intrinsic muscles of the hand are affected, and the hand assumes the claw shape. Sensibility is usually altered over the medial side of the arm and forearm, and there is paralysis of the sympathetic.

Infra-clavicular injuries, as already stated, are most often produced by a sub-coracoid dislocation of the humerus; the medial cord is that most frequently injured, and the muscles paralysed are those supplied by the ulnar nerve, with, in addition, those intrinsic muscles of the hand supplied by the median. Sensibility is affected over the medial surface of the forearm and ulnar area of the hand. Injury of the lateral and posterior cords is very rare.

Treatment is carried out on the lines already laid down for nerve injuries in general. It is impossible to diagnose between complete and incomplete rupture of the nerve cords, until sufficient time has elapsed to allow of the establishment of the reaction of degeneration. If this is present at the end of fourteen days, operation should not be delayed. Access to the cords of the plexus is obtained by a dissection similar to that employed for the subclavian artery, and the nerves are sought for as they emerge from under cover of the scalenus anterior, and are then traced until the seat of injury is found. In the case of the first dorsal nerve, it may be necessary temporarily to resect the clavicle. The usual after-treatment must be persisted in until recovery ensues, and care must be taken that the paralysed muscles do not become over-stretched. The prognosis is less favourable in the supra-clavicular lesions than in those below the clavicle, which nearly always recover without surgical intervention.

In the *brachial birth-paralysis* met with in infants, the lesion is due to over-stretching of the plexus, and is nearly always of the Erb-Duchenne type. The injury is usually unilateral, it occurs with almost equal frequency in breech and in vertex presentations, and the left arm is more often affected than the right. The lesion is seldom recognised at birth. The first symptom noticed is tenderness in the supra-clavicular region, the child crying when this part is touched or the arm is moved. The attitude may be that of the Erb-Duchenne type, or the whole of the muscles of the upper limb may be flaccid, and the arm hangs powerless. A considerable proportion of the cases recover spontaneously. The arm is to be kept at rest, with the affected muscles relaxed, and, as soon as tenderness has disappeared, daily massage and passive movements are employed. The reaction of degeneration can rarely be satisfactorily tested before the child is three months old, but if it is present, an operation should be performed. After operation, the shoulder should be elevated so that no traction is exerted on the affected cords.

The long thoracic nerve (nerve of Bell), which supplies the serratus anterior, is rarely injured. In those whose occupation entails carrying weights upon the shoulder it may be contused, and the resulting paralysis of the serratus is usually combined with paralysis of the lower part of the trapezius, the branches from the third and fourth cervical nerves which supply this muscle also being exposed to pressure as they pass across the root of the neck. There is complaint of pain above the clavicle, and winging of the scapula; the patient is unable to raise the arm in front of the body above the level of the shoulder or to perform any forward pushing movements; on attempting either of these the winging of the scapula is at once increased. If the scapula is compared with that on the sound side, it is seen that, in addition to the lower angle being more prominent, the spine is more horizontal and the lower angle nearer the middle line. The majority of these cases recover if the limb is placed at absolute rest, the elbow supported, and massage and galvanism persevered with. If the paralysis persists, the sterno-costal portion of the pectoralis major may be transplanted to the lower angle of the scapula.

The long thoracic nerve may be cut across while clearing out the axilla in operating for cancer of the breast. The displacement of the scapula is not so marked as in the preceding type, and the patient is able to perform pushing movements below the level of the shoulder. If the reaction of degeneration develops, an operation may be performed, the ends of the nerve being sutured, or the distal end grafted into the posterior cord of the brachial plexus.

The Axillary (Circumflex) Nerve.—In the majority of cases in which paralysis of the deltoid follows upon an injury of the shoulder, it is due to a lesion of the fifth cervical nerve, as has already been described in injuries of the brachial plexus. The axillary nerve itself as it passes round the neck of the humerus is most liable to be injured from the pressure of a crutch, or of the head of the humerus in sub-glenoid dislocation, or in fracture of the neck of the scapula or of the humerus. In miners, who work for long periods lying on the side, the muscle may be paralysed by direct pressure on the terminal filaments of the nerve, and the nerve may also be involved as a result of disease in the sub-deltoid bursa.

The deltoid is wasted, and the acromion unduly prominent. In recent cases paralysis of the muscle is easily detected. In cases of long standing it is not so simple, because other muscles, the spinati, the clavicular fibres of the pectoral and the serratus, take its place and elevate the arm; there is always loss of sensation on the lateral aspect of the shoulder. There is rarely any call for operative treatment, as the paralysis is usually compensated for by other muscles.

When the *supra-scapular nerve* is contused or stretched in injuries of the shoulder, the spinati muscles are paralysed and wasted, the spine of the scapula is unduly prominent, and there is impairment in the power of abducting the arm and rotating it laterally.

The *musculo-cutaneous nerve* is very rarely injured; when cut across, there is paralysis of the coraco-brachialis, biceps, and part of the brachialis, but no movements are abolished, the forearm being flexed, in the pronated position, by the brachio-radialis and long radial extensor of the wrist; in the supinated position, by that portion of the brachialis supplied by the radial nerve. Supination is feebly performed by the supinator muscle. Protopathic and epicritic sensibility are lost over the radial side of the forearm.

Radial (Musculo-Spiral) Nerve.—From its anatomical relationships this trunk is more exposed to injury than any other nerve in the body. It is frequently compressed against the humerus in sleeping with the arm resting on the back of a chair, especially in the deep sleep of alcoholic intoxication (drunkard's palsy). It may be pressed upon by a crutch in the axilla, by the dislocated head of the humerus, or by violent compression of the arm, as when an elastic tourniquet is applied too tightly. The most serious and permanent injuries of this nerve are associated with fractures of the humerus, especially those from direct violence attended with comminution of the bone. The nerve may be crushed or torn by one of the fragments at the time of the injury, or at a later period may be compressed by callus.

Clinical Features.—Immediately after the injury it is impossible to tell whether the nerve is torn across or merely compressed. The patient may complain of numbness and tingling in the distribution of the superficial branch of the nerve, but it is a striking fact, that so long as the nerve is divided below the level at which it gives off the dorsal cutaneous nerve of the forearm (external cutaneous branch), there is no loss of sensation. When it is divided above the origin of the dorsal cutaneous branch, or when the dorsal branch of the musculo-cutaneous nerve is also divided, there is a loss of sensibility on the dorsum of the hand.

The motor symptoms predominate, the muscles affected being the extensors of the wrist and fingers, and the supinators. There is a characteristic "dropwrist"; the wrist is flexed and pronated, and the patient is unable to dorsiflex the wrist or fingers (Fig. 90). If the hand and proximal phalanges are supported, the second and third phalanges may be partly extended by the interossei and lumbricals. There is also considerable impairment of power in the muscles which antagonise those that are paralysed, so that the grasp of the hand is feeble, and the patient almost loses the use of it; in some cases this would appear to be due to the median nerve having been injured at the same time.

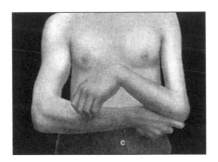

FIG. 90. Drop-wrist following Fracture of Shaft of Humerus.

If the lesion is high up, as it is, for example, in crutch paralysis, the triceps and anconeus may also suffer.

Treatment.—The slighter forms of injury by compression recover under massage, douching, and electricity. If there is drop-wrist, the hand and forearm are placed on a palmar splint, with the hand dorsiflexed to nearly a right angle, and this position is maintained until voluntary dorsiflexion at the wrist returns to the normal. Recovery is sometimes delayed for several months.

In the more severe injuries associated with fracture of the humerus and attended with the reaction of degeneration, it is necessary to cut down upon the nerve and free it from the pressure of a fragment of bone or from callus or adhesions. If the nerve is torn across, the ends must be sutured, and if this is impossible owing to loss of tissue, the gap may be bridged by a graft taken from the superficial branch of the radial nerve, or the ends may be implanted into the median.

Finally, in cases in which the paralysis is permanent and incurable, the disability may be relieved by operation. A fascial graft can be employed to act as a ligament permanently extending the wrist; it is attached to the third and fourth metacarpal bones distally and to the radius or ulna proximally. The flexor carpi radialis can then be joined up with the extensor digitorum communis by passing its tendon through an aperture in the interosseous membrane, or better still, through the pronator quadratus, as there is less likelihood of the formation of adhesions when the tendon passes through muscle than through interosseous membrane. The palmaris longus is anastomosed with the abductor pollicis longus (extensor ossis metacarpi pollicis), thus securing a fair amount of abduction of the thumb. The flexor carpi ulnaris may also be anastomosed with the common extensor of the fingers. The extensors of the wrist may be shortened, so as to place the hand in the position of dorsal flexion, and thus improve the attitude and grasp of the hand.

The superficial branch of the radial (radial nerve) *and the deep branch* (posterior interosseous), apart from suffering in lesions of the radial, are liable to be contused or torn is dislocation of the head of the radius, and in fracture of the neck of the bone. The deep branch may be divided as it passes through the supinator in operations on old fractures and dislocations in the region of the elbow. Division of the superficial branch in the upper two-thirds of the forearm produces no loss of sensibility; division in the lower third after the nerve has become associated with branches from the musculo-cutaneous is followed by a loss of sensibility on the radial side of the hand and thumb. Wounds on the dorsal surface of the wrist and forearm are often followed by loss of sensibility over a larger area, because the musculo-cutaneous nerve is divided as well, and some of the fibres of the lower lateral cutaneous branch of the radial.

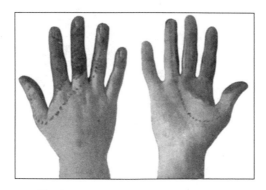

FIG. 91. To illustrate the Loss of Sensation produced by Division of the Median Nerve. The area of complete cutaneous insensibility is shaded black. The parts insensitive to light touch and to intermediate degrees of temperature are enclosed within the dotted line. (After Head and Sherren.)

The Median Nerve is most frequently injured in wounds made by broken glass in the region of the wrist. It may also be injured in fractures of the lower end of the humerus, in fractures of both bones of the forearm, and as a result of pressure by splints. After *division at the elbow*, there is impairment of mobility which affects the thumb, and to a less extent the index finger: the terminal phalanx of the thumb cannot be flexed owing to the paralysis of the flexor pollicis longus, and the index can only be flexed at its metacarpo-phalangeal joint by the interosseous muscles attached to it. Pronation of the forearm is feeble, and is completed by the weight of the hand. After *division at the wrist*, the abductor-opponens group of muscles and the two lateral lumbricals only are affected; the abduction of the thumb can be feebly imitated by the short extensor and the long abductor (ext. ossis metacarpi pollicis), while opposition may be simulated by contraction of the long flexor and the short abductor of the thumb; the paralysis of the two medial lumbricals produces no symptoms that can be recognised. It is important to remember that when the median nerve is divided at the wrist, deep touch can be appreciated over the whole of the area supplied by the nerve; the injury, therefore, is liable to be over looked. If, however, the tendons are divided as well as the nerve, there is insensibility to deep touch. The areas of epicritic and of protopathic insensibility are illustrated in Fig. 91. The division of the nerve at the elbow, or even at the axilla, does not increase the extent of the loss of epicritic or protopathic sensibility, but usually affects deep sensibility.

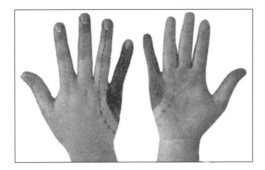

FIG. 92. To illustrate Loss of Sensation produced by complete Division of Ulnar Nerve. Loss of all forms of cutaneous sensibility is represented by the shaded area. The parts insensitive to light touch and to intermediate degrees of heat and cold are enclosed within the dotted line. (Head and Sherren.)]

The Ulnar Nerve.—The most common injury of this nerve is its division in transverse accidental wounds just above the wrist. In the arm it may be contused, along with the radial, in crutch paralysis; in the region of the elbow it may be injured in fractures or dislocations, or it may be accidentally divided in the operation for excising the elbow-joint.

When it is injured *at or above the elbow*, there is paralysis of the flexor carpi ulnaris, the ulnar half of the flexor digitorum profundus, all the interossei, the two medial lumbricals, and the adductors of the thumb. The hand assumes a characteristic attitude: the index and middle fingers are extended at the metacarpo-phalangeal joints owing to paralysis of the interosseous muscles attached to them; the little and ring fingers are hyper-extended at these joints in consequence of the paralysis of the lumbricals; all the fingers are flexed at the inter-phalangeal joints, the flexion being most marked in the little and ring fingers—claw-hand or *main en griffe*. On flexing the wrist, the hand is tilted to the radial side, but the paralysis of the flexor carpi ulnaris is often compensated for by the action of the palmaris longus. The little and ring fingers can be flexed to a slight degree by the slips of the flexor sublimis attached to them and supplied by the median nerve; flexion of the terminal phalanx of the little finger is almost impossible. Adduction and abduction movements of the fingers are lost. Adduction of the thumb is carried out, not by the paralysed adductor pollicis, but the movement may be simulated by the long flexor and extensor muscles of the thumb. Epicritic sensibility is lost over the little finger, the ulnar half of the ring finger, and that part of the palm and dorsum of the hand to the ulnar side of a line drawn longitudinally through the ring finger and continued upwards. Protopathic sensibility is lost over an area which varies in different cases. Deep sensibility is usually lost over an area almost as extensive as that of protopathic insensibility.

When the nerve is *divided at the wrist*, the adjacent tendons are also frequently severed. If divided below the point at which its dorsal branch is given off, the sensory paralysis is much less marked, and the injury is therefore liable to be overlooked until the wasting of muscles and typical *main en griffe* ensue. The loss of sensibility after division of the nerve before the dorsal branch is given off resembles that after division at the elbow, except that in uncomplicated cases deep sensibility is usually retained. If the tendons are divided as well, however, deep touch is also lost.

Care must be taken in all these injuries to prevent deformity; a splint must be worn, at least during the night, until the muscles regain their power of voluntary movement, and then exercises should be instituted.

Dislocation of the ulnar nerve at the elbow results from sudden and violent flexion of the joint, the muscular effort causing stretching or laceration of the fascia that holds the nerve in its groove; it is predisposed to if the groove is shallow as a result of imperfect development of the medial condyle of the humerus, and by cubitus valgus.

The nerve slips forward, and may be felt lying on the medial aspect of the condyle. It may retain this position, or it may slip backwards and forwards with the movements of the arm. The symptoms at the time of the displacement are some disability at the elbow, and pain and tingling along the nerve, which are exaggerated by movement and by pressure. The symptoms may subside altogether, or a neuritis may develop, with severe pain shooting up the nerve.

The dislocated nerve is easily replaced, but is difficult to retain in position. In recent cases the arm may be placed in the extended position with a pad over the condyle, care being taken to avoid pressure on the nerve. Failing relief, it is better to make a bed for the nerve by dividing the deep fascia behind the medial condyle and to stitch the edges of the fascia over the nerve. This operation has been successful in all the recorded cases.

The Sciatic Nerve.—When this nerve is compressed, as by sitting on a fence, there is tingling and powerlessness in the limb as a whole, known as "sleeping" of the limb, but these phenomena are evanescent. *Injuries to the great sciatic nerve* are rare except in war. Partial division is more common than complete, and it is noteworthy that the fibres destined for the peroneal nerve are more often and more severely injured than those for the tibial (internal popliteal). After complete division, all the muscles of the leg are paralysed; if the section is in the upper part of the thigh, the hamstrings are also paralysed. The limb is at first quite powerless, but the patient usually recovers sufficiently to be able to walk with a little support, and although the hamstrings are paralysed the knee can be flexed by the sartorius and gracilis. The chief feature is drop-foot. There is also loss of sensation below the knee except along the course of the long saphenous nerve on the medial side of the leg and foot. Sensibility to deep touch is only lost over a comparatively small area on the dorsum of the foot.

The Common Peroneal (external popliteal) nerve is exposed to injury where it winds round the neck of the fibula, because it is superficial and lies against the unyielding bone. It may be compressed by a tourniquet, or it may be bruised or torn in fractures of the upper end of the bone. It has been divided in accidental wounds,—by a scythe, for example,—in incising for cellulitis, and in performing subcutaneous tenotomy of the biceps tendon. Cases have been observed of paralysis of the nerve as a result of prolonged acute flexion of the knee in certain occupations.

When the nerve is divided, the most obvious result is "drop-foot"; the patient is unable to dorsiflex the foot and cannot lift his toes off the ground, so that in walking he is obliged to jerk the foot forwards and laterally. The loss of sensibility depends upon whether the nerve is divided above or below the origin of the large cutaneous branch which comes off just before it passes round the neck of the fibula. In course of time the foot becomes inverted and the toes are pointed—pes equino-varus—and trophic sores are liable to form.

The Tibial (internal popliteal) nerve is rarely injured.

The Cranial nerves are considered with affections of the head and neck (Vol. II.).

NEURALGIA

The term neuralgia is applied clinically to any pain which follows the course of a nerve, and is not referable to any discoverable cause. It should not be applied to pain which results from pressure on a nerve by a tumour, a mass of callus, an aneurysm, or by any similar gross lesion. We shall only consider here those forms of neuralgia which are amenable to surgical treatment.

Brachial Neuralgia.—The pain is definitely located in the distribution of one of the branches or nerve roots, is often intermittent, and is usually associated with tingling and disturbance of tactile sensation. The root of the neck should be examined to exclude pressure as the cause of the pain by a cervical rib, a tumour, or an aneurysm. When medical treatment fails, the nerve-trunks may be injected with saline solution or recourse may be had to operative measures, the affected cords being exposed and stretched through an incision in the posterior triangle of the neck. If this fails to give relief, the more serious operation of resecting the posterior roots of the affected nerves within the vertebral canal may be considered.

Neuralgia of the sciatic nerve—**sciatica**—is the most common form of neuralgia met with in surgical practice.

It is chiefly met with in adults of gouty or rheumatic tendencies who suffer from indigestion, constipation, and oxaluria—in fact, the same type of patients who are liable to lumbago, and the two affections are frequently associated. In hospital practice it is commonly met with in coal-miners and others who assume a squatting position at work. The onset of the pain may follow over-exertion and exposure to cold and wet, especially in those who do not take regular exercise. Any error of diet or indulgence in beer or wine may contribute to its development.

The essential symptom is paroxysmal or continuous pain along the course of the nerve in the buttock, thigh, or leg. It may be comparatively slight, or it may be so severe as to prevent sleep. It is aggravated by movement, so that the patient walks lame or is obliged to lie up. It is aggravated also by any movement which tends to put the nerve on the stretch, as in bending down to put on the shoes, such movements also causing tingling down the nerve, and sometimes numbness in the foot. This may be demonstrated by flexing the thigh on the abdomen, the knee being kept extended; there is no pain if the same manoeuvre is repeated with the knee flexed. The nerve is sensitive to pressure, the most tender points being its emergence from the greater sciatic foramen, the hollow between the trochanter and the ischial tuberosity, and where the common peroneal nerve winds round the neck of the fibula. The muscles of the thigh are often wasted and are liable to twitch.

The clinical features vary a good deal in different cases; the affection is often obstinate, and may last for many weeks or even months.

In the sciatica that results from neuritis and perineuritis, there is marked tenderness on pressure due to the involvement of the nerve filaments in the sheath of the nerve, and there may be patches of cutaneous anæsthesia, loss of tendon reflexes, localised wasting of muscles, and vaso-motor and trophic changes. The presence of the reaction of degeneration confirms the diagnosis of neuritis. In long-standing cases the pain and discomfort may lead to a postural scoliosis (*ischias-scoliotica*).

Diagnosis.—Pain referred along the course of the sciatic nerve on one side, or, as is sometimes the case, on both sides, is a symptom of tumours of the uterus, the rectum, or the pelvic bones. It may result also from the pressure of an abscess or an aneurysm either inside the pelvis or in the buttock, and is sometimes associated with disease of the spinal medulla, such as tabes. Gluteal fibrositis may be mistaken for sciatica. It is also necessary to exclude such conditions as disease in the hip or sacro-iliac joint, especially tuberculous disease and arthritis deformans, before arriving at a diagnosis of sciatica. A digital examination of the rectum or vagina is of great value in excluding intra-pelvic tumours.

Treatment is both general and local. Any constitutional tendency, such as gout or rheumatism, must be counteracted, and indigestion, oxaluria, and constipation should receive appropriate treatment. In acute cases the patient is confined to bed between blankets, the limb is wrapped in thermogene wool, and the knee is flexed over a pillow; in some cases relief is experienced from the use of a long splint, or slinging the leg in a Salter's cradle. A rubber hot-bottle may be applied over the seat of greatest pain. The bowels should be well opened by castor oil or by calomel followed by a saline. Salicylate of soda in full doses, or aspirin, usually proves effectual in relieving pain, but when this is very intense it may call for injections of heroin or morphin. Potassium iodide is of benefit in chronic cases.

Relief usually results from bathing, douching, and massage, and from repeated gentle stretching of the nerve. This may be carried out by passive movements of the limb—the hip being flexed while the knee is kept extended; and by active movements—the patient flexing the limb at the hip, the knee being maintained in the extended position. These exercises, which may be preceded by massage, are carried out night and morning, and should be practised systematically by those who are liable to sciatica.

Benefit has followed the injection into the nerve itself, or into the tissues surrounding it, of normal saline solution; from 70-100 c.c. are injected at one time. If the pain recurs, the injection may require to be repeated on many occasions at different points up and down the nerve. Needling or acupuncture consists in piercing the nerve at intervals in the buttock and thigh with long steel needles. Six or eight needles are inserted and left in position for from fifteen to thirty minutes.

In obstinate and severe cases the nerve may be *forcibly stretched*. This may be done bloodlessly by placing the patient on his back with the hip flexed to a right angle, and then gradually extending the knee until it is in a straight line with the thigh (Billroth). A general anæsthetic is usually required. A more effectual method is to expose the nerve through an incision at the fold of the buttock, and forcibly pull upon it. This operation is most successful when the pain is due to the nerve being involved in adhesions.

Trigeminal Neuralgia.—A severe form of epileptiform neuralgia occurs in the branches of the fifth nerve, and is one of the most painful affections to which human flesh is liable. So far as its pathology is known, it is believed to be due to degenerative changes in the semilunar (Gasserian) ganglion. It is met with in adults, is almost invariably unilateral, and develops without apparent cause. The pain, which occurs in paroxysms, is at first of moderate severity, but gradually becomes agonising. In the early stages the paroxysms occur at wide intervals, but later they recur with such frequency as to be almost continuous. They are usually excited by some trivial cause, such as moving the jaws in eating or speaking, touching the face as in washing, or exposure to a draught of cold air. Between the paroxysms the patient is free from pain, but is in constant terror of its return, and the face wears an expression of extreme suffering and anxiety. When the paroxysm is accompanied by twitching of the facial muscles, it is called *spasmodic tic*.

The skin of the affected area may be glazed and red, or may be pale and moist with inspissated sweat, the patient not daring to touch or wash it.

There is excessive tenderness at the points of emergence of the different branches on the face, and pressure over one or other of these points may excite a paroxysm. In typical cases the patient is unable to take any active part in life. The attempt to eat is attended with such severe pain that he avoids taking food. In some cases the suffering is so great that the patient only obtains sleep by the use of hypnotics, and he is often on the verge of suicide.

Diagnosis.—There is seldom any difficulty in recognising the disease. It is important, however, to exclude the hysterical form of neuralgia, which is characterised by its occurrence earlier in life, by the pain varying in situation, being frequently bilateral, and being more often constant than paroxysmal.

Treatment.—Before having recourse to the measures described below, it is advisable to give a thorough trial to the medical measures used in the treatment of neuralgia.

The Injection of Alcohol into the Nerve.—The alcohol acts by destroying the nerve fibres, and must be brought into direct contact with them; if the nerve has been properly struck the injection is followed by complete anæsthesia in the distribution of the nerve. The relief may last for from six months to three years; if the pain returns, the injection may be repeated. The strength of the alcohol should be 85 per cent., and the amount injected about 2 c.c.; a general, or preferably a local, anæsthetic (novocain) should be employed (Schlösser); the needle is 8 cm. long, and 0.7 mm. in diameter. The severe pain which the alcohol causes may be lessened, after the needle has penetrated to the necessary depth, by passing a few cubic centimetres of a 2 per cent. solution of *novocain-suprarenin* through it before the alcohol is injected. The treatment by injection of alcohol is superior to the resection of branches of the nerve, for though relapses occur after the treatment with alcohol, renewed freedom from pain may be obtained by its repetition. The ophthalmic division should not, however, be treated in this manner, for the alcohol may escape into the orbit and endanger other nerves in this region. Harris recommends the injection of alcohol into the semilunar ganglion.

Operative Treatment.—This consists in the removal of the affected nerve or nerves, either by resection—*neurectomy*; or by a combination of resection with twisting or tearing of the nerve from its central connections—*avulsion*. To prevent the regeneration of the nerve after these operations, the canal of exit through the bone should be obliterated; this is best accomplished by a silver screw-nail driven home by an ordinary screw-driver (Charles H. Mayo).

When the neuralgia involves branches of two or of all three trunks, or when it has recurred after temporary relief following resection of individual branches, the *removal of the semilunar ganglion*, along with the main trunks of the maxillary and mandibular divisions, should be considered.

The operation is a difficult and serious one, but the results are satisfactory so far as the cure of the neuralgia is concerned. There is little or no disability from the unilateral paralysis of the muscles of mastication; but on account of the insensitiveness of the cornea, the eye must be protected from irritation, especially during the first month or two after the operation; this may be done by fixing a large watch-glass around the edge of the orbit with adhesive plaster.

If the ophthalmic branch is not involved, neither it nor the ganglion should be interfered with; the maxillary and mandibular divisions should be divided within the skull, and the foramen rotundum and foramen ovale obliterated.

THE SKIN AND SUBCUTANEOUS TISSUE

Structure of Skin • *Blisters*
Callosities • *Corns* • *Chilblains*
Boils • *Carbuncle* • *Abscess* • *Veldt Sores*
Tuberculosis of Skin: Inoculation Tubercle
Lupus: Varieties • *Sporotrichosis* • *Elephantiasis*
Sebaceous Cysts or Wens • *Moles* • *Horns*
New Growths: Fibroma; Papilloma; Adenoma; Epithelioma; Rodent Cancer; Melanotic Cancer; Sarcoma
Affections of Cicatrices • *Varieties of Scars*
Keloid • *Tumours* • *Affections of Nails*

Structure of Skin.—The skin is composed of a superficial cellular layer—the epidermis, and the corium or true skin. The *epidermis* is differentiated from without inwards into the stratum corneum, the stratum lucidum, the stratum granulosum, and the rete Malpighii or germinal layer, from which all the others are developed. The *corium* or *true skin* consists of connective tissue, in which ramify the blood vessels, lymphatics, and nerves. That part of the corium immediately adjoining the epidermis is known as the papillary portion, and contains the terminal loops of the cutaneous blood vessels and the terminations of the cutaneous nerves. The deeper portion of the true skin is known as the reticular portion, and is largely composed of adipose tissue.

Blisters result from the exudation of serous fluid beneath the horny layer of the epidermis. The fluid may be clear, as in the blisters of a recent burn, or blood-stained, as in the blisters commonly accompanying fractures of the leg. It may become purulent as a result of infection, and this may be the starting-point of lymphangitis or cellulitis.

The skin should be disinfected and the blisters punctured. When infected, the separated horny layer must be cut away with scissors to allow of the necessary purification.

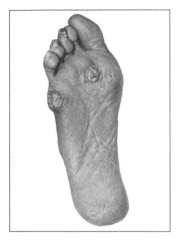

FIG. 93. Callosities and Corns on the Sole and Plantar Aspect of the Toes in a woman who was also the subject of flat-foot.

Callosities are prominent, indurated masses of the horny layer of the epidermis, where it has been exposed to prolonged friction and pressure. They occur on the fingers and hand as a result of certain occupations and sports, but are most common under the balls of the toes or heel. A bursa may form beneath a callosity, and if it becomes inflamed may cause considerable suffering; if suppuration ensues, a sinus may form, resembling a perforating ulcer of the foot.

The *treatment* of callosities on the foot consists in removing pressure by wearing properly fitting boots, and in applying a ring pad around the callosity; another method is to fit a sock of spongiopilene with a hole cut out opposite the callosity. After soaking in hot water, the overgrown horny layer is pared away, and the part painted daily with a saturated solution of salicylic acid in flexile collodion.

Corns.—A corn is a localised overgrowth of the horny layer of the epidermis, which grows downwards, pressing upon and displacing the sensitive papillæ of the corium. Corns are due to the friction and pressure of ill-fitting boots, and are met with chiefly on the toes and sole of the foot. A corn is usually hard, dry, and white; but it may be sodden from moisture, as in "soft corns" between the toes. A bursa may form beneath a corn, and if inflamed constitutes one form of bunion. When suppuration takes place in relation to a corn, there is great pain and disability, and it may prove the starting-point of lymphangitis.

The *treatment* consists in the wearing of properly fitting boots and stockings, and, if the symptoms persist, the corn should be removed. This is done after the manner of chiropodists by digging out the corn with a suitably shaped knife. A more radical procedure is to excise, under local anæsthesia, the portion of skin containing the corn and the underlying bursa. The majority of so-called corn solvents consist of a solution of salicylic acid in collodion; if this is painted on daily, the epidermis dies and can then be pared away. The unskilful paring of corns may determine the occurrence of senile gangrene in those who are predisposed to it by disease of the arteries.

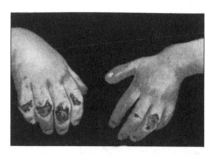

FIG. 94. Ulcerated Chilblains on Fingers of a Child.

Chilblains.—Chilblain or *erythema pernio* is a vascular disturbance resulting from the alternate action of cold and heat on the distal parts of the body. Chilblains are met with chiefly on the fingers and toes in children and anæmic girls. In the mild form there is a sensation of burning and itching, the part becomes swollen, of a dusky red colour, and the skin is tense and shiny. In more severe cases the burning and itching are attended with pain, and the skin becomes of a violet or wine-red colour. There is a third degree, closely approaching frost-bite, in which the skin tends to blister and give way, leaving an indolent raw surface popularly known as a "broken chilblain."

Those liable to chilblains should take open-air exercise, nourishing food, cod-liver oil, and tonics. Woollen stockings and gloves should be worn in cold weather, and sudden changes of temperature avoided. The symptoms may be relieved by ichthyol ointment, glycerin and belladonna, or a mixture of Venice turpentine, castor oil, and collodion applied on lint which is wrapped round the toe. Another favourite application is one of equal parts of tincture of capsicum and compound liniment of camphor, painted over the area night and morning. Balsam of Peru or resin ointment spread on gauze should be applied to broken chilblains. The most effective treatment is Bier's bandage applied for about six hours twice daily; it can be worn while the patient is following his occupation; in chronic cases this may be supplemented with hot-air baths.

Boils and Carbuncles.—These result from infection with the staphylococcus aureus, which enters the orifices of the ducts of the skin under the influence of friction and pressure, as was demonstrated by the well-known experiment of Garrè, who produced a crop of pustules and boils on his own forearm by rubbing in a culture of the staphylococcus aureus.

A **boil** results when the infection is located in a hair follicle or sebaceous gland. A hard, painful, conical swelling develops, to which, so long as the skin retains its normal appearance, the term "blind boil" is applied. Usually, however, the skin becomes red, and after a time breaks, giving exit to a drop or two of thick pus. After an interval of from six to ten days a soft white slough is discharged; this is known as the "core," and consists of the necrosed hair follicle or sebaceous gland. After the separation of the core the boil heals rapidly, leaving a small depressed scar.

Boils are most frequently met with on the back of the neck and the buttocks, and on other parts where the skin is coarse and thick and is exposed to friction and pressure. The occurrence of a number or a succession of boils is due to spread of the infection, the cocci from the original boil obtaining access to adjacent hair follicles. The spread of boils may be unwittingly promoted by the use of a domestic poultice or the wearing of infected underclothing.

While boils are frequently met with in debilitated persons, and particularly in those suffering from diabetes or Bright's disease, they also occur in those who enjoy vigorous health. They seldom prove dangerous to life except in diabetic subjects, but when they occur on the face there is a risk of lymphatic and of general pyogenic infection. Boils may be differentia ted from syphilitic lesions of the skin by their acute onset and progress, and by the absence of other evidence of syphilis; and from the malignant or anthrax pustule by the absence of the central black eschar and of the circumstances which attend upon anthrax infection.

Treatment.—The skin of the affected area should be painted with iodine, and a Klapp's suction bell applied thrice daily. If pus forms, the skin is frozen with ethyl-chloride and a small incision made, after which the application of the suction bell is persevered with. The further treatment consists in the use of diluted boracic or resin ointment. In multiple boils on the trunk and limbs, lysol or boracic baths are of service; the underclothing should be frequently changed, and that which is discarded must be disinfected. In patients with recurrence of boils about the neck, re-infection frequently takes place from the scalp, to which therefore treatment should be directed.

Any impaired condition of health should be corrected; when, there is sugar or albumen in the urine the conditions on which these depend must receive appropriate treatment. When there are successive crops of boils, recourse should be had to vaccines. In refractory cases benefit has followed the subcutaneous injection of lipoid solution containing tin.

Carbuncle may be looked upon as an aggrega-tion of boils, and is characterised by a densely hard base and a brownish-red discoloration of the skin. It is usually about the size of a crown-piece, but it may continue to enlarge until it attains the size of a dinner-plate. The patient is ill and feverish, and the pain may be so severe as to prevent sleep. As time goes on several points of suppuration appear, and when these burst there are formed a number of openings in the skin, giving it a cribriform appearance; these openings exude pus. The different open-ings ultimately fuse and the large adherent

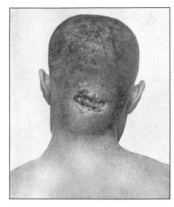

FIG. 95. Carbuncle of seven-teen days' duration in a woman æt. 57.

greyish-white slough is exposed. The separation of the slough is a tedious process, and the patient may become exhausted by pain, discharge, and toxin absorption. When the slough is finally thrown off, a deep gap is left, which takes a long time to heal. A large carbuncle is a grave disease, especially in a weakly person suffering from diabetes or chronic alcoholism; we have on several occasions seen diabetic coma supervene and the patient die without recovering consciousness. In the majority of cases the patient is laid aside for several months. It is most common in male adults over forty years of age, and is usually situated on the back between the shoulders. When it occurs on the face or anterior part of the neck it is especially dangerous, because of the greater risk of dissemination of the infection.

A carbuncle is to be differentiated from an ulcerated gumma and from anthrax pustule.

Treatment.—Pain is relieved by full doses of opium or codein, and these drugs are specially indicated when sugar is present in the urine. Vaccines may be given a trial. The diet should be liberal and easily digested, and strychnin and other stimulants may be of service. Locally the treatment is carried out on the same lines as for boils.

In some cases it is advisable to excise the carbuncle or to make incisions across it in different directions, so that the resulting wound presents a stellate appearance.

Acute Abscesses of the Skin and Subcutaneous Tissue in Young Children.—In young infants, abscesses are not infrequently met with scattered over the trunk and limbs, and are probably the result of infection of the sebaceous glands from dirty underclothing. The abscesses should be opened, and the further spread of infection prevented by cleansing of the skin and by the use of clean under-linen. Similar abscesses are met with on the scalp in association with eczema, impetigo, and pediculosis.

Veldt Sore.—This sore usually originates in an abrasion of the epidermis, such as a sun blister, the bite of an insect, or a scratch. A pustule forms and bursts, and a brownish-yellow scab forms over it. When this is removed, an ulcer is left which has little tendency to heal. These sores are most common about the hands, arms, neck, and feet, and are most apt to occur in those who have had no opportunities of washing, and who have lived for a long time on tinned foods.

Tuberculosis of the Skin.—Interest attaches chiefly to the primary forms of tuberculosis of the skin in which the bacilli penetrate from without—inoculation tubercle and lupus.

Inoculation Tubercle.—The appearances vary with the conditions under which the inoculation takes place. As observed on the fingers of adults, the affection takes the form of an indolent painless swelling, the epidermis being red and glazed, or warty, and irregularly fissured. Sometimes the epidermis gives way, forming an ulcer with flabby granulations. The infection rarely spreads to the lymphatics, but we have seen inoculation tubercle of the index-finger followed by a large cold abscess on the median side of the upper arm and by a huge mass of breaking down glands in the axilla.

In children who run about barefooted in towns, tubercle may be inoculated into wounds in the sole or about the toes, and although the local appearances may not be characteristic, the nature of the infection is revealed by its tendency to spread up the limb along the lymph vessels, giving rise to abscesses and fungating ulcers in relation to the femoral glands.

Tuberculous Lupus.—This is an extremely chronic affection of the skin. It rarely extends to the lymph glands, and of all tuberculous lesions is the least dangerous to life. The commonest form of lupus—*lupus vulgaris*—usually commences in childhood or youth, and is most often met with on the nose or cheek. The early and typical appearance is that of brownish-yellow or pink nodules in the skin, about the size of hemp seed. Healing frequently occurs in the centre of the affected area while the disease continues to extend at the margin.

When there is actual destruction of tissue and ulceration—the so-called "*lupus excedens*" or "*ulcerans*"—healing is attended with cicatricial contraction, which may cause unsightly deformity. When the cheek is affected, the lower eyelid may be drawn down and everted; when the lips are affected, the mouth may be distorted or seriously diminished in size. When the nose is attacked, both the skin and mucous surfaces are usually involved, and the nasal orifices may be narrowed or even obliterated; sometimes the soft parts, including the cartilages, are destroyed, leaving only the bones covered by tightly stretched scar tissue.

The disease progresses slowly, healing in some places and spreading at others. The patient complains of a burning sensation, but little of pain, and is chiefly concerned about the disfigurement. Nothing is more characteristic of lupus than the appearance of fresh nodules in parts which have already healed. In the course of years large tracts of the face and neck may become affected. From the lips it may spread to the gum and palate, giving to the mucous membrane the appearance of a raised, bright-red, papillary or villous surface. When the disease affects the gums, the teeth may become loose and fall out.

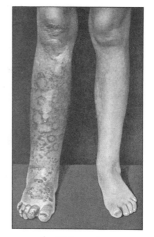

FIG. 96. Tuberculous Elephantiasis in a woman æt. 35

On parts of the body other than the face, the disease is even more chronic, and is often attended with a considerable production of dense fibrous tissue—the so-called *fibroid lupus*. Sometimes there is a warty thickening of the epidermis—*lupus verrucosus*. In the fingers and toes it may lead to a progressive destruction of tissue like that observed in leprosy, and from the resulting loss of portions of the digits it has been called *lupus mutilans*. In the lower extremity a remarkable form of the disease is sometimes met with, to which the term *lupus elephantiasis* (Fig. 96) has been applied. It commences as an ordinary lupus of the toes or dorsum of the foot, from which the tuberculous infection spreads to the lymph vessels, and the limb as a whole becomes enormously swollen and unshapely.

Finally, a long-standing lupus, especially on the cheek, may become the seat of epithelioma—*lupus epithelioma*—usually of the exuberant or cauliflower type, which, like other epitheliomas that originate in scar tissue, presents little tendency to infect the lymphatics.

The *diagnosis* of lupus is founded on the chronic progress and long duration, and the central scarring with peripheral extension of the disease. On the face it is most liable to be confused with syphilis and with rodent cancer. The syphilitic lesion belongs to the tertiary period, and although presenting a superficial resemblance to tuberculosis, its progress is more rapid, so that within a few months it may involve an area of skin as wide as would be affected by lupus in as many years. Further, it readily yields to anti-syphilitic treatment. In cases of tertiary syphilis in which the nose is destroyed, it will be noticed that the bones have suffered most, while in lupus the destruction of tissue involves chiefly the soft parts.

Rodent cancer is liable to be mistaken for lupus, because it affects the same parts of the face; it is equally chronic, and may partly heal. It begins later in life, however, the margin of the ulcer is more sharply defined, and often presents a "rolled" appearance.

Treatment.—When the disease is confined to a limited area, the most rapid and certain cure is obtained by *excision*; larger areas are scraped with the sharp spoon. The *ray treatment* includes the use of luminous, Röntgen, or radium rays, and possesses the advantage of being comparatively painless and of being followed by the least amount of scarring and deformity.

Encouraging results have also been obtained by the application of carbon dioxide snow.

Multiple subcutaneous tuberculous nodules are met with chiefly in children. They are indolent and painless, and rarely attract attention until they break down and form abscesses, which are usually about the size of a cherry, and when these burst sinuses or ulcers result. If the overlying skin is still intact, the best treatment is excision. If the abscess has already infected the skin, each focus should be scraped and packed.

Sporotrichosis is a mycotic infection due to the sporothrix Shenkii. It presents so many features resembling syphilis and tubercle that it is frequently mistaken for one or other of these affections. It occurs chiefly in males between fifteen and forty-five, who are farmers, fruit and vegetable dealers, or florists. There is usually a history of trauma of the nature of a scratch or a cut, and after a long incubation period there develop a series of small, hard, round nodules in the skin and subcutaneous tissue which, without pain or temperature, soften into cold abscesses and leave indolent ulcers or sinuses. The infection is of slow progress and follows the course of the lymphatics. From the gelatinous pus the organism is cultivated without difficulty, and this is the essential step in arriving at a diagnosis. The disease yields in a few weeks to full doses of iodide of potassium.

Elephantiasis.—This term is applied to an excessive enlargement of a part depending upon an overgrowth of the skin and subcutaneous cellular tissue, and it may result from a number of causes, acting independently or in combination. The condition is observed chiefly in the extremities and in the external organs of generation.

Elephantiasis from Lymphatic or Venous Obstruction.—Of this the best-known example is *tropical elephantiasis* (E. arabum), which is endemic in Samoa, Barbadoes, and other places. It attacks the lower extremity or the genitals in either sex (Figs. 97, 98). The disease is usually ushered in with fever, and signs of lymphangitis in the part affected. After a number of such attacks, the lymph vessels appear to become obliterated, and the skin and subcutaneous cellular tissue, being bathed in stagnant lymph—which possibly contains the products of streptococci—take on an overgrowth, which continues until the part assumes gigantic proportions. In certain cases the lymph trunks have been found to be blocked with the parent worms of the filaria Bancrofti. Cases of elephantiasis of the lower extremity are met with in this country in which there are no filarial parasites in the lymph vessels, and these present features closely resembling the tropical variety, and usually follow upon repeated attacks of lymphangitis or erysipelas.

The part affected is enormously increased in size, and causes inconvenience from its bulk and weight. In contrast to ordinary dropsy, there is no pitting on pressure, and the swelling does not disappear on elevation of the limb. The skin becomes rough and warty, and may hang down in pendulous folds. Blisters form on the surface and yield an abundant exudate of clear lymph. From neglect of cleanliness, the skin becomes the seat of eczema or even of ulceration attended with foul discharge.

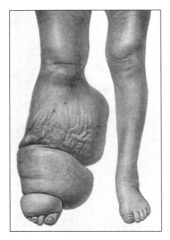

FIG. 97. Elephantiasis in a woman æt. 45.

Samson Handley has sought to replace the blocked lymph vessels by burying in the subcutaneous tissue of the swollen part a number of stout silk threads—*lymphangioplasty*. By their capillary action they drain the lymph to a healthy region above, and thus enable it to enter the circulation. It has been more successful in the face and upper limb than in the lower extremity. If the tissues are infected with pus organisms, a course of vaccines should precede the operation.

A similar type of elephantiasis may occur after extirpation of the lymph glands in the axilla or groin; in the leg in long-standing standing varix and phlebitis with chronic ulcer; in the arm as a result of extensive cancerous disease of the lymphatics in the axilla secondarily to cancer of the breast; and in extensive tuberculous disease of the lymphatics. The last-named is chiefly observed in the lower limb in young adult women, and from its following upon lupus of the toes or foot it has been called *lupus elephantiasis*. The tuberculous infection spreads slowly up the limb by way of the lymph vessels, and as these are obliterated the skin and cellular tissues become hypertrophied, and the surface is studded over with fungating tuberculous masses of a livid blue colour. As the more severe forms of the disease may prove dangerous to life by pyogenic complications inducing gangrene of the limb, the question of amputation may have to be considered.

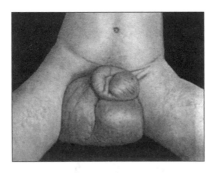

FIG. 98. Elephantiasis of Penis and Scrotum in native of Demerara. (Mr. Annandale's case.)

368

Belonging to this group also is a form of *congenital elephantiasis* resulting from the circular constriction of a limb *in utero* by amniotic bands.

Elephantiasis occurring apart from lymphatic or venous obstruction is illustrated by *elephantiasis nervorum*, in which there is an overgrowth of the skin and cellular tissue of an extremity in association with neuro-fibromatosis of the cutaneous nerves (Fig. 89); and by *elephantiasis Græcorum*—a form of leprosy in which the skin of the face becomes the seat of tumour-like masses consisting of leprous nodules. It is also illustrated by *elephantiasis involving the scrotum* as a result of prolonged irritation by the urine in cases in which the penis has been amputated and the urine has infiltrated the scrotal tissues over a period of years.

Sebaceous Cysts.—Atheromatous cysts or wens are formed in relation to the sebaceous glands and hair follicles. They are commonly met with in adults, on the scalp (Fig. 99), face, neck, back, and external genitals. Sometimes they are multiple, and they may be met with in several members of the same family. They are smooth, rounded, or discoid cysts, varying in size from a split-pea to a Tangerine orange. In consistence they are firm and elastic, or fluctuating, and are incorporated with the overlying skin, but movable on the deeper structures. The orifice of the partly blocked sebaceous follicle is sometimes visible, and the contents of the cyst can be squeezed through the opening. The wall of the cyst is composed of a connective-tissue capsule lined by stratified squamous epithelium. The contents consist of accumulated epithelial cells, and are at first dry and pearly white in appearance, but as a result of fatty degeneration they break down into a greyish-yellow pultaceous and semi-fluid material having a peculiar stale odour. It is probable that the decomposition of the contents is the result of the presence of bacteria, and that from the surgical point of view they should be regarded as infective. A sebaceous cyst may remain indefinitely without change, or may slowly increase in size, the skin over it becoming stretched and closely adherent to the cyst wall as a result of friction and pressure. The contents may ooze from the orifice of the duct and dry on the skin surface, leading to the formation of a sebaceous horn (Fig. 100). As a result of injury the cyst may undergo sudden enlargement from hæmorrhage into its interior.

Recurrent attacks of inflammation frequently occur, especially in wens of the face and scalp. Suppuration may ensue and be followed by cure of the cyst, or an offensive fungating ulcer forms which may be mistaken for epithelioma. True cancerous transformation is rare.

Wens are to be *diagnosed* from dermoids, from fatty tumours, and from cold abscesses. Dermoids usually appear before adult life, and as they nearly always lie beneath the fascia, the skin is movable over them. A fatty tumour is movable, and is often lobulated. The confusion with a cold abscess is most likely to occur in wens of the neck or back, and it may be impossible without the use of an exploring needle to differentiate between them.

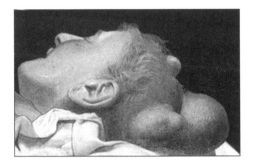

FIG. 99. Multiple Sebaceous Cysts or Wens; the larger ones are of many years' duration.

Treatment.—The removal of wens is to be recommended while they are small and freely movable, as they are then easily shelled out after incising the overlying skin; sometimes splitting the cyst makes its removal easier. Local anæsthesia is to be preferred. It is important that none of the cyst wall be left behind. In large and adherent wens an ellipse of skin is removed along with the cyst. When inflamed, it may be impossible to dissect out the cyst, and the wall should be destroyed with carbolic acid, the resulting wound being treated by the open method.

Moles.—The term mole is applied to a pigmented, and usually hairy, patch of skin, present at or appearing shortly after birth. The colour varies from brown to black, according to the amount of melanin pigment present. The lesion consists in an overgrowth of epidermis which often presents an alveolar arrangement. Moles vary greatly in size: some are mere dots, others are as large as the palm of the hand, and occasionally a mole covers half the face. In addition to being unsightly, they bleed freely when abraded, are liable to ulcerate from friction and pressure, and occasionally become the starting-point of melanotic cancer. Rodent cancer sometimes originates in the slightly pigmented moles met with on the face. Overgrowths in relation to the cutaneous nerves, especially the plexiform neuroma, occasionally originate in pigmented moles. Soldau believes that the pigmentation and overgrowth of the epidermis in moles are associated with, and probably result from, a fibromatosis of the cutaneous nerves.

Treatment.—The quickest way to get rid of a mole is to excise it; if the edges of the gap cannot be brought together with sutures, recourse should be had to grafting. In large hairy moles of the face whose size forbids excision, radium or the X-rays should be employed. Excellent results have been obtained by refrigeration with solid carbon dioxide. In children and women with delicate skin, applications of from ten to thirty seconds suffice. In persons with coarse skin an application of one minute may be necessary, and it may have to be repeated.

Horns.—The *sebaceous* horn results from the accumulation of the dried contents of a wen on the surface of the skin: the sebaceous material after drying up becomes cornified, and as fresh material is added to the base the horn increases in length (Fig. 100). The *wart* horn grows from a warty papilloma of the skin. *Cicatrix* horns are formed by the heaping up of epidermis in the scars that result from burns. *Nail* horns are overgrown nails (keratomata of the nail bed), and are met with chiefly in the great toe of elderly bedridden patients. If an ulcer forms at the base of a horn, it may prove the starting-point of epithelioma, and for this reason, as well as for others, horns should be removed.

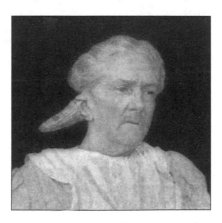

FIG. 100. Sebaceous Horn growing from Auricle. (Dr. Kenneth Maclachan's case.)

New Growths in the Skin and Subcutaneous Tissue.—The *Angioma* has been described with diseases of blood vessels. *Fibroma.*—Various types of fibroma occur in the skin. A soft pedunculated fibroma, about the size of a pea, is commonly met with, especially on the neck and trunk; it is usually solitary, and is easily removed with scissors. The multiple, soft fibroma known as *molluscum fibrosum*, which depends upon a neuro-fibromatosis of the cutaneous nerves, is described with the tumours of nerves. Hard fibromas occurring singly or in groups may be met with, especially in the skin of the buttock, and may present a local malignancy, recurring after removal like the "recurrent fibroid" of Paget. The "painful subcutaneous nodule" is a solitary fibroma related to one of the cutaneous nerves. The hard fibroma known as *keloid* is described with the affections of scars.

Papilloma.—The *common wart* or verruca is an outgrowth of the surface epidermis. It may be sessile or pedunculated hard or soft. The surface may be smooth, or fissured and foliated like a cauliflower, or it may be divided up into a number of spines. Warts are met with chiefly on the hands, and are often multiple, occurring in clusters or in successive crops. Multiple warts appear to result from some contagion, the nature of which is unknown; they sometimes occur in an epidemic form among school-children, and show a remarkable tendency to disappear spontaneously. The solitary flat-topped wart which occurs on the face of old people may, if irritated, become the seat of epithelioma. A warty growth of the epidermis is a frequent accompaniment of moles and of that variety of lupus known as *lupus verrucosus*.

Treatment.—In the multiple warts of children the health should be braced up by a change to the seaside. A dusting-powder, consisting of boracic acid with 5 per cent. salicylic acid, may be rubbed into the hands after washing and drying. The persistent warts of young adults should be excised after freezing with chloride of ethyl. When cutting is objected to, they may be painted night and morning with salicylic collodion, the epidermis being dehydrated with alcohol before each application.

Venereal warts occur on the genitals of either sex, and may form large cauliflower-like masses on the inner surface of the prepuce or of the labia majora. Although frequently co-existing with gonorrhoea or syphilis, they occur independently of these diseases, being probably acquired by contact with another individual suffering from warts (C. W. Cathcart). They give rise to considerable irritation and suffering, and when cleanliness is neglected there may be an offensive discharge.

In the female, the cauliflower-like masses are dissected from the labia; in the male, the prepuce is removed and the warts on the glans are snipped off with scissors. In milder cases, the warts usually disappear if the parts are kept absolutely dry and clean. A useful dusting-powder is one consisting of calamine and 5 per cent. salicylic acid; the exsiccated sulphate of iron, in the form of a powder, may be employed in cases which resist this treatment.

Adenoma.—This is a comparatively rare tumour growing from the glands of the skin. One variety, known as the "tomato tumour," which apparently originates from *the sweat glands* , is met with on the scalp and face in women past middle life. These growths are often multiple; the individual tumours vary in size, and the skin, which is almost devoid of hairs, is glistening and tightly stretched over them. A similar tumour may occur on the nose. The *sebaceous adenoma*, which originates from the sebaceous glands, forms a projecting tumour on the face or scalp, and when the skin is irritated it may ulcerate and fungate. The treatment consists in the removal of the tumour along with the overlying skin.

The exuberant masses on the nose known as "rhinophyma," "lipoma nasi," or "potato nose" are of the nature of sebaceous adenoma, and are removed by shaving them off with a knife until the normal shape of the nose is restored Healing takes place with remarkable rapidity.

Cancer.—There are several types of primary cancer of the skin, the most important being squamous epithelioma, rodent cancer, and melanotic cancer.

Epithelioma occurs in a variety of forms. When originating in a small ulcer or wart-for example on the face in old people—it presents the features of a chronic indurated ulcer. A more exuberant and rapidly growing form of epithelial cancer, described by Hutchinson as the *crateriform ulcer*, commences on the face as a small red pimple which rapidly develops into an elevated mass shaped like a bee-hive,

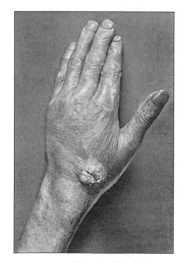

FIG. 101. Paraffin Epithelioma.

373

and breaks down in the centre. Epithelioma may develop anywhere on the body in relation to long-standing ulcers, especially that resulting from a burn or from lupus; this form usually presents an exuberant outgrowth of epidermis not unlike a cauliflower. An interesting example of epithelioma has been described by Neve of Kashmir. The natives in that province are in the habit of carrying a fire-basket suspended from the waist, which often burns the skin and causes a chronic ulcer, and many of these ulcers become the seat of epithelioma, due, in Neve's opinion, to the actual contact of the sooty pan with the skin.

The term *trade epithelioma* has been applied to that form met with in those who follow certain occupations, such as paraffin workers and chimney-sweeps. The most recent member of this group is the *X-ray carcinoma*, which is met with in those who are constantly exposed to the irritation of the X-rays; there is first a chronic dermatitis with warty overgrowth of the surface epithelium, pigmentation, and the formation of fissures and warts. The trade epithelioma varies a good deal in malignancy, but it tends to cause death in the same manner as other epitheliomas.

Epithelial cancer has also been observed in those who have taken arsenic over long periods for medicinal purposes.

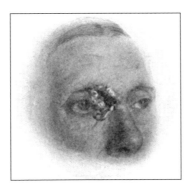

FIG. 102. Rodent Cancer of Inner Canthus.

Rodent Cancer (Rodent Ulcer).—This is a cancer originating in the sweat glands or sebaceous follicles, or in the foetal residues of cutaneous glands. The cells are small and closely packed together in alveoli or in reticulated columns; cell nests are rare. It is remarkably constant in its seat of origin, being nearly always located on the lateral aspect of the nose or in the vicinity of the lower eyelid (Fig. 102). It is rare on the trunk or limbs. It commences as a small flattened nodule in the skin, the epidermis over it being stretched and shining. The centre becomes depressed, while the margins extend in the form of an elevated ridge. Sooner or later the epidermis gives way in the centre, exposing a smooth raw surface devoid of granulations.

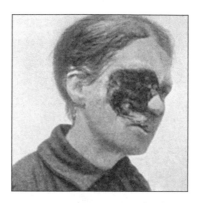

FIG. 103. Rodent Cancer of fifteen years' duration, which has destroyed the contents of the Orbit. (Sir Montagu Cotterill's case)

The margin, while in parts irregular, is typically represented by a well-defined "rolled" border which consists of the peripheral portion of the cancer that has not broken down. The central ulcer may temporarily heal. There is itching but little pain, and the condition progresses extremely slowly; rodent cancers which have existed for many years are frequently met with. The disease attacks and destroys every structure with which it comes in contact, such as the eyelids, the walls of the nasal cavities, and the bones of the face; hence it may produce the most hideous deformities (Fig. 103). The patient may succumb to hæmorrhage or to infective complications such as erysipelas or meningitis.

Secondary growths in the lymph glands, while not unknown, are extremely rare. We have only seen them once—in a case of rodent cancer in the groin.

Diagnosis.—Lupus is the disease most often mistaken for rodent cancer. Lupus usually begins earlier in life, it presents apple-jelly nodules, and lacks the rounded, elevated border. Syphilitic lesions progress more rapidly, and also lack the characteristic margin. The differentiation from squamous epithelioma is of considerable importance, as the latter affection spreads more rapidly, involves the lymph glands early, and is much more dangerous to life.

Treatment.—In rodent cancers of limited size—say less than one inch in diameter—free excision is the most rapid and certain method of treatment. The alternative is the application of radium or of the Röntgen rays, which, although requiring many exposures, results in cure with the minimum of disfigurement. If the cancer already covers an extensive area, or has invaded the cavity of the orbit or nose, radium or X-rays yield the best results. The effect is soon shown by the ingrowth of healthy epithelium from the surrounding skin, and at the same time the discharge is lessened. Good results are also reported from the application of carbon dioxide snow, especially when this follows upon a course of X-ray treatment.

Paget's disease of the nipple is an epithelioma occurring in women over forty years of age: a similar form of epithelioma is sometimes met with at the umbilicus or on the genitals.

Melanotic Cancer.—Under this head are included all new growths which contain an excess of melanin pigment. Many of these were formerly described as melanotic sarcoma. They nearly always originate in a pigmented mole which has been subjected to irritation. The primary growth may remain so small that its presence is not even suspected, or it may increase in size, ulcerate, and fungate. The amount of pigment varies: when small in amount the growth is brown, when abundant it is a deep black. The most remarkable feature is the rapidity with which the disease becomes disseminated along the lymphatics, the first evidence of which is an enlargement of the lymph glands. As the primary growth is often situated on the sole of the foot or in the matrix of the nail of the great toe, the femoral and inguinal glands become enlarged in succession, forming tumours much larger than the primary growth. Sometimes the dissemination involves the lymph vessels of the limb, forming a series of indurated pigmented cords and nodules (Fig. 104). Lastly, the dissemination may be universal throughout the body, and this usually occurs at a comparatively early stage. The secondary growths are deeply pigmented, being usually of a coal-black colour, and melanin pigment may be present in the urine. When recurrence takes place in or near the scar left by the operation, the cancer nodules are not necessarily pigmented.

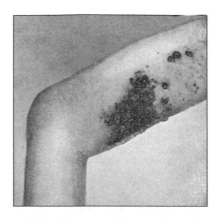

FIG. 104. Diffuse Melanotic Cancer of Lymphatics of Skin secondary to a Growth in the Sole of the Foot.

To extirpate the disease it is necessary to excise the tumour, with a zone of healthy skin around it and a somewhat large zone of the underlying subcutaneous tissue and deep fascia. Hogarth Pringle recommends that a broad strip of subcutaneous fascia up to and including the nearest anatomical group of glands should be removed with the tumour in one continuous piece.

Secondary Cancer of the Skin.—Cancer may spread to the skin from a subjacent growth by direct continuity or by way of the lymphatics. Both of these processes are so well illustrated in cases of mammary cancer that they will be described in relation to that disease.

Sarcoma of various types is met with in the skin. The fibroma, after excision, may recur as a fibro-sarcoma. The alveolar sarcoma commences as a hard lump and increases in size until the epidermis gives way and an ulcer is formed.

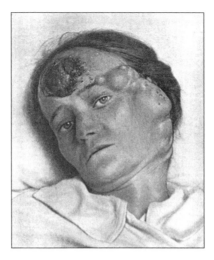

FIG. 105. Melanotic Cancer of Forehead with Metastases in Lymph Vessels and Glands. (Mr. D. P. D. Wilkie's case.)

A number of fresh tumours may spring up around the original growth. Sometimes the primary growth appears in the form of multiple nodules which tend to become confluent. Excision, unless performed early, is of little avail, and in any case should be followed up by exposure to radium.

AFFECTIONS OF CICATRICES

A cicatrix or scar consists of closely packed bundles of white fibres covered by epidermis; the skin glands and hair follicles are usually absent. The size, shape, and level of the cicatrix depend upon the conditions which preceded healing.

A healthy scar, when recently formed, has a smooth, glossy surface of a pinkish colour, which tends to become whiter as a result of obliteration of the blood vessels concerned in its formation.

Weak Scars.—A scar is said to be weak when it readily breaks down as a result of irritation or pressure. The scars resulting from severe burns and those over amputation stumps are especially liable to break down from trivial causes. The treatment is to excise the weak portion of the scar and bring the edges of the gap together.

Contracted scars frequently cause deformity either by displacing parts, such as the eyelid or lip, or by fixing parts and preventing the normal movements—for example, a scar on the flexor aspect of a joint may prevent exten-

378

sion of the forearm (Fig. 63). These are treated by dividing the scar, correcting the deformity, and filling up the gap with epithelial grafts, or with a flap of the whole thickness of the skin. When deformity results from *depression of a scar*, as is not uncommon after the healing of a sinus, the treatment is to excise the scar. Depressed scars may be raised by the injection of paraffin into the subcutaneous tissue.

Painful Scars.—Pain in relation to a scar is usually due to nerve fibres being compressed or stretched in the cicatricial tissue; and in some cases to ascending neuritis. The treatment consists in excising the scar or in stretching or excising a portion of the nerve affected.

Pigmented or Discoloured Scars.—The best-known examples are the blue coloration which results from coal-dust or gunpowder, the brown scars resulting from chronic ulcer with venous congestion of the leg, and the variously coloured scars caused by tattooing. The only satisfactory method of getting rid of the coloration is to excise the scar; the edges are brought together by sutures, or the raw surface is covered with skin-grafts according to the size of the gap.

Hypertrophied Scars.—Scars occasionally broaden out and become prominent, and on exposed parts this may prove a source of disappointment after operations such as those for goitre or tuberculous glands in the neck. There is sometimes considerable improvement from exposure to the X-rays.

Keloid.—This term is applied to an overgrowth of scar tissue which extends beyond the area of the original wound, and the name is derived from the fact that this extension occurs in the form of radiating processes, suggesting the claws of a crab. It is essentially a fibroma or new growth of fibrous tissue, which commences in relation to the walls of the smaller blood vessels; the bundles of fibrous tissue are for the most part parallel with the surface, and the epidermis is tightly stretched over them. It is more frequent in the negro and in those who are, or have been, the subjects of tuberculous disease.

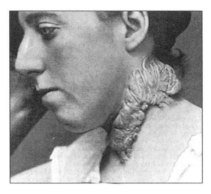

FIG. 106. Recurrent Keloid in scar left by operation for tuberculous glands in a girl æt. 7.

Keloid may attack scars of any kind, such as those resulting from leech-bites, acne pustules, boils or blisters; those resulting from operation or accidental wounds; and the scars resulting from burns, especially when situated over the sternum, appear to be specially liable. The scar becomes more and more conspicuous, is elevated above the surface, of a pinkish or brownish-pink pink colour, and sends out irregular prolongations around its margins. The patient may complain of itching and burning, and of great sensitiveness of the scar, even to contact with the clothing.

There is a natural hesitation to excise keloid because of the fear of its returning in the new scar. The application of radium is, so far as we know, the only means of preventing such return. The irritation associated with keloid may be relieved by the application of salicylic collodion or of salicylic and creosote plaster.

Epithelioma is liable to attack scars in old people, especially those which result from burns sustained early in childhood and have never really healed. From the absence of lymphatics in scar tissue, the disease does not spread to the glands until it has invaded the tissues outside the scar; the prognosis is therefore better than in epithelioma in general. It should be excised widely; in the lower extremity when there is also extensive destruction of tissue from an antecedent chronic ulcer or osteomyelitis, it may be better to amputate the limb.

AFFECTION OF THE NAILS

Injuries.—When a nail is contused or crushed, blood is extravasated beneath it, and the nail is usually shed, a new one growing in its place. A splinter driven underneath the nail causes great pain, and if organisms are carried in along with it, may give rise to infective complications. The free edge of the nail should be clipped away to allow of the removal of the foreign body and the necessary disinfection.

Trophic Changes.—The growth of the nails may be interfered with in any disturbance of the general health. In nerve lesions, such as a divided nerve-trunk, the nails are apt to suffer, becoming curved, brittle, or furrowed, or they may be shed.

Onychia is the term applied to an infection of the soft parts around the nail or of the matrix beneath it. The commonest form of onychia has already been referred to with whitlow. There is a superficial variety resulting from the extension of a purulent blister beneath the nail lifting it up from its bed, the pus being visible through the nail. The nail as well as the raised horny layer of the epidermis should be removed. A deeper and more troublesome onychia results from infection at the nail-fold; the infection spreads slowly beneath the fold until it reaches the matrix, and a drop or two of pus forms beneath the nail, usually in the region of the lunule. This affection entails a disability of the finger which may last for weeks unless it is properly treated. Treatment by hyperæmia, using a suction bell, should first be tried, and, failing improvement, the nail-fold and lunule should be frozen, and a considerable portion removed with the knife; if only a small portion of the nail is removed, the opening is blocked by granulations springing from the matrix. A new nail is formed, but it is liable to be misshapen.

Tuberculous onychia is met with in children and adolescents. It appears as a livid or red swelling at the root of the nail and spreading around its margins. The epidermis, which is thin and shiny, gives way, and the nail is usually shed.

Syphilitic affections of the nails assume various aspects. A primary chancre at the edge of the nail may be mistaken for a whitlow, especially if it is attended with much pain. Other forms of onychia occur during secondary syphilis simultaneously with the skin eruptions, and may prove obstinate and lead to shedding of the nails. They also occur in inherited syphilis. In addition to general treatment, an ointment containing 5 per cent. of oleate of mercury should be applied locally.

Ingrowing Toe-nail.—This is more accurately described as an overgrowth of the soft tissues along the edge of the nail. It is most frequently met with in the great toe in young adults with flat-foot whose feet perspire freely, who wear ill-fitting shoes, and who cut their toe-nails carelessly or tear them with their fingers. Where the soft tissues are pressed against the edge of the nail, the skin gives way and there is the formation of exuberant granulations and of discharge which is sometimes foetid. The affection is a painful one and may unfit the patient for work. In mild cases the condition may be remedied by getting rid of contributing causes and by disinfecting the skin and nail; the nail is cut evenly, and the groove between it and the skin packed with an antiseptic dusting-powder, such as boracic acid. In more severe cases it may be necessary to remove an ellipse of tissue consisting of the edge of the nail, together with the subjacent matrix and the redundant nail-fold.

Subungual exostosis is an osteoma growing from the terminal phalanx of the great toe (Fig. 107). It raises the nail and may be accompanied by ulceration of the skin over the most prominent part of the growth. The soft parts, including the nail, should be reflected towards the dorsum in the form of a flap, the base of the exostosis divided with the chisel, and the exostosis removed.

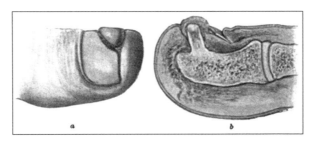

FIG. 107. Subungual Exostosis growing from Distal Phalanx of Great Toe, showing Ulceration of Skin and Displacement of Nail. *a.* Surface view. *b.* On section.

Malignant disease in relation to the nails is rare. Squamous epithelioma and melanotic cancer are the forms met with. Treatment consists in amputating the digit concerned, and in removing the associated lymph glands.

• XVIII •

THE MUSCLES, TENDONS, AND TENDON SHEATHS

Injuries: Contusion; Sprain; Rupture
Hernia of Muscle ✦ *Dislocation of Tendons*
Wounds ✦ *Avulsion of Tendon*
Diseases of Muscles and Tendons: Atrophy;
"Muscular Rheumatism" ✦ *Fibrositis; Contracture; Myositis;*
Calcification and Ossification; Tumours ✦ *Diseases of Tendon Sheaths:*
Teno-synovitis

INJURIES

Contusion of Muscle.—Contusion of muscle, which consists in bruising of its fibres and blood vessels, may be due to violence acting from without, as in a blow, a kick, or a fall; or from within, as by the displacement of bone in a fracture or dislocation.

The symptoms are those common to all contusions, and the patient complains of severe pain on attempting to use the muscle, and maintains an attitude which relaxes it. If the sheath of the muscle also is torn, there is subcutaneous ecchymosis, and the accumulation of blood may result in the formation of a hæmatoma.

Restoration of function is usually complete; but when the nerve supplying the muscle is bruised at the same time, as may occur in the deltoid, wasting and loss of function may be persistent. In exceptional cases the process of repair may be attended with the formation of bone in the substance of the muscle, and this may likewise impair its function.

A contused muscle should be placed at rest and supported by cotton wool and a bandage; after an interval, massage and appropriate exercises are employed.

Sprain and Partial Rupture of Muscle.—This lesion consists in overstretching and partial rupture of the fibres of a muscle or its aponeurosis. It is of common occurrence in athletes and in those who follow laborious occupations. It may follow upon a single or repeated effort—especially in those who are out of training. Familiar examples of muscular sprain are the "labourer's" or "golfer's back," affecting the latissimus dorsi or the sacrospinalis (erector spinæ); the "tennis-player's elbow," and the "sculler's sprain," affecting the muscles and ligaments about the elbow; the "angler's elbow," affecting the common origin of the extensors and supinators; the "sprinter's sprain," affecting the flexors of the hip; and the "jumper's and dancer's sprain," affecting the muscles of the calf. The patient complains of pain, often sudden in onset, of tenderness on pressure, and of inability to carry out the particular movement by which the sprain was produced. The disability varies in different cases, and it may incapacitate the patient from following his occupation or sport for weeks or, if imperfectly treated, even for months.

The *treatment* consists in resting the muscle from the particular effort concerned in the production of the sprain, in gently exercising it in other directions, in the use of massage, and the induction of hyperæmia by means of heat. In neglected cases, that is, where the muscle has not been exercised, the patient shrinks from using it and the disablement threatens to be permanent; it is sometimes said that adhesions have formed and that these interfere with the recovery of function. The condition may be overcome by graduated movements or by a sudden forcible movement under an anæsthetic. These cases afford a fruitful field for the bone-setter.

Rupture of Muscle or Tendon.—A muscle or a tendon may be ruptured in its continuity or torn from its attachment to bone. The site of rupture in individual muscles is remarkably constant, and is usually at the junction of the muscular and tendinous portions. When rupture takes place through the belly of a muscle, the ends retract, the amount of retraction depending on the length of the muscle, and the extent of its attachment to adjacent aponeurosis or bone. The biceps in the arm, and the sartorius in the thigh, furnish examples of muscles in which the separation between the ends may be considerable.

The gap in the muscle becomes filled with blood, and this in time is replaced by connective tissue, which forms a bond of union between the ends. When the space is considerable the connecting medium consists of fibrous tissue, but when the ends are in contact it contains a number of newly formed muscle fibres. In the process of repair, one or both ends of the muscle or tendon may become fixed by adhesions to adjacent structures, and if the distal portion of a muscle is deprived of its nerve supply it may undergo degeneration and so have its function impaired.

Rupture of a muscle or tendon is usually the result of a sudden, and often involuntary, movement. As examples may be cited the rupture of the quadriceps extensor in attempting to regain the balance when falling backwards; of the gastrocnemius, plantaris, or tendo-calcaneus in jumping or dancing; of the adductors of the thigh in gripping a horse when it swerves—"rider's sprain"; of the abdominal muscles in vomiting, and of the biceps in sudden movements of the arm. Sometimes the effort is one that would scarcely be thought likely to rupture a muscle, as in the case recorded by Pagenstecher, where a professional athlete, while sitting at table, ruptured his biceps in a sudden effort to catch a falling glass. It would appear that the rupture is brought about not so much by the contraction of the muscle concerned, as by the contraction of the antagonistic muscles taking place before that of the muscle which undergoes rupture is completed. The violent muscular contractions of epilepsy, tetanus, or delirium rarely cause rupture.

The *clinical features* ar e usually characteristic. The patient experiences a sudden pain, with the sensation of being struck with a whip, and of something giving way; sometimes a distant snap is heard. The limb becomes powerless. At the seat of rupture there is tenderness and swelling, and there may be ecchymosis. As the swelling subsides, a gap may be felt between the retracted ends, and this becomes wider when the muscle is thrown into contraction. If untreated, a hard, fibrous cord remains at the seat of rupture.

Treatment.—The ends are approximated by placing the limb in an attitude which relaxes the muscle, and the position is maintained by bandages, splints, or special apparatus. When it is impossible thus to approximate the ends satisfactorily, the muscle or tendon is exposed by incision, and the ends brought into accurate contact by catgut sutures. This operation of primary suture yields the most satisfactory results, and is most successful when it is done within five or six days of the accident. Secondary suture after an interval of months is rendered difficult by the retraction of the ends and by their adhesion to adjacent structures.

Rupture of the biceps of the arm may involve the long or the short head, or the belly of the muscle. Most interest attaches to rupture of the long tendon of origin. There is pain and tenderness in front of the upper end of the humerus, the patient is unable to abduct or to elevate the arm, and he may be unable to flex the elbow when the forearm is supinated. The long axis of the muscle, instead of being parallel with the humerus, inclines downwards and outwards. When the patient is asked to contract the muscle, its belly is seen to be drawn towards the elbow.

The *adductor longus* may be ruptured, or torn from the pubes, by a violent effort to adduct the limb. A swelling forms in the upper and medial part of the thigh, which becomes smaller and harder when the muscle is thrown into contraction.

The *quadriceps femoris* is usually ruptured close to its insertion into the patella, in the attempt to avoid falling backwards. The injury is sometimes bilateral. The injured limb is rendered useless for progression, as it suddenly gives way whenever the knee is flexed. Treatment is conducted on the same lines as in transverse fracture of the patella; in the majority of cases the continuity of the quadriceps should be re-established by suture within five or six days of the accident.

The *tendo calcaneus* (Achillis) is comparatively easily ruptured, and the symptoms are sometimes so slight that the nature of the injury may be overlooked. The limb should be put up with the knee flexed and the toes pointed. This may be effected by attaching one end of an elastic band to the heel of a slipper, and securing the other to the lower third of the thigh. If this is not sufficient to bring the ends into apposition they should be approximated by an open operation.

The *plantaris* is not infrequently ruptured from trivial causes, such as a sudden movement in boxing, tennis, or hockey. A sharp stinging pain like the stroke of a whip is felt in the calf; there is marked tenderness at the seat of rupture, and the patient is unable to raise the heel without pain. The injury is of little importance, and if the patient does not raise the heel from the ground in walking, it is recovered from in a couple of weeks or so, without it being necessary to lay him up.

Hernia of Muscle.—This is a rare condition, in which, owing to the fascia covering a muscle becoming stretched or torn, the muscular substance is protruded through the rent. It has been observed chiefly in the adductor longus. An oval swelling forms in the upper part of the thigh, is soft and prominent when the muscle is relaxed, less prominent when it is passively extended, and disappears when the muscle is thrown into contraction. It is liable to be mistaken, according to its situation, for a tumour, a cyst, a pouched vein, or a femoral or obturator hernia. Treatment is only called for when it is causing inconvenience, the muscle being exposed by a suitable incision, the herniated portion excised, and the rent in the sheath closed by sutures.

Dislocation of Tendons.—Tendons which run in grooves may be displaced as a result of rupture of the confining sheath. This injury is met with chiefly in the tendons at the ankle and in the long tendon of the biceps.

Dislocation of the *peronei tendons* may occur, for example, from a violent twist of the foot. There is severe pain and considerable swelling on the lateral aspect of the ankle; the peroneus longus by itself, or together with the brevis, can be felt on the lateral aspect or in front of the lateral malleolus; the patient is unable to move the foot. By a little manipulation the tendons are replaced in their grooves, and are retained there by a series of strips of plaster. At the end of three weeks massage and exercises are employed.

In other cases there is no history of injury, but whenever the foot is everted the tendon of the peroneus longus is liable to be jerked forwards out of its groove, sometimes with an audible snap. The patient suffers pain and is disabled until the tendon is replaced. Reduction is easy, but as the displacement tends to recur, an operation is required to fix the tendon in its place. An incision is made over the tendon; if the sheath is slack or torn, it is tightened up or closed with catgut sutures; or an artificial sheath is made by raising up a quadrilateral flap of periosteum from the lateral aspect of the fibula, and stitching it over the tendon.

Similarly the *tibialis posterior* may be displaced over the medial malleolus as a result of inversion of the foot.

The *long tendon of the biceps* may be dislocated laterally—or more frequently medially—as a result of violent or repeated rotation movements of the arm, such as are performed in wringing clothes. The patient is aware of the displacement taking place, and is unable to extend the forearm until the displaced tendon has been reduced by abducting the arm. In recurrent cases the patient may be able to dislocate the tendon at will, but the disability is so inconsiderable that there is rarely any occasion for interference.

Wounds of Muscles and Tendons.—When a muscle is cut across in a wound, its ends should be brought together with sutures. If the ends are allowed to retract, and especially if the wound suppurates, they become united by scar tissue and fixed to bone or other adjacent structure. In a limb this interferes with the functions of the muscle; in the abdominal wall the scar tissue may stretch, and so favour the development of a ventral hernia.

Tendons may be cut across accidentally, especially in those wounds so commonly met with above the wrist as a result, for example, of the hand being thrust through a pane of glass. It is essential that the ends should be sutured to each other, and as the proximal end is retracted the original wound may require to be enlarged in an upward direction. When primary suture has been omitted, or has failed in consequence of suppuration, the separated ends of the tendon become adherent to adjacent structures, and the function of the associated muscle is impaired or lost. Under these conditions the operation of secondary suture is indicated.

A free incision is necessary to discover and isolate the ends of the tendon; if the interval is too wide to admit of their being approximated by sutures, means must be taken to lengthen the tendon, or one from some other part may be inserted in the gap. A new sheath may be provided for the tendon by resecting a portion of the great saphenous vein.

Injuries of the tendons of the fingers are comparatively common. One of the best known is the partial or complete rupture of the aponeurosis of the extensor tendon close to its insertion into the terminal phalanx—*drop-* or *mallet-finger*. This may result from comparatively slight violence, such as striking the tip of the extended finger against an object, or the violence may be more severe, as in attempting to catch a cricket ball or in falling. The terminal phalanx is flexed towards the palm and the patient is unable to extend it. The treatment consists in putting up the finger with the middle joint strongly flexed. In neglected cases, a perfect functional result can only be obtained by operation; under a local anæsthetic, the ruptured tendon is exposed and is sutured to the base of the phalanx, which may be drilled for the passage of the sutures.

Subcutaneous rupture of one or other *of the digital tendons* in the hand or at the wrist can be remedied only by operation. When some time has elapsed since the accident, the proximal end may be so retracted that it cannot be brought down into contact with the distal end, in which case a slip may be taken from an adjacent tendon; in the case of one of the extensors of the thumb, the extensor carpi radialis longus may be detached from its insertion and stitched to the distal end of the tendon of the thumb.

Subcutaneous *rupture of the tendon of the extensor pollicis longus* at the wrist takes place just after its emergence from beneath the annular ligament; the actual rupture may occur painlessly, more frequently a sharp pain is felt over the back of the wrist. The prominence of the tendon, which normally forms the ulnar border of the snuff-box, disappears. This lesion is chiefly met with in drummer-boys and is the cause of drummer's palsy. The only chance of restoring function is in uniting the ruptured tendon by open operation.

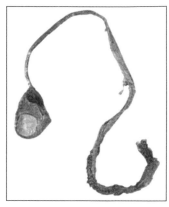

FIG. 108. Avulsion of Tendon with Terminal Phalanx of Thumb. (Surgical Museum, University of Edinburgh.)

Avulsion of Tendons.—This is a rare injury, in which the tendons of a finger or toe are torn from their attachments along with a portion of the digit concerned. In the hand, it is usually brought about by the fingers being caught in the reins of a runaway horse, or being seized in a horse's teeth, or in machinery. It is usually the terminal phalanx that is separated, and with it the tendon of the deep flexor, which ruptures at its junction with the belly of the muscle (Fig. 108). The treatment consists in disinfecting the wound, closing the tendon-sheath, and trimming the mutilated finger so as to provide a useful stump.

DISEASES OF MUSCLES AND TENDONS

Congenital absence of muscles is sometimes met with, usually in association with other deformities. The pectoralis major, for example, may be absent on one or on both sides, without, however, causing any disability, as other muscles enlarge and take on its functions.

Atrophy of Muscle.—Simple atrophy, in which the muscle elements are merely diminished in size without undergoing any structural alteration, is commonly met with as a result of disuse, as when a patient is confined to bed for a long period.

In cases of joint disease, the muscles acting on the joint become atrophied more rapidly than is accounted for by disuse alone, and this is attributed to an interference with the trophic innervation of the muscles reflected from centres in the spinal medulla. It is more marked in the extensor than in the flexor groups of muscles. Those affected become soft and flaccid, exhibit tremors on attempted movement, and their excitability to the faradic current is diminished.

Neuropathic atrophy is associated with lesions of the nervous system. It is most pronounced in lesions of the motor nerve-trunks, probably because vaso-motor and trophic fibres are involved as well as those that are purely motor in function. It is attended with definite structural alterations, the muscle elements first undergoing fatty degeneration, and then being absorbed, and replaced to a large extent by ordinary connective tissue and fat. At a certain stage the muscles exhibit the reaction of degeneration. In the common form of paralysis resulting from poliomyelitis, many fibres undergo fatty degeneration and are replaced by fat, while at the same time there is a regeneration of muscle fibres.

Fibrositis or "**Muscular Rheumatism.**"—This clinical term is applied to a group of affections of which lumbago is the best-known example. The group includes lumbago, stiff-neck, and pleurodynia—conditions which have this in common, that sudden and severe pain is excited by movement of the affected part. The lesion consists in inflammatory hyperplasia of the connective tissue; the new tissue differs from normal fibrous tissue in its tendency to contract, in being swollen, painful and tender on pressure, and in the fact that it can be massaged away (Stockman). It would appear to involve mainly the fibrous tissue of muscles, although it may extend from this to aponeuroses, ligaments, periosteum, and the sheaths of nerves. The term *fibrositis* was applied to it by Gowers in 1904.

In *lumbago—lumbo-sacral fibrositis*—the pain is usually located over the sacrum, the sacro-iliac joint, or the aponeurosis of the lumbar muscles on one or both sides. The amount of tenderness varies, and so long as the patient is still he is free from pain. The slightest attempt to alter his position, however, is attended by pain, which may be so severe as to render him helpless for the moment. The pain is most marked on rising from the stooping or sitting posture, and may extend down the back of the hip, especially if, as is commonly the case, lumbago and gluteal fibrosis coexist. Once a patient has suffered from lumbago, it is liable to recur, and an attack may be determined by errors of diet, changes of weather, exposure to cold or unwonted exertion. It is met with chiefly in male adults, and is most apt to occur in those who are gouty or are the subjects of oxaluric dyspepsia.

Gluteal fibrositis usually follows exposure to wet, and affects the gluteal muscles, particularly the medius, and their aponeurotic coverings. When the condition has lasted for some time, indurated strands or nodules can be detected on palpating the relaxed muscles. The patient complains of persistent aching and stiffness over the buttock, and sometimes extending down the lateral aspect of the thigh. The pain is aggravated by such movements as bring the affected muscles into action. It is not referred to the line of the sciatic nerve, nor is there tenderness on pressing over the nerve, or sensations of tingling or numbness in the leg or foot.

If untreated, the morbid process may implicate the sheath of the sciatic nerve and cause genuine sciatic neuralgia (Llewellyn and Jones). A similar condition may implicate the fascia lata of the thigh, or the calf muscles and their aponeuroses—*crural fibrositis.*

In *painful stiff-neck*, or "rheumatic torticollis," the pain is located in one side of the neck, and is excited by some inadvertent movement. The head is held stiffly on one side as in wry-neck, the patient contracting the sterno-mastoid. There may be tenderness over the vertebral spines or in the lines of the cervical nerves, and the sterno-mastoid may undergo atrophy. This affection is more often met with in children.

In *pleurodynia—intercostal fibrositis*—the pain is in the line of the intercostal nerves, and is excited by movement of the chest, as in coughing, or by any bodily exertion. There is often marked tenderness.

A similar affection is met with in the *shoulder and arm—brachial fibrositis*—especially on waking from sleep. There is acute pain on attempting to abduct the arm, and there may be localised tenderness in the region of the axillary nerve.

Treatment.—The general treatment is concerned with the diet, attention to the stomach, bowels, and kidneys and with the correction of any gouty tendencies that may be present. Remedies such as salicylates are given for the relief of pain, and for this purpose drugs of the aspirin type are to be preferred, and these may be followed by large doses of iodide of potassium. Great benefit is derived from massage, and from the induction of hyperæmia by means of heat. Cupping or needling, or, in exceptional cases, hypodermic injections of antipyrin or morphin, may be called for. To prevent relapses of lumbago, the patient must take systematic exercises of all kinds, especially such as bring out the movements of the vertebral column and hip-joints.

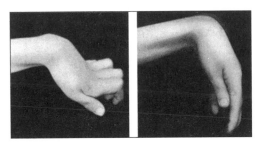

FIG. 109. Volkmann's Ischæmic Contracture. When the wrist is flexed to a right angle it is possible to extend the fingers. (Photographs lent by Mr. Lawford Knaggs)

Contracture of Muscles.—Permanent shortening of muscles results from the prolonged approximation of their points of attachment, or from structural changes in their substance produced by injury or by disease. It is a frequent accompaniment and sometimes a cause of deformities, in the treatment of which lengthening of the shortened muscles or their tendons may be an essential step.

Myositis.—*Ischæmic Myositis.*—Volkmann was the first to describe a form of myositis followed by contracture, resulting from interference with the arterial blood supply. It is most frequently observed in the flexor muscles of the forearm in children and young persons under treatment for fractures in the region of the elbow, the splints and bandages causing compression of the blood vessels. There is considerable effusion of blood, the skin is tense, and the muscles, vessels, and nerves are compressed; this is further increased if the elbow is flexed and splints and tight bandages are applied. The muscles acquire a board-like hardness and no longer contract under the will, and passive motion is painful and restricted. Slight contracture of the fingers is usually the first sign of the malady; in time the muscles undergo further contraction, and this brings about a claw-like deformity of the hand. The affected muscles usually show the reaction of degeneration. In severe cases the median and ulnar nerves are also the seat of cicatricial changes (ischæmic neuritis).

By means of splints, the interphalangeal, metacarpo-phalangeal, and wrist joints should be gradually extended until the deformity is over-corrected (R. Jones). Murphy advises resection of the radius and ulna sufficient to admit of dorsiflexion of the joints and lengthening of the flexor tendons.

Various forms of *pyogenic* infection are met with in muscle, most frequently in relation to pyæmia and to typhoid fever. These may result in overgrowth of the connective-tissue framework of the muscle and degeneration of its fibres, or in suppuration and the formation of one or more abscesses in the muscle substance. Repair may be associated with contracture.

A *gonorrhoeal* form of myositis is sometimes met with; it is painful, but rarely goes on to suppuration.

In the early secondary period of *syphilis*, the muscles may be the seat of dull, aching, nocturnal pains, especially in the neck and back. *Syphilitic contracture* is a condition which has been observed chiefly in the later secondary period; the biceps of the arm and the hamstrings in the thigh are the muscles more commonly affected. The striking feature is a gradually increasing difficulty of extending the limb at the elbow or knee, and progressive flexion of the joint. The affected muscle is larger and firmer than normal, and its electric excitability is diminished. In tertiary syphilis, individual muscles may become the seat of interstitial myositis or of gummata, and these affections readily yield to anti-syphilitic remedies.

Tuberculous disease in muscle, while usually due to extension from adjacent tissues, is sometimes the result of a primary infection through the blood-stream. Tuberculous nodules are found disseminated throughout the muscle; the surrounding tissues are indurated, and central caseation may take place and lead to abscess formation and sinuses. We have observed this form of tuberculous disease in the gastrocnemius and in the psoas—in the latter muscle apart from tuberculous disease in the vertebræ.

Tendinitis.—German authors describe an inflammation of tendon as distinguished from inflammation of its sheath, and give it the name tendinitis. It is met with most frequently in the tendo-calcaneus in gouty and rheumatic subjects who have overstrained the tendon, especially during cold and damp weather. There is localised pain which is aggravated by walking, and the tendon is sensitive and swollen from a little above its insertion to its junction with the muscle. Gouty nodules may form in its substance. Constitutional measures, massage, and douching should be employed, and the tendon should be protected from strain.

Calcification and Ossification in Muscles, Tendons, and Fasciæ.—*Myositis ossificans.*—Ossifications in muscles, tendons, fasciæ, and ligaments, in those who are the subjects of arthritis deformans, are seldom recognised clinically, but are frequently met with in dissecting-rooms and museums. Similar localised ossifications are met with in Charcot's disease of joints, and in fractures which have repaired with exuberant callus. The new bone may be in the form of spicules, plates, or irregular masses, which, when connected with a bone, are called *false exostoses* (Fig. 110).

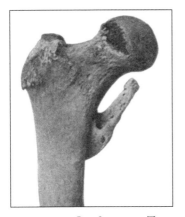

FIG. 110. Ossification in Tendon of Ilio-psoas Muscle.

Traumatic Ossification in Relation to Muscle.—Various forms of ossification are met with in muscle as the result of a single or of repeated injury. Ossification in the crureus or vastus lateralis muscle has been frequently observed as a result of a kick from a horse. Within a week or two a swelling appears at the site of injury, and becomes progressively harder until its consistence is that of bone. If the mass of new bone moves with the affected muscle, it causes little inconvenience. If, as is commonly the case, it is fixed to the femur, the action of the muscle is impaired, and the patient complains of pain and difficulty in flexing the knee. A skiagram shows the extent of the mass and its relationship to the femur. The treatment consists in excising the bony mass.

Difficulty may arise in differentiating such a mass of bone from sarcoma; the ossification in muscle is uniformly hard, while the sarcoma varies in consistence at different parts, and the X-ray picture shows a clear outline of the bone in the vicinity of the ossification in muscle, whereas in sarcoma the involvement of the bone is shown by indentations and irregularity in its contour.

A similar ossification has been observed in relation to the insertion of the brachialis muscle as a sequel of dislocation of the elbow. After reduction of the dislocation, the range of movement gradually diminishes and a hard swelling appears in front of the lower end of the humerus. The lump continues to increase in size and in three to four weeks the disability becomes complete. A radiogram shows a shadow in the muscle, attached at one part as a rule to the coronoid process. During the next three or four months, the lump in front of the elbow remains stationary in size; a gradual decrease then ensues, but the swelling persists, as a rule, for several years.

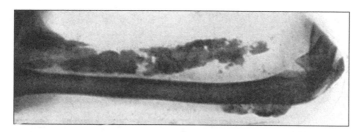

FIG. 111. Calcification and Ossification in Biceps and Triceps.(From a radiogram lent by Dr. C. A. Adair Dighton.)

Ossification in the adductor longus was first described by Billroth under the name of "rider's bone." It follows bruising and partial rupture of the muscle, and has been observed chiefly in cavalry soldiers. If it causes inconvenience the bone may be removed by operation.

Ossification in the deltoid and pectoral muscles has been observed in foot-soldiers in the German army, and has received the name of "drill-bone"; it is due to bruising of the muscle by the recoil of the rifle.

Progressive Ossifying Myositis.—This is a rare and interesting disease, in which the muscles, tendons, and fasciæ throughout the body become the seat of ossification. It affects almost exclusively the male sex, and usually begins in childhood or youth, sometimes after an injury, sometimes without apparent cause. The muscles of the back, especially the trapezius and latissimus, are the first to be affected, and the initial complaint is limitation of movement.

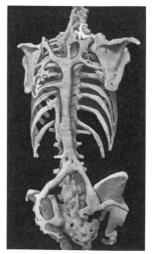

FIG. 112. Ossification in Muscles of Trunk in a case of generalised Ossifying Myositis. (Photograph lent by Dr. Rustomjee.)

The affected muscles show swellings which are rounded or oval, firm and elastic, sharply defined, without tenderness and without discoloration of the overlying skin. Skiagrams show that a considerable deposit of lime salts may precede the formation of bone, as is seen in Fig. 111. In course of time the vertebral column becomes rigid, the head is bent forward, the hips are flexed, and abduction and other movements of the arms are limited. The disease progresses by fits and starts, until all the striped muscles of the body are replaced by bone, and all movements, even those of the jaws, are abolished. The subjects of this disease usually succumb to pulmonary tuberculosis.

There is no means of arresting the disease, and surgical treatment is restricted to the removal or division of any mass of bone that interferes with an important movement.

A remarkable feature of this disease is the frequent presence of a deformity of the great toe, which usually takes the form of hallux valgus, the great toe coming to lie beneath the second one; the shortening is usually ascribed to absence of the first phalanx, but it has been shown to depend also on a synostosis and imperfect development of the phalanges. A similar deformity of the thumb is sometimes met with.

Microscopical examination of the muscles shows that, prior to the deposition of lime salts and the formation of bone, there occurs a proliferation of the intra-muscular connective tissue and a gradual replacement and absorption of the muscle fibres. The bone is spongy in character, and its development takes place along similar lines to those observed in ossification from the periosteum.

Tumours of Muscle.—With the exception of congenital varieties, such as the rhabdomyoma, tumours of muscle grow from the connective-tissue framework and not from the muscle fibres. Innocent tumours, such as the fibroma, lipoma, angioma, and neuro-fibroma, are rare. Malignant tumours may be primary in the muscle, or may result from extension from adjacent growths—for example, implication of the pectoral muscle in cancer of the breast—or they may be derived from tumours situated elsewhere. The diagnosis of an intra-muscular tumour is made by observing that the swelling is situated beneath the deep fascia, that it becomes firm and fixed when the muscle contracts, and that, when the muscle is relaxed, it becomes softer, and can be moved in the transverse axis of the muscle, but not in its long axis.

Clinical interest attaches to that form of slowly growing fibro-sarcoma—*the recurrent fibroid of Paget*—which is most frequently met with in the muscles of the abdominal wall. A rarer variety is the ossifying chondro-sarcoma, which undergoes ossification to such an extent as to be visible in skiagrams.

In primary sarcoma the treatment consists in removing the muscle. In the limbs, the function of the muscle that is removed may be retained by transplanting an adjacent muscle in its place.

Hydatid cysts of muscle resemble those developing in other tissues.

DISEASES OF TENDON SHEATHS

Tendon sheaths have the same structure and function as the synovial membranes of joints, and are liable to the same diseases. Apart from the tendon sheaths displayed in anatomical dissections, there is a loose peritendinous and perimuscular cellular tissue which is subject to the same pathological conditions as the tendon sheaths proper.

Teno-synovitis.—The toxic or infective agent is conveyed to the tendon sheaths through the blood-stream, as in the gouty, gonorrhoeal, and tuberculous varieties, or is introduced directly through a wound, as in the common pyogenic form of teno-synovitis.

Teno-synovitis Crepitans.—In the simple or traumatic form of teno-synovitis, although the most prominent etiological factor is a strain or over-use of the tendon, there would appear to be some other, probably a toxic, factor in its production, otherwise the affection would be much more common than it is: only a small proportion of those who strain or over-use their tendons become the subjects of teno-synovitis. The opposed surfaces of the tendon and its sheath are covered with fibrinous lymph, so that there is friction when they move on one another.

The *clinical features* are pain on movement, tenderness on pressure over the affected tendon, and a sensation of crepitation or friction when the tendon is moved in its sheath. The crepitation may be soft like the friction of snow, or may resemble the creaking of new leather—"saddle-back creaking." There may be swelling in the long axis of the tendon, and redness and oedema of the skin. If there is an effusion of fluid into the sheath, the swelling is more marked and crepitation is absent. There is little tendency to the formation of adhesions.

In the upper extremity, the sheath of the long tendon of the biceps may be affected, but the condition is most common in the tendons about the wrist, particularly in the extensors of the thumb, and it is most frequently met with in those who follow occupations which involve prolonged use or excessive straining of these tendons—for example, washerwomen or riveters. It also occurs as a result of excessive piano-playing, fencing, or rowing.

At the ankle it affects the peronei, the extensor digitorum longus, or the tibialis anterior. It is most often met with in relation to the tendo-calcaneus—*Achillo-dynia*—and results from the pressure of ill-fitting boots or from the excessive use and strain of the tendon in cycling, walking, or dancing. There is pain in raising the heel from the ground, and creaking can be felt on palpation.

The *treatment* consists in putting the affected tendon at rest, and with this object a splint may be helpful; the usual remedies for inflammation are indicated: Bier's hyperæmia, lead and opium fomentations, and ichthyol and glycerine. The affection readily subsides under treatment, but is liable to relapse on a repetition of the exciting cause.

Gouty Teno-synovitis.—A deposit of urate of soda beneath the endothelial covering of tendons or of that lining their sheaths is commonly met with in gouty subjects. The accumulation of urates may result in the formation of visible nodular swellings, varying in size from a pea to a cherry, attached to the tendon and moving with it. They may be merely unsightly, or they may interfere with the use of the tendon. Recurrent attacks of inflammation are prone to occur. We have removed such gouty masses with satisfactory results.

Suppurative Teno-synovitis.—This form usually follows upon infected wounds of the fingers—especially of the thumb or little finger—and is a frequent sequel to whitlow; it may also follow amputation of a finger. Once the infection has gained access to the sheath, it tends to spread, and may reach the palm or even the forearm, being then associated with cellulitis. In moderately acute cases the tendon and its sheath become covered with granulations, which subsequently lead to the formation of adhesions; while in more acute cases the tendon sloughs. The pus may burst into the cellular tissue outside the sheath, and the suppuration is liable to spread to neighbouring sheaths or to adjacent bones or joints—for example, those of the wrist.

The *treatment* consists in inducing hyperæmia and making small incisions for the escape of pus. The site of incision is determined by the point of greatest tenderness on pressure. After the inflammation has subsided, active and passive movements are employed to prevent the formation of adhesions between the tendon and its sheath. If the tendon sloughs, the dead portion should be cut away, as its separation is extremely slow and is attended with prolonged suppuration.

Gonorrhoeal Teno-synovitis.—This is met with especially in the tendon sheaths about the wrist and ankle. It may occur in a mild form, with pain, impairment of movement, and oedema, and sometimes an elongated, fluctuating swelling, the result of serous effusion into the sheath. This condition may alternate with a gonorrhoeal affection of one of the larger joints. It may subside under rest and soothing applications, but is liable to relapse. In the more severe variety the skin is red, and the swelling partakes of the characters of a phlegmon with threatening suppuration; it may result in crippling from adhesions. Even if pus forms in the sheath, the tendon rarely sloughs. The treatment consists in inducing hyperæmia by Bier's method; and a vaccine may be employed with satisfactory results.

Tuberculous Disease of Tendon Sheaths.—This is a comparatively common affection, and is analogous to tuberculous disease of the synovial membrane of joints. It may originate in the sheath, or may spread to it from an adjacent bone.

The commonest form—hydrops—is that in which the synovial sheath is distended with a viscous fluid, and the fibrinous material on the free surface becomes detached and is moulded into melon-seed bodies by the movement of the tendon. The sheath itself is thickened by the growth of tuberculous granulation tissue. The bodies are smooth and of a dull-white colour, and vary greatly in size and shape. There may be an overgrowth of the fatty fringes of the synovial sheath, a condition described as "arborescent lipoma."

The *clinical features* vary with the tendon sheath affected. In the common flexor sheath of the hand an hour-glass-shaped swelling is formed, bulging above and below the transverse carpal (anterior annular) ligament—formerly known as *compound palmar ganglion*. There is little or no pain, but the fingers tend to be stiff and weak, and to become flexed. On palpation, it is usually possible to displace the contents of the sheath from one compartment to the other, and this may yield fluctuation, and, what is more characteristic, a peculiar soft crepitant sensation from the movement of the melon-seed bodies. In the sheath of the peronei or other tendons about the ankle, the swelling is sausage-shaped, and is constricted opposite the annular ligament.

The onset and progress of the affection are most insidious, and the condition may remain stationary for long periods. It is aggravated by use or strain of the tendons involved. In exceptional cases the skin is thinned and gives way, resulting in the formation of a sinus.

Treatment.—In the common flexor sheath of the palm, an attempt may be made to cure the condition by removing the contents through a small incision and filling the cavity with iodoform glycerine, followed by the use of Bier's bandage. If this fails, the distended sheath is laid open, the contents removed, the wall scraped, and the wound closed.

A less common form of tuberculous disease is that in which the sheath becomes the seat of *a diffuse tuberculous thickening*, not unlike the white swelling met with in joints, and with a similar tendency to caseation. A painless swelling of an elastic character forms in relation to the tendon sheath. It is hour-glass-shaped in the common flexor sheath of the palm, elongated or sausage-shaped in the extensors of the wrist and in the tendons at the ankle. The tuberculous granulation tissue is liable to break down and lead to the formation of a cold abscess and sinuses, and in our experience is often associated with disease in an adjacent bone or joint. In the peronei tendons, for example, it may result from disease of the fibula or of the ankle-joint.

When conservative measures fail, excision of the affected sheath should be performed; the whole of the diseased area being exposed by free incision of the overlying soft parts, the sheath is carefully isolated from the surrounding tissues and is cut across above and below. Any tuberculous tissue on the tendon itself is removed with a sharp spoon. Associated bone or joint lesions are dealt with at the same time. In the after-treatment the functions of the tendons must be preserved by voluntary and passive movements.

Syphilitic Affections of Tendon Sheaths.—These closely resemble the syphilitic affections of the synovial membrane of joints. During the secondary period the lesion usually consists in effusion into the sheath; gummata are met with during the tertiary period.

Arborescent lipoma has been found in the sheaths of tendons about the wrist and ankle, sometimes in a multiple and symmetrical form, unattended by symptoms and disappearing under anti-syphilitic treatment.

Tumours of Tendon Sheaths.—Innocent tumours, such as *lipoma, fibroma,* and *myxoma*, are rare. Special mention should be made of the *myeloma* which is met with at the wrist or ankle as an elongated swelling of slow development, or over the phalanx of a finger as a small rounded swelling. The tumour tissue, when exposed by dissection, is of a chocolate or chamois-yellow colour, and consists almost entirely of giant cells. The treatment consists in dissecting the tumour tissue off the tendons, and this is usually successful in bringing about a permanent cure.

All varieties of *sarcoma* are met with, but their origin from tendon sheaths is not associated with special features.

THE BURSÆ

A bursa is a closed sac lined by endothelium and containing synovia. Some are normally present—for instance, that between the skin and the patella, and that between the aponeurosis of the gluteus maximus and the great trochanter. *Adventitious bursæ* are developed as a result of abnormal pressure—for example, over the tarsal bones in cases of club-foot.

Injuries of Bursæ.—As a result of contusion, especially in bleeders, hæmorrhage may occur into the cavity of a bursa and give rise to a *bursal hæmatoma*. Such a hæmatoma may mask a fracture of the bone beneath—for example, fracture of the olecranon.

Diseases of Bursæ.—The lining membrane of bursæ resembles that of joints and tendon sheaths, and is liable to the same forms of disease.

Infective bursitis frequently follows abrasions, scratches, and wounds of the skin over the prepatellar or olecranon bursa, and in neglected cases the infection transgresses the wall of the bursa and gives rise to a spreading cellulitis.

Traumatic or Trade Bursitis.—This term may be conveniently applied to those affections of bursæ which result from repeated slight traumatism incident to particular occupations. The most familiar examples of these are the enlargement of the prepatellar bursa met with in housemaids—the "housemaid's knee" (Fig. 113); the enlargement of the olecranon bursa—"miner's elbow"; and of the ischial bursa—"weaver's" or "tailor's bottom" (Fig. 116). These affections are characterised by an effusion of fluid into the sac of the bursa with thickening of its lining membrane. While friction and pressure are the most evident factors in their production, it is probable that there is also some toxic agent concerned, otherwise these affections would be much more common than they are. Of the countless housemaids in whom the pre-patellar bursa is subjected to friction and pressure, only a small proportion become the subjects of housemaid's knee.

Clinical Features.—As these are best illustrated in the different varieties of prepatellar bursitis, it is convenient to take this as the type. In a number of cases the inflammation is acute and the patient is unable to use the limb; the part is hot, swollen, and tender, and fluctuation can be detected in the bursa. In the majority the condition is chronic, and the chief feature is the gradual accumulation of fluid constituting the *bursal hydrops* or *hygroma*. When the affection has lasted some time, or has frequently relapsed, the wall of the bursa becomes thickened by fibrous tissue, which may be deposited irregularly, so that septa, bands, or fringes are formed, not unlike those met with in arthritis deformans. These fringes may be detached and form loose bodies like those met with in joints; less frequently there are fibrinous bodies of the melon-seed type, sometimes moulded into circular discs like wafers. The presence of irregular thickenings of the wall, or of loose bodies, may be recognised on palpation, especially in superficial bursæ, if the sac is not tensely filled with fluid. The thickening of the wall may take place in a uniform and concentric fashion, resulting in the formation of a fibrous tumour—*the solid bursal tumour*—a small cavity remaining in the centre which serves to distinguish it from a new growth or neoplasm.

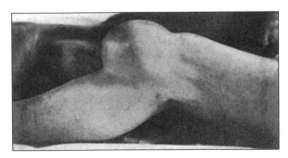

FIG. 113. Hydrops of Prepatellar Bursa in a housemaid.

The *treatment* varies according to the variety and stage of the affection. In recent cases the symptoms subside under rest and the application of fomentations. Hydrops may be got rid of by blistering, by tapping, or by incision and drainage. When the wall is thickened, the most satisfactory treatment is to excise the bursa; the overlying skin being reflected in the shape of a horseshoe flap or being removed along with the bursa.

Other Diseases of Bursæ are associated with *gonorrhoeal infection*, and with *rheumatism*, especially that following scarlet fever, and are apt to be persistent or to relapse after apparent cure. In the *gouty* form, urate of soda is deposited in the wall of the bursa, and may result in the formation of chalky tumours, sometimes of considerable size (Fig. 114).

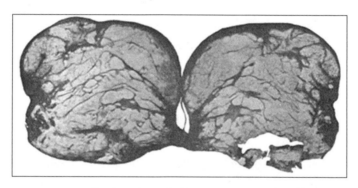

FIG. 114. Section through Bursa over external malleolus, showing deposit of urate of soda. (Cf. Fig. 117.)

Tuberculous disease of bursæ closely resembles that of tendon sheaths. It may occur as an independent affection, or may be associated with disease in an adjacent bone or joint. It is met with chiefly in the prepatellar and subdeltoid bursæ, or in one of the bursæ over the great trochanter. The clinical features are those of an indolent hydrops, with or without melon-seed bodies, or of uniform thickening of the wall of the bursa; the tuberculous granulation tissue may break down into a cold abscess, and give rise to sinuses. The best treatment is to excise the affected bursa, or, when this is impracticable, to lay it freely open, remove the tuberculous tissue with the sharp spoon or knife, and treat the cavity by the open method.

Syphilitic dise ase is rarely recognised except in the form of bursal and peri-bursal gummata in front of the knee-joint.

New growths include the fibroma, the myxoma, the myeloma or giant-celled tumour, and various forms of sarcoma.

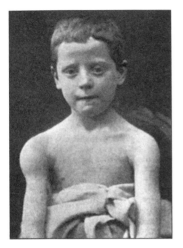

FIG. 115. Tuberculous Disease of Sub-deltoid Bursa.
(From a photograph lent by Sir George T. Beatson.)

Diseases of Individual Bursæ.—The *olecranon bursa* is frequently the seat of pyogenic infection and of traumatic or trade bursitis, the latter being known as "miner's" or "student's elbow."

The *sub-deltoid* or *sub-acromial bursa,* which usually presents a single cavity and does not normally communicate with the shoulder-joint, is indispensable in abduction and rotation of the humerus. When the arm is abducted, the fixed lower part or floor of the bursa is carried under the acromion, and the upper part or roof is rolled up in the same direction, hence tenderness over the inflamed bursa may disappear when the arm is abducted (Dawbarn's sign). It is liable to traumatic affections from a fall on the shoulder, pressure, or over-use of the limb. Pain, located commonly at the insertion of the deltoid, is a constant symptom and is especially annoying at night, the patient being unable to get into a comfortable position. Tenderness may be elicited over the anatomical limits of the bursa, and is usually most marked over the great tuberosity, just external to the inter-tubercular (bicipital) groove. When adhesions are present, abduction beyond 10 degrees is impossible. Demonstrable effusion is not uncommon, but is disguised by the overlying tissues. If left to himself, the patient tends to maintain the limb in the "sling position," and resists movements in the direction of abduction and rotation. In the treatment of this affection the arm should be maintained at a right angle to the body, the arm being rotated medially (Codman). When pain does not prevent it, movements of the arm and massage are persevered with. In neglected cases, when adhesions have formed and the shoulder is fixed, it may be necessary to break down the adhesions under an anæsthetic.

The bursa is also liable to infective conditions, such as acute rheumatism, gonorrhoea, suppuration, or tubercle. In tuberculous disease a large fluctuating swelling may form and acquire the characters of a cold abscess (Fig. 115).

The bursa underneath the tendon of the *subscapularis* muscle when inflamed causes alteration in the attitude of the shoulder and impairment of its movements.

An adventitious bursa forms over the *acromion* process in porters and others who carry weights on the shoulder, and may be the seat of traumatic bursitis.

The bursa under the *tendon of insertion of the biceps*, when the seat of disease, is attended with pain and swelling about a finger's breadth below the bend of the elbow; there is pain and difficulty in effecting the combined movement of flexion and supination, slight limitation of extension, and restriction of pronation.

In the lower extremity, a large number of normal and adventitious bursæ are met with and may be the seat of bursitis. That over the *tuberosity of the ischium*, when enlarged as a trade disease, is known as "weaver's" or "tailor's bottom." It may form a fluctuating swelling of great size, projecting on the buttock and extending down the thigh, and causing great inconvenience in sitting (Fig. 116). It sometimes contains a number of loose bodies.

There are two bursæ over the *great trochanter*, one superficial to, the other beneath the aponeurosis of the gluteus maximus; the latter is not infrequently infected by tuberculous disease that has spread from the trochanter.

The bursa *between the psoas muscle and the capsule of the hip-joint* may be the seat of tuberculous disease, and give rise to clinical features not unlike those of disease of the hip-joint. The limb is flexed, abducted and rotated out; there is a swelling in the upper part of Scarpa's triangle, but the movements are not restricted in directions which do not entail putting the ilio-psoas muscle on the stretch.

Cartilaginous and partly ossified loose bodies may accumulate in the ilio-psoas bursa and distend it, both in a downward direction towards the hip-joint, with which it communicates, and upwards, projecting towards the abdomen.

The bursa beneath the quadriceps extensor—*subcrural bursa*—usually communicates with the knee-joint and shares in its diseases. When shut off from the joint it may suffer independently, and when distended with fluid forms a horse-shoe swelling above the patella.

In front of the patella and its ligament is the *prepatellar bursa*, which may have one, two, or three compartments, usually communicating with one another. It is the seat of the affection known as "housemaid's knee," which is very common and is sometimes bilateral, and, less frequently, of tuberculous disease which usually originates in the patella.

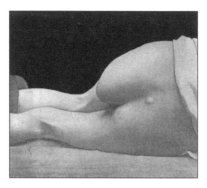

FIG. 116. Great Enlargement of the Ischial Bursa.
(Mr. Scot-Skirving's case.)

The bursa *between the ligamentum patellæ and the tibia* is rarely the seat of disease. When it is, there is pain and tenderness referred to the ligament, the patient is unable to extend the limb completely, the tuberosity of the tibia is apparently enlarged, and there is a fluctuating swelling on either side of the ligament, most marked in the extended position of the limb.

Of the numerous bursæ in the popliteal space, that *between the semi-mem-branosus and the medial head of the gastrocnemius* is most frequently the seat of disease, which is usually of the nature of a simple hydrops, forming a fluctuating egg-or sausage-shaped swelling at the medial side of the popliteal space. It is flaccid in the flexed, and tense in the extended position. As a rule it causes little inconvenience, and may be left alone. Otherwise it should be dissected out, and if, as is frequently the case, there is a communication with the knee-joint, this should be closed with sutures.

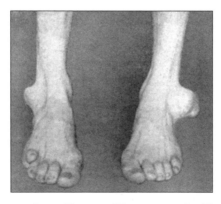

FIG. 117. Gouty Disease of Bursæ in a tailor. The bursal tumours were almost entirely composed of urate of soda. (Cf. Fig. 114.)

An adventitious bursa may form over the *lateral malleolus*, especially in tailors, giving rise to the condition known as "tailor's ankle" (Fig. 117).

The bursa *between the tendo-calcaneus (Achillis) and the upper part of the calcaneus* may become inflamed—especially as a result of post-scarlatinal rheumatism or gonorrhoea. The affection is known as Achillo-bursitis. There is severe pain in the region of the insertion of the tendo-calcaneus, the movements at the ankle-joint are restricted, and the patient may be unable to walk. There is a tender swelling on either side of the tendon. When, in spite of palliative treatment, the affection persists or relapses, it is best to excise the bursa. The tendo-calcaneus is detached from the calcaneus, the bursa dissected out, and the tendon replaced. If there is a bony projection from the calcaneus, it should be shaved off with the chisel.

The bursa that is sometimes met with on the under aspect of the calcaneus—*the subcalcanean bursa*—when inflamed, gives rise to pain and tenderness in the sole of the foot. This affection may be associated with a spinous projection from the bone, which is capable of being recognised in a skiagram. The soft parts of the heel are turned forwards as a flap, the bursa is dissected out, and the projection of bone, if present, is removed.

The enlargement of adventitious bursæ over the head of the first metatarsal in hallux valgus; over the tarsus, metatarsus, and digits in the different forms of club-foot; over the angular projection in Pott's disease of the spine; over the end of the bone in amputation stumps, and over hard tumours such as chondroma and osteoma, are described elsewhere.

• XX •

DISEASES OF BONE

Anatomy and Physiology
Regeneration of Bone
Transplantation of Bone
Diseases of Bone • Definition of Terms
Pyogenic Diseases: Acute Osteomyelitis and Periostitis; Chronic and
Relapsing Osteomyelitis; Abscess of Bone • Tuberculous Disease
Syphilitic Disease • Hydatids; Rickets; Osteomalacia
Ostitis Deformans of Paget
Osteomyelitis Fibrosa • Affections of Bones in Diseases of the Nervous
System • Fragilitas Ossium
Tumours and Cysts of Bone.

Surgical Anatomy.—During the period of growth, a long bone such as the tibia consists of a shaft or *diaphysis*, and two extremities or *epiphyses*. So long as growth continues there intervenes between the shaft and each of the epiphyses a disc of actively growing cartilage—*the epiphysial cartilage*; and at the junction of this cartilage with the shaft is a zone of young, vascular, spongy bone known as the *metaphysis* or *epiphysial junction*. The shaft is a cylinder of compact bone enclosing the medullary canal, which is filled with yellow marrow. The extremities, which include the ossifying junctions, consist of spongy bone, the spaces of which are filled with red marrow. The articular aspect of the epiphysis is invested with a thick layer of hyaline cartilage, known as the *articular cartilage*, which would appear to be mainly nourished from the synovia.

The external investment—the *periosteum*—is thick and vascular during the period of growth, but becomes thin and less vascular when the skeleton has attained maturity. Except where muscles are attached it is easily separated from the bone; at the extremities it is intimately connected with the epiphysial cartilage and with the epiphysis, and at the margin of the latter it becomes continuous with the capsule of the adjacent joint. It consists of two layers, an outer fibrous and an inner cellular layer; the cells, which are called osteoblasts, are continuous with those lining the Haversian canals and the medullary cavity.

The arrangement of the *blood vessels* determines to some extent the incidence of disease in bone. The nutrient artery, after entering the medullary canal through a special foramen in the cortex, bifurcates, and one main division runs towards each of the extremities, and terminates at the ossifying junction in a series of capillary loops projected against the epiphysial cartilage. This arrangement favours the lodgment of any organisms that may be circulating in the blood, and partly accounts for the frequency with which diseases of bacterial origin develop in the region of the ossifying junction. The diaphysis is also nourished by numerous blood vessels from the periosteum, which penetrate the cortex through the Haversian canals and anastomose with those derived from the nutrient artery. The epiphyses are nourished by a separate system of blood vessels, derived from the arteries which supply the adjacent joint. The veins of the marrow are of large calibre and are devoid of valves.

The *nerves* enter the marrow along with the arteries, and, being derived from the sympathetic system, are probably chiefly concerned with the innervation of the blood vessels, but they are also capable of transmitting sensory impulses, as pain is a prominent feature of many bone affections.

It has long been believed that *the function of the periosteum* is to form new bone, but this view has been questioned by Sir William Macewen, who maintains that its chief function is to limit the formation of new bone. His experimental observations appear to show that new bone is exclusively formed by the cellular elements or osteoblasts: these are found on the surface of the bone, lining the Haversian canals and in the marrow. We believe that it will avoid confusion in the study of the diseases of bone if the osteoblasts on the surface of the bone are still regarded as forming the deeper layer of the periosteum.

The formation of new bone by the osteoblasts may be *defective* as a result of physiological conditions, such as old age and disease of a part, and defective formation is often associated with atrophy, or more strictly speaking, absorption, of the existing bone, as is well seen in the edentulous jaw and in the neck of the femur of a person advanced in years. Defective formation associated with atrophy is also illustrated in the bones of the lower limbs of persons who are unable to stand or walk, and in the distal portion of a bone which is the seat of an ununited fracture. The same combination is seen in an exaggerated degree in the bones of limbs that are paralysed; in the case of adults, atrophy of bone predominates; in children and adolescents, defective formation is the more prominent feature, and the affected bones are attenuated, smooth on the surface, and abnormally light.

On the other hand, the formation of new bone may be *exaggerated*, the osteoblasts being excited to abnormal activity by stimuli of different kinds: for example, the secretion of certain glandular organs, such as the pituitary and thyreoid; the diluted toxins of certain micro-organisms, such as the staphylococcus aureus and the spirochæte of syphilis; a condition of hyperæmia, such as that produced artificially by the application of a Bier's bandage or that which accompanies a chronic leg-ulcer.

The new bone is laid down on the surface, in the Haversian canals, or in the cancellous spaces and medullary canal, or in all three situations. The new bone on the surface sometimes takes the form of a diffuse *encrustation* of porous or spongy bone as in secondary syphilis, sometimes as a uniform increase in the girth of the bone—*hyperostosis*, sometimes as a localised heaping up of bone or *node*, and sometimes in the form of spicules, spoken of as *osteophytes*. When the new bone is laid down in the Haversian canals, cancellous spaces and medulla, the bone becomes denser and heavier, and is said to be *sclerosed*; in extreme instances this may result in obliteration of the medullary canal. Hyperostosis and sclerosis are frequently met with in combination, a condition that is well illustrated in the femur and tibia in tertiary syphilis; if the subject of this condition is confined to bed for several months before his death, the sclerosis may be undone, and rarefaction may even proceed beyond the normal, the bone becoming lighter and richer in fat, although retaining its abnormal girth.

The *function of the epiphysial cartilage* is to provide for the growth of the shaft in length. While all epiphysial cartilages contribute to this result, certain of them functionate more actively and for a longer period than others. Those at the knee, for example, contribute more to the length of limb than do those at the hip or ankle, and they are also the last to unite. In the upper limb the more active epiphyses are at the shoulder and wrist, and these also are the last to unite.

The activity of the epiphysial cartilage may be modified as a result of disease. In rickets, for example, the formation of new bone may take place unequally, and may go on more rapidly in one half of the disc than in the other, with the result that the axis of the shaft comes to deviate from the normal, giving rise to knock-knee or bow-knee. In bacterial diseases originating in the marrow, if the epiphysial junction is directly involved in the destructive process, its bone-forming functions may be retarded or abolished, and the subsequent growth of the bone be seriously interfered with. On the other hand, if it is not directly involved but is merely influenced by the proximity of an infective focus, its bone-forming functions may be stimulated by the diluted toxins and the growth of the bone in length exaggerated. In paralysed limbs the growth from the epiphyses is usually little short of the normal. The result of interference with growth is more injurious in the lower than in the upper limb, because, from the functional point of view, it is essential that the lower extremities should be approximately of equal length. In the forearm or leg, where there are two parallel bones, if the growth of one is arrested the continued growth of the other results in a deviation of the hand or foot to one side.

In certain diseases, such as rickets and inherited syphilis, and in developmental anomalies such as achondroplasia, *dwarfing* of the skeleton results from defective growth of bone at the ossifying junctions. Conversely, excessive growth of bone at the ossifying junctions results in abnormal height of the skeleton or *giantism* as a result, for example, of increased activity of the pituitary in adolescents, and in eunuchs who have been castrated in childhood or adolescence; in the latter, union of the epiphyses at the ends of the long bones is delayed beyond the usual period at which the skeleton attains maturity.

Regeneration of Bone.—When bone has been lost or destroyed as a result of injury or disease, it is capable of being reproduced, the extent to which regeneration takes place varying under different conditions. The chief part in the regeneration of bone is played by the osteoblasts in the adjacent marrow and in the deeper layer of the periosteum. The shaft of a long bone may be reproduced after having been destroyed by disease or removed by operation. The flat bones of the skull and the bones of the face, which are primarily developed in membrane, have little capacity of regeneration; hence, when bone has been lost or removed in these situations, there results a permanent defect.

Wounds or defects in articular cartilage are repaired by fibrous or osseous tissue derived from the subjacent cancellous spaces.

Transplantation of Bone—Bone-grafting.—Clinical experience is conclusive that a portion of bone which has been completely detached from its surroundings—for example, a trephine circle, or a flap of bone detached with the saw, or the loose fragments in a compound fracture—may become, if replaced in position, firmly and permanently incorporated with the surrounding bone. Embedded foreign bodies, on the other hand, such as ivory pegs or decalcified bone, exhibit, on removal after a sufficient interval, evidence of having been eroded, in the shape of worm-eaten depressions and perforations, and do not become united or fused to the surrounding bone. It follows from this that the implanting of living bone is to be preferred to the implanting of dead bone or of foreign material. We believe that transplanted living bone when placed under favourable conditions survives and becomes incorporated with the bone with which it is in contact, and does not merely act as a scaffolding. We believe also that the retention of the periosteum on the graft is not essential, but, by favouring the establishment of vascular connections, it contributes to the survival of the graft and the success of the transplantation. Macewen maintains that bone grafts "take" better if broken up into small fragments; we regard this as unnecessary. Bone grafts yield better functional results when they are immovably fixed to the adjacent bone by suture, pegs, or plates. As in all grafting procedures, asepsis is essential.

Transplanted bone retains its vitality when embedded in the soft parts, but is gradually absorbed and replaced by fibrous tissue.

DISEASES OF BONE

The morbid processes met with in bone originate in the same way and lead to the same results as do similar processes in other tissues. The structural peculiarities of bone, however, and the important changes which take place in the skeleton during the period of growth, modify certain of the clinical and pathological features.

Definition of Terms.—Any diseased process that affects the periosteum is spoken of as *periostitis*; the term *osteomyelitis* is employed when it is located in the marrow. The term *epiphysitis* has been applied to an inflammatory process in two distinct situations—namely, the ossifying nucleus in the epiphysis, and the ossifying junction or metaphysis between the epiphysial cartilage and the diaphysis. We shall restrict the term to inflammation in the first of these situations. Inflammation at the ossifying junction is included under the term osteomyelitis.

The term *rarefying ostitis* is applied to any process that is attended with excessive absorption of the framework of a bone, whereby it becomes more porous or spongy than it was before, a condition known as *osteoporosis*.

The term *caries* is employed to indicate any diseased process associated with crumbling away of the trabecular framework of a bone. It may be considered as the equivalent of ulceration or molecular destruction in the soft parts. The carious process is preceded by the formation of granulation tissue in the marrow or periosteum, which eats away and replaces the bone in contact with it. The subsequent degeneration and death of the granulation tissue under the necrotic influence of bacterial toxins results in disintegration and crumbling away of the trabecular framework of the portion of bone affected. Clinically, carious bone yields a soft grating sensation under the pressure of the probe. The macerated bone presents a rough, eroded surface.

The term *dry caries* (*caries sicca*) is applied to that variety which is unattended with suppuration.

Necrosis is the term applied to the death of a tangible portion of bone, and the dead portion when separated is called a *sequestrum*. The term *exfoliation* is sometimes employed to indicate the separation or throwing off of a superficial sequestrum. The edges and deep surface of the sequestrum present a serrated or worm-eaten appearance due to the process of erosion by which the dead bone has been separated from the living.

BACTERIAL DISEASES

The most important diseases in this group are the pyogenic, the tuberculous, and the syphilitic.

PYOGENIC DISEASES OF BONE.—These diseases result from infection with pyogenic organisms, and two varieties or types are recognised according to whether the organisms concerned reach their seat of action by way of the blood-stream, or through an infection of the soft parts in contact with the bone.

INFECTIONS THROUGH THE BLOOD-STREAM

Diseases caused by the Staphylococcus Aureus.—As the majority of pyogenic diseases are due to infection with the staphylococcus aureus, these will be described first.

Acute osteomyelitis is a suppurative process beginning in the marrow and tending to spread to the periosteum. The disease is common in children, but is rare after the skeleton has attained maturity. Boys are affected more often than girls, in the proportion of three to one, probably because they are more liable to exposure, to injury, and to violent exertion.

Etiology.—Staphylococci gain access to the blood-stream in various ways, it may be through the skin or through a mucous surface.

Such conditions as, for example, a blow, some extra exertion such as a long walk, or exposure to cold, as in wading, may act as localising factors.

The long bones are chiefly affected, and the commonest sites are: either end of the tibia and the lower end of the femur; the other bones of the skeleton are affected in rare instances.

Pathology.—The disease commences and is most intense in the marrow of the ossifying junction at one end of the diaphysis; it may commence at both ends simultaneously—*bipolar osteomyelitis*; or, commencing at one end, may spread to the other.

The changes observed are those of intense engorgement of the marrow, going on to greenish-yellow purulent infiltration. Where the process is most advanced—that is, at the ossifying junction—there are evidences of absorption of the framework of the bone; the marrow spaces and Haversian canals undergo enlargement and become filled with greenish-yellow pus. This rarefaction of the spongy bone is the earliest change seen with the X-rays.

The process may remain localised to the ossifying junction, but usually spreads along the medullary canal for a varying distance, and also extends to the periosteum by way of the enlarged Haversian canals. The pus accumulates under the periosteum and lifts it up from the bone. The extent of spread in the medullary canal and beneath the periosteum is in close correspondence. The periosteum of the diaphysis is easily separated—hence the facility with which the pus spreads along the shaft; but in the region of the ossifying junction it is raised with difficulty because of its intimate connection with the epiphysial cartilage. Less frequently there is more than one collection of pus under the periosteum, each being derived from a focus of suppuration in the subjacent marrow. The pus perforates the periosteum, and makes its way to the surface by the easiest anatomical route, and discharges externally, forming one or more sinuses through which fresh infection may take place. The infection may spread to the adjacent joint, either directly through the epiphysis and articular cartilage, or along the deep layer of the periosteum and its continuation—the capsular ligament. When the epiphysis is intra-articular, as, for example, in the head of the femur, the pus when it reaches the surface of the bone necessarily erupts directly into the joint.

While the occurrence of purely periosteal suppuration is regarded as possible, we are of opinion that the embolic form of staphylococcal osteomyelitis always originates in the marrow.

The portion of the diaphysis which has sustained the action of the concentrated toxins has its vitality further impaired as a result of the stripping of the periosteum and thrombosis of the blood vessels of the marrow, so that *necrosis* of bone is one of the most striking results of the disease, and as this takes place rapidly, that is, in a day or two, the term *acute necrosis*, formerly applied to the disease, was amply justified.

When there is marked rarefaction of the bone at the ossifying junction, the epiphysis is liable to be separated—*epiphysiolysis*. The separation usually takes place through the young bone of the ossifying junction, and the surfaces of the diaphysis and epiphysis are opposed to each other by irregular eroded surfaces bathed in pus. The separated epiphysis may be kept in place by the periosteum, but when this has been detached by the formation of pus beneath it, the epiphysis is liable to be displaced by muscular action or by some movement of the limb, or it is the diaphysis that is displaced, for example, the lower end of the diaphysis of the femur may be projected into the popliteal space.

The epiphysial cartilage usually continues its bone-forming functions, but when it has been seriously damaged or displaced, the further growth of the bone in length may be interfered with. Sometimes the separated and displaced epiphysis dies and constitutes a sequestrum.

The adjacent joint may become filled at an early stage with a serous effusion, which may be sterile. When the cocci gain access to the joint, the lesion assumes the characters of a purulent arthritis, which, from its frequency during the earlier years of life, has been called *the acute arthritis of infants*.

Separation of an epiphysis nearly always results in infection and destruction of the adjacent joint.

Osteomyelitis is rare in the bones of the carpus and tarsus, and the associated joints are usually infected from the outset. In flat bones, such as the skull, the scapula, or the ilium, suppuration usually occurs on both aspects of the bone as well as in the marrow.

Clinical Features.—The constitutional symptoms, which are due to the associated toxæmia, vary considerably in different cases. In mild cases they may be so slight as to escape recognition. In exceptionally severe cases the patient may succumb before there are obvious signs of the localisation of the staphylococci in the bone marrow. In average cases the temperature rises rapidly with a rigor and runs an irregular course with morning remissions, there is marked general illness accompanied by headache, vomiting, and sometimes delirium.

The local manifestations are pain and tenderness in relation to one of the long bones; the pain may be so severe as to prevent sleep and to cause the child to cry out. Tenderness on pressure over the bone is the most valuable diagnostic sign. At a later stage there is an ill-defined swelling in the region of the ossifying junction, with oedema of the overlying skin and dilatation of the superficial veins.

The swelling appears earlier and is more definite in superficial bones such as the tibia, than in those more deeply placed such as the upper end of the femur. It may be less evident to the eye than to the fingers, and is best appreciated by gently stroking the bone from the middle of its shaft towards the end. The maximum thickening and tenderness usually correspond to the junction of the diaphysis with the epiphysis, and the swelling tails off gradually along the shaft. As time goes on there is redness of the skin, especially over a superficial bone, such as the tibia, the swelling becomes softer, and gives evidence of fluctuation. This stage may be reached at the end of twenty-four hours, or not for some days.

Suppuration spreads towards the surface, until, some days later, the skin sloughs and pus escapes, after which the fever usually remits and the pain and other symptoms are relieved. The pus may contain blood and droplets of fat derived from the marrow, and in some cases minute particles of bone are present also. The presence of fat and bony particles in the pus confirms the medullary origin of the suppuration.

If an incision is made, the periosteum is found to be raised from the bone; the extent of the bare bone will be found to correspond fairly accurately with the extent of the lesion in the marrow.

Local Complications.—The adjacent joint may exhibit symptoms which vary from those of a simple effusion to those of a purulent *arthritis*. The joint symptoms may count for little in the clinical picture, or, as in the case of the hip, may so predominate as to overshadow those of the bone lesion from which they originated.

Separation and displacement of the epiphysis usually reveals itself by an alteration in the attitude of the limb; it is nearly always associated with suppuration in the adjacent joint.

When *pathological fracture* of the shaft occurs, as it may do, from some muscular effort or strain, it is attended with the usual signs of fracture.

Dislocation of the adjacent joint has been chiefly observed at the hip; it may result from effusion into the joint and stretching of the ligaments, or may be the sequel of a purulent arthritis; the signs of dislocation are not so obvious as might be expected, but it is attended with an alteration in the attitude of the limb, and the displacement of the head of the bone is readily shown in a skiagram.

General Complications.—In some cases a *multiplicity of lesions* in the bones and joints imparts to the disease the features of pyæmia. The occurrence of endocarditis, as indicated by alterations in the heart sounds and the development of murmurs, may cause widespread infective embolism, and metastatic suppurations in the kidneys, heart-wall, and lungs, as well as in other bones and joints than those primarily affected. The secondary suppurations are liable to be overlooked unless sought for, as they are rarely attended with much pain.

In these multiple forms of osteomyelitis the toxæmic symptoms predominate; the patient is dull and listless, or he may be restless and talkative, or actually delirious. The tongue is dry and coated, the lips and teeth are covered with sordes, the motions are loose and offensive, and may be passed involuntarily. The temperature is remittent and irregular, the pulse small and rapid, and the urine may contain blood and albumen. Sometimes the skin shows erythematous and purpuric rashes, and the patient may cry out as in meningitis. The post-mortem appearances are those of pyæmia.

Differential Diagnosis.—Acute osteomyelitis is to be diagnosed from infections of the soft parts, such as erysipelas and cellulitis, and, in the case of the tibia, from erythema nodosum. Tenderness localised to the ossifying junction is the most valuable diagnostic sign of osteomyelitis.

When there is early and pronounced general intoxication, there is likely to be confusion with other acute febrile illnesses, such as scarlet fever. In all febrile conditions in children and adolescents, the ossifying junctions of the long bones should be examined for areas of pain and tenderness.

Osteomyelitis has many features in common with acute articular rheumatism, and some authorities believe them to be different forms of the same disease (Kocher). In acute rheumatism, however, the joint symptoms predominate, there is an absence of suppuration, and the pains and temperature yield to salicylates.

The *prognosis* varies with the type of the disease, with its location—the vertebræ, skull, pelvis, and lower jaw being specially unfavourable—with the multiplicity of the lesions, and with the development of endocarditis and internal metastases.

Treatment.—This is carried out on the same lines as in other pyogenic infections.

In the earliest stages of the disease, the induction of hyperæmia is indicated, and should be employed until the diagnosis is definitely established, and in the meantime preparations for operation should be made. An incision is made down to and through the periosteum, and whether pus is found or not, the bone should be opened in the vicinity of the ossifying junction by means of a drill, gouge, or trephine. If pus is found, the opening in the bone is extended along the shaft as far as the periosteum has been separated, and the infected marrow is removed with the spoon. The cavity is then lightly packed with rubber dam, or, as recommended by Bier, the skin edges are brought together by sutures which are loosely tied to afford sufficient space between them for the exit of discharge, and the hyperæmic treatment is continued.

When there is widespread suppuration in the marrow, and the shaft is extensively bared of periosteum and appears likely to die, it may be resected straight away or after an interval of a day or two. Early resection of the shaft is also indicated if the opening of the medullary canal is not followed by relief of symptoms. In the leg and forearm, the unaffected bone maintains the length and contour of the limb; in the case of the femur and humerus, extension with weight and pulley along with some form of moulded gutter splint is employed with a similar object.

Amputation of the limb is reserved for grave cases, in which life is endangered by toxæmia, which is attributed to the primary lesion. It may be called for later if the limb is likely to be useless, as, for example, when the whole shaft of the bone is dead without the formation of a new case, when the epiphyses are separated and displaced, and the joints are disorganised.

Flat bones, such as the skull or ilium, must be trephined and the pus cleared out from both aspects of the bone. In the vertebræ, operative interference is usually restricted to opening and draining the associated abscess.

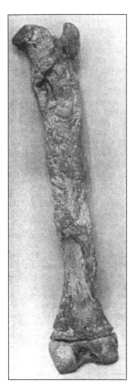

FIG. 118. Shaft of Femur after Acute Osteomyelitis. The shaft has undergone extensive necrosis, and a shell of new bone has been formed by the periosteum.

Nature's Effort at Repair.—*In cases which are left to nature*, and in which necrosis of bone has occurred, those portions of the periosteum and marrow which have retained their vitality resume their osteogenetic functions, often to an exaggerated degree. Where the periosteum has been lifted up by an accumulation of pus, or is in contact with bone that is dead, it proceeds to form new bone with great activity, so that the dead shaft becomes surrounded by a sheath or case of new bone, known as the *involucrum* (Fig. 118). Where the periosteum has been perforated by pus making its way to the surface, there are defects or holes in the involucrum, called *cloacæ*. As these correspond more or less in position to the sinuses in the skin, in passing a probe down one of the sinuses it usually passes through a cloaca and strikes the dead bone lying in the interior. If the periosteum has been extensively destroyed, new bone may only be formed in patches, or not at all. The dead bone is separated from the living by the agency of granulation tissue with its usual complements of phagocytes and osteoclasts, so that the sequestrum presents along its margins and on its deep surface a pitted, grooved, and worm-eaten appearance, except on the periosteal aspect, which is unaltered. Ultimately the dead bone becomes loose and lies in a cavity a little larger than itself; the wall of the cavity is formed by the new case, lined with granulation tissue. The separation of the sequestrum takes place more rapidly in the spongy bone of the ossifying junction than in the compact bone of the shaft.

When foci of suppuration have been scattered up and down the medullary cavity, and the bone has died in patches, several sequestra may be included by the new case; each portion of dead bone is slowly separated, and comes to lie in a cavity lined by granulations.

Even at a distance from the actual necrosis there is formation of new bone by the marrow; the medullary canal is often obliterated, and the bone becomes heavier and denser—sclerosis; and the new bone which is deposited on the original shaft results in an increase in the girth of the bone—hyperostosis.

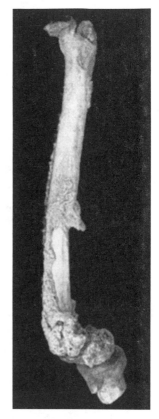

Pathological fracture of the shaft may occur at the site of necrosis, when the new case is incapable of resisting the strain put upon it, and is most frequently met with in the shaft of the femur. Short of fracture, there may be bending or curving of the new case, and this results in deformity and shortening of the limb (Fig. 119).

The *extrusion of a sequestrum* may occur, provided there is a cloaca large enough to allow of its escape, but the surgeon has usually to interfere by performing the operation of sequestrectomy. Displacement or partial extrusion of the dead bone may cause complications, as when a sequestrum derived from the trigone of the femur perforates the popliteal artery or the cavity of the knee-joint, or a sequestrum of the pelvis perforates the wall of the urinary bladder.

The extent to which bone which has been lost is reproduced varies in different parts of the skeleton: while the long bones, the scapula, the mandible, and other bones which are developed in cartilage are almost completely re-formed, bones which are entirely developed in membrane, such as the flat bones of the skull and the maxilla, are not reproduced.

FIG. 119. Femur and Tibia showing results of Acute Osteomyelitis affecting Trigone of Femur; sequestrum partly surrounded by new case; backward displacement of lower epiphysis and implication of knee-joint.

It may be instructive to describe *the X-ray appearances of a long bone that has passed through an attack of acute osteomyelitis* severe enough to have caused necrosis of part of the diaphysis. The shadow of the dead bone is seen in the position of the original shaft which it represents; it is of the same shape and density as the original shaft, while its margins present an irregular contour from the erosion concerned in its separation.

The sequestrum is separated from the living bone by a clear zone which corresponds to the layer of granulations lining the cavity in which it lies. This clear zone separating the shadow of the dead bone from that of the living bone by which it is surrounded is conclusive evidence of a sequestrum. The medullary canal in the vicinity of the sequestrum being obliterated, is represented by a shadow of varying density, continuous with that of the surrounding bone. The shadow of the new case or involucrum with its wavy contour is also in evidence, with its openings or cloacæ, and is mainly responsible for the increase in the diameter of the bone.

The skiagram may also show separation and displacement of the adjacent epiphysis and destruction of the articular surfaces or dislocation of the joint.

Sequelæ of Acute Suppurative Osteomyelitis.—The commonest sequel is the presence of a sequestrum with one or more discharging sinuses; owing to the abundant formation of scar tissue these sinuses have rigid edges which are usually depressed and adherent to the bone.

The Recognition and Removal of Sequestra.—So long as there is dead bone there will be suppuration from the granulations lining the cavity in which it lies, and a discharge of pus from the sinuses, so that the mere persistence of discharge after an attack of osteomyelitis, is presumptive evidence of the occurrence of necrosis. Where there are one or more sinuses, the passage of a probe which strikes bare bone affords corroboration of the view that the bone has perished. When the dead bone has been separated from the living, the X-rays yield the most exact information.

The traditional practice is to wait until the dead bone is entirely separated before undertaking an operation for its removal, from fear, on the one hand, of leaving portions behind which may keep up the discharge, and, on the other, of removing more bone than is necessary. This practice need not be adhered to, as by operating at an earlier stage healing is greatly hastened. If it is decided to wait for separation of the dead bone, drainage should be improved, and the infective element combated by the induction of hyperæmia.

The operation for the removal of the dead bone (*sequestrectomy*) consists in opening up the periosteum and the new case sufficiently to allow of the removal of all the dead bone, including the most minute sequestra. The limb having been rendered bloodless, existing sinuses are enlarged, but if these are inconveniently situated—for example, in the centre of the popliteal space in necrosis of the femoral trigone—it is better to make a fresh wound down to the bone on that aspect of the limb which affords best access, and which entails the least injury of the soft parts. The periosteum, which is thick and easily separable, is raised from the new case with an elevator, and with the chisel or gouge enough of the new bone is taken away to allow of the removal of the sequestrum. Care must be taken not to leave behind any fragment of dead bone, as this will interfere with healing, and may determine a relapse of suppuration.

The dead bone having been removed, the lining granulations are scraped away with a spoon, and the cavity is disinfected.

There are different ways of dealing with a *bone cavity*. It may be packed with gauze (impregnated with "bipp" or with iodoform), which is changed at intervals until healing takes place from the bottom; it may be filled with a flap of bone and periosteum raised from the vicinity, or with bone grafts; or the wall of bone on one side of the cavity may be chiselled through at its base, so that it can be brought into contact with the opposite wall. The method of filling bone cavities devised by Mosetig-Moorhof, consists in disinfecting and drying the cavity by a current of hot air, and filling it with a mixture of powdered iodoform (60 parts) and oil of sesame and spermaceti (each 40 parts), which is fluid at a temperature of 112° F.; the soft parts are then brought together without drainage. As the cavity fills up with new bone the iodoform is gradually absorbed. Iodoform gives a dark shadow with the X-rays, so that the process of its absorption can be followed in skiagrams taken at intervals.

These procedures may be carried out at the same time as the sequestrum is removed, or after an interval. In all of them, asepsis is essential for success.

The *deformities* resulting from osteomyelitis are more marked the earlier in life the disease occurs. Even under favourable conditions, and with the continuous effort at reconstruction of the bone by Nature's method, the return to normal is often far from perfect, and there usually remains a variable amount of hyperostosis and sclerosis and sometimes curving of the bone. Under less favourable conditions, the late results of osteomyelitis may be more serious. *Shortening* is not uncommon from interference with growth at the ossifying junction. *Exaggerated growth* in the length of a bone is rare, and has been observed chiefly in the bones of the leg. Where there are two parallel bones—as in the leg, for example—the growth of the diseased bone may be impaired, and the other continuing its normal growth becomes disproportionately long; less frequently the growth of the diseased bone is exaggerated, and it becomes the longer of the two. In either case, the longer bone becomes curved. An *obliquity* of the bone may result when one half of the epiphysial cartilage is destroyed and the other half continues to form bone, giving rise to such deformities as knock-knee and club-hand.

Deformity may also result from vicious union of a pathological fracture, permanent displacement of an epiphysis, contracture, ankylosis, or dislocation of the adjacent joint.

Relapsing Osteomyelitis.—As the term indicates, the various forms of relapsing osteomyelitis date back to an antecedent attack, and their occurrence depends on the capacity of staphylococci to lie latent in the marrow.

Relapse may take place within a few months of the original attack, or not for many years. Cases are sometimes met with in which relapses recur at regular intervals for several years, the tendency, however, being for the attacks to become milder as the virulence of the organisms becomes more and more attenuated.

Clinical Features.—Osteomyelitis in a patient over twenty-five is nearly always of the relapsing variety. In some cases the bone becomes enlarged, with pain and tenderness on pressure; in others there are the usual phenomena which attend suppuration, but the pus is slow in coming to the surface, and the constitutional symptoms are slight. The pus may escape by new channels, or one of the old sinuses may re-open. Radiograms usually furnish useful information as to the condition of the bone, both as it is altered by the original attack and by the changes that attend the relapse of the infective process.

Treatment.—In cases of thickening of the bone with persistent and severe pain, if relief is not afforded by the repeated application of blisters, the thickened periosteum should be incised, and the bone opened up with the chisel or trephine. In cases attended with suppuration, the swelling is incised and drained, and if there is a sequestrum, it must be removed.

Circumscribed Abscess of Bone—"Brodie's Abscess."—The most important form of relapsing osteomyelitis is the circumscribed abscess of bone first described by Benjamin Brodie. It is usually met with in young adults, but we have met with it in patients over fifty. Several years may intervene between the original attack of osteomyelitis and the onset of symptoms of abscess.

Morbid Anatomy.[7]—The abscess is nearly always situated in the central axis of the bone in the region of the ossifying junction, although cases are occasionally met with in which it lies nearer the middle of the shaft. In exceptional cases there is more than one abscess (Fig. 120). The tibia is the bone most commonly affected, but the lower end of the femur, or either end of the humerus, may be the seat of the abscess. In the quiescent stage the lesion is represented by a small cavity in the bone, filled with clear serum, and lined by a fibrous membrane which is engaged in forming bone. Around the cavity the bone is sclerosed, and the medullary canal is obliterated. When the infection becomes active, the contents of the cavity are transformed into a greenish-yellow pus from which the staphylococcus can be isolated, and the cavity is lined by a thin film of granulation tissue which erodes the surrounding

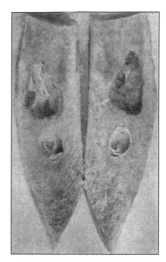

FIG. 120. Segment of Tibia resected for Brodie's Abscess. The specimen shows two separate abscesses in the centre of the shaft, the lower one quiescent, the upper one active and increasing in size.

bone and so causes the abscess to increase in size. If the erosion proceeds uniformly, the cavity is spherical or oval; if it is more active at some points than others, diverticula or tunnels are formed, and one of these may finally erupt through the shell of the bone or into an adjacent joint. Small irregular sequestra are occasionally found within the abscess cavity. In long-standing cases it is common to find extensive obliteration of the medullary canal, and a considerable increase in the girth of the bone.

The size of the abscess ranges from that of a cherry to that of a walnut, but specimens in museums show that, if left to Nature, the abscess may attain much greater dimensions.

The affected bone is not only thicker and heavier than normal, but may also be curved or otherwise deformed as a result of the original attack of osteomyelitis.

The *clinical features* are almost exclusively local. Pain, due to tension within the abscess, is the dominant symptom. At first it is vague and difficult to localise, later it is referred to the interior of the bone, and is described as "boring." It is aggravated by use of the limb, and there are often, espe-

[7] Alexis Thomson, *Edin. Med. Journ.*, 1906.

cially during the night, exacerbations in which the pain becomes excruciating. In the early stages there are periods of days or weeks during which the symptoms abate, but as the abscess increases these become shorter, until the patient is hardly ever free from pain. Localised tenderness can almost always be elicited by percussion, or by compressing the bone between the fingers and thumb. The pain induced by the traction of muscles attached to the bone, or by the weight of the body, may interfere with the function of the limb, and in the lower extremity cause a limp in walking. The limb may be disabled from *involvement of the adjacent joint*, in which there may be an intermittent hydrops which comes and goes coincidently with exacerbations of pain; or the abscess may perforate the joint and set up an acute arthritis.

The *diagnosis* of Brodie's abscess from other affections met with at the ends of long bones, and particularly from tuberculosis, syphilis, and new growths, is made by a consideration of the previous history, especially with reference to an antecedent attack of osteomyelitis. When the adjacent joint is implicated, the surgeon may be misled by the patient referring all the symptoms to the joint.

The X-ray picture is usually diagnostic chiefly because all the lesions which are liable to be confused with Brodie's abscess—gumma, tubercle, myeloma, chondroma, and sarcoma—give a well-marked central clear area; the sclerosis around Brodie's abscess gives a dense shadow in which the central clear area is either not seen at all or only faintly (Fig. 121).

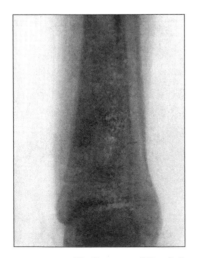

FIG. 121. Radiogram of Brodie's Abscess in Lower End of Tibia.

Treatment.—If an abscess is suspected, there should be no hesitation in exploring the interior of the bone. It is exposed by a suitable incision; the periosteum is reflected and the bone is opened up by a trephine or chisel, and the presence of an abscess may be at once indicated by the escape of pus. If, owing to the small size of the abscess or the density of the bone surrounding it, the pus is not reached by this procedure, the bone should be drilled in different directions.

Other Forms of Acute Osteomyelitis.—Among the less severe forms of osteomyelitis resulting from the action of attenuated organisms are the *serous* variety, in which an effusion of serous fluid forms under the periosteum; and *growth fever*, in which the child complains of vague evanescent pains (growing pains), and of feeling tired and disinclined to play; there may be some rise of temperature in the evening.

Infection with the *staphylococcus albus*, the *streptococcus*, or the *pneumococcus* also causes a mild form of osteomyelitis which may go on to suppuration.

Necrosis with out suppuration, described by Paget under the name "quiet necrosis," is a rare disease, and would appear to be associated with an attenuated form of staphylococcal infection (Tavel). It occurs in adults, being met with up to the age of fifty or sixty, and is characterised by the insidious development of a swelling which involves a considerable extent of a long bone. The pain varies in intensity, and may be continuous or intermittent, and there is tenderness on pressure. The shaft is increased in girth as a result of its being surrounded by a new case of bone. The resemblance to sarcoma may be very close, but the swelling is not as defined as in sarcoma, nor does it ever assume the characteristic "leg of mutton" shape. In both diseases there is a tendency to pathological fracture. It is difficult also in the absence of skiagrams to differentiate the condition from syphilitic and from tuberculous disease. If the diagnosis is not established after examination with the X-rays, an exploratory incision should be made; if dead bone is found, it is removed.

In typhoid fever the bone marrow is liable to be invaded by *the typhoid bacillus*, which may set up osteomyelitis soon after its lodgment, or it may lie latent for a considerable period before doing so. The lesions may be single or multiple, they involve the marrow or the periosteum or both, and they may or may not be attended with suppuration. They are most commonly met with in the tibia and in the ribs at the costo-chondral junctions.

The bone lesions usually occur during the seventh or eighth week of the fever, but have been known to occur much later. The chief complaint is of vague pains, at first referred to several bones, later becoming localised in one; they are aggravated by movement, or by handling the bone, and are worst at night. There is redness and oedema of the overlying soft parts, and swelling with vague fluctuation, and on incision there escapes a yellow creamy pus, or a brown syrupy fluid containing the typhoid bacillus in pure culture. Necrosis is exceptional.

When the abscess develops slowly, the condition resembles tuberculous disease, from which it may be diagnosed by the history of typhoid fever, and by obtaining a positive Widal reaction.

The prognosis is favourable, but recovery is apt to be slow, and relapse is not uncommon.

It is usually sufficient to incise the periosteum, but when the disease occurs in a rib it may be necessary to resect a portion of bone.

Pyogenic Osteomyelitis due to Spread of Infection from the Soft Parts.— There still remain those forms of osteomyelitis which result from infection through a wound involving the bone—for example, compound fractures, gunshot injuries, osteotomies, amputations, resections, or operations for un-united fracture. In all of these the marrow is exposed to infection by such organisms as are present in the wound. A similar form of osteomyelitis may occur apart from a wound—for example, infection may spread to the jaws from lesions of the mouth; to the skull, from lesions of the scalp or of the cranial bones themselves—such as a syphilitic gumma or a sarcoma which has fungated externally; or to the petrous temporal, from suppuration in the middle ear.

The most common is an osteomyelitis commencing in the marrow exposed in a wound infected with pyogenic organisms. In amputation stumps, fungating granulations protrude from the sawn end of the bone, and if necrosis takes place, the sequestrum is annular, affecting the cross-section of the bone at the saw-line; or tubular, extending up the shaft, and tapering off above. The periosteum is more easily detached, is thicker than normal, and is actively engaged in forming bone. In the macerated specimen, the new bone presents a characteristic coral-like appearance, and may be perforated by cloacæ (Fig. 122).

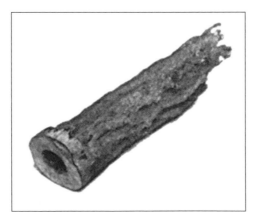

FIG. 122. Tubular Sequestrum resulting from Septic Osteomyelitis in Amputation Stump.

Like other pyogenic infections, it may terminate in pyæmia, as a result of septic phlebitis in the marrow.

The *clinical features* of osteomyelitis in *an amputation stump* are those of ordinary pyogenic infection; the involvement of the bone may be suspected from the clinical course, the absence of improvement from measures directed towards overcoming the sepsis in the soft parts, and the persistence of suppuration in spite of free drainage, but it is not recognised unless the bone is exposed by opening up the stump or the changes in the bone are shown by the X-rays. The first change is due to the deposit of new bone on the periosteal surface; later, there is the shadow of the sequestrum.

Healing does not take place until the sequestrum is extruded or removed by operation.

In compound fractures, if a fragment dies and forms a sequestrum, it is apt to be walled in by new bone; the sinuses continue to discharge until the sequestrum is removed. Even after healing has taken place, relapse is liable to occur, especially in gun-shot injuries. Months or years afterwards, the bone may become painful and tender. The symptoms may subside under rest and elevation of the limb and the application of

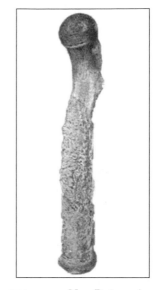

FIG. 123. New Periosteal Bone on surface of Femur from Amputation Stump. Osteomyelitis supervened on the amputation, and resulted in necrosis at the sawn section of the bone. (Anatomical Museum, University of Edinburgh.)

a compress, or an abscess forms and bursts with comparatively little suffering. The contents may be clear yellow serum or watery pus; sometimes a small spicule of bone is discharged. Valuable information, both for diagnosis and treatment, is afforded by skiagrams.

TUBERCULOUS DISEASE

The tuberculous diseases of bone result from infection of the marrow or periosteum by tubercle bacilli conveyed through the arteries; it is exceedingly rare for tubercle to appear in bone as a primary infection, the bacilli being usually derived from some pre-existing focus in the bronchial glands or elsewhere. According to the observations of John Fraser, 60 per cent. of the cases of bone and joint tubercle in children are due to the bovine bacillus, 37 per cent. to the human variety, and in 3 per cent. both types are present.

Tuberculous disease in bone is characterised by its insidious onset and slow progress, and by the frequency with which it is associated with disease of the adjacent joint.

Periosteal tuberculosis is met with in the ribs, sternum, vertebral column, skull, and less frequently in the long bones of the limbs. It may originate in the periosteum, or may spread thence from the marrow, or from synovial membrane.

In superficial bones, such as the sternum, the formation of tuberculous granulation tissue in the deeper layer of the periosteum, and its subsequent caseation and liquefaction, is attended by the insidious development of a doughy swelling, which is not as a rule painful, although tender on pressure. While the swelling often remains quiescent for some time, it tends to increase in size, to become boggy or fluctuating, and to assume the characters of a cold abscess. The pus perforates the fibrous layer of the periosteum, invading and infecting the overlying soft parts, its spread being influenced by the anatomical arrangement of the tissues. The size of the abscess affords no indication of the extent of the bone lesion from which it originates. As the abscess reaches the surface, the skin becomes of a dusky red or livid colour, is gradually thinned out, and finally sloughs, forming a sinus. A probe passed into the sinus strikes carious bone. Small sequestra may be found embedded in the granulation tissue. The sinus persists as long as any active tubercle remains in the tissues, and is apt to form an avenue for pyogenic infection.

In deeply seated bones, such as the upper end of the femur, the formation of a cold abscess in the soft parts is often the first evidence of the disease.

Diagnosis.—Before the stage of cold abscess is reached, the localised swelling is to be differentiated from a gumma, from chronic forms of staphylococcal osteomyelitis, from enlarged bursa or ganglion, from sub-periosteal lipoma, and from sarcoma. Most difficulty is met with in relation to periosteal sarcoma, which must be differentiated either by the X-ray appearances or by an exploratory incision.

X-ray appearances in periosteal tubercle: the surface of the cortical bone in the area of disease is roughened and irregular by erosion, and in the vicinity there may be a deposit of new bone on the surface, particularly if a sinus is present and mixed infection has occurred; in *syphilis* the shadow of the bone is denser as a result of sclerosis, and there is usually more new bone on the surface—hyperostosis; in *periosteal sarcoma* there is greater erosion and consequently greater irregularity in the contour of the cortical bone, and frequently there is evidence of formation of bone in the form of characteristic spicules projecting from the surface at a right angle.

The early recognition of periosteal lesions in the articular ends of bones is of importance, as the disease, if left to itself, is liable to spread to the adjacent joint.

The *treatment* is that of tuberculous lesions in general; if conservative measures fail, the choice lies between the injection of iodoform, and removal of the infected tissues with the sharp spoon. In the ribs it is more satisfactory to remove the diseased portion of bone along with the wall of the associated abscess or sinus. If all the tubercle has been removed and there is no pyogenic infection, the wound is stitched up with the object of obtaining primary union; otherwise it is treated by the open method.

Tuberculous Osteomyelitis.—Tuberculous lesions in the marrow occur as isolated or as multiple foci of granulation tissue, which replace the marrow and erode the trabeculæ of bone in the vicinity (Fig. 124). The individual focus varies in size from a pea to a walnut. The changes that ensue resemble in character those in other tissues, and the extent of the destruction varies according to the way in which the tubercle bacillus and the marrow interact upon one another. The granulation tissue may undergo caseation and liquefaction, or may become encapsulated by fibrous tissue—"encysted tubercle."

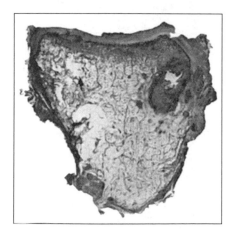

FIG. 124. Tuberculous Osteomyelitis of Os Magnum, excised from a boy æt. 8. Note well-defined caseous focus, with several minute foci in surrounding marrow.

433

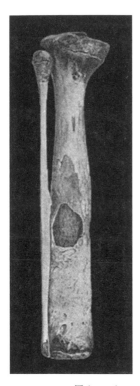

FIG. 125. Tuberculous Disease of Child's Tibia, showing sequestrum in medullary cavity, and increase in girth from excess of new bone.

Sometimes the tuberculous granulation tissue spreads in the marrow, assuming the characters of a diffuse infiltration—diffuse tuberculous osteomyelitis. The trabecular framework of the bone undergoes erosion and absorption—rarefying ostitis—and either disappears altogether or only irregular fragments or sequestra of microscopic dimensions remain in the area affected. Less frequently the trabecular framework is added to by the formation of new bone, resulting in a remarkable degree of sclerosis, and if, following upon this, there is caseation of the tubercle and death of the affected portion of bone, there results a sequestrum often of considerable size and characteristic shape, which, because of the sclerosis and surrounding endarteritis, is exceedingly slow in separating. When the sequestrum involves an articular surface it is often wedge-shaped; in other situations it is rounded or truncated and lies in the long axis of the medullary canal (Fig. 125). Finally, the sequestrum lies loose in a cavity lined by tuberculous granulation tissue, and is readily identified in a radiogram. This type of sclerosis preceding death of the bone is highly characteristic of tuberculosis..

Clinical Features.—As a rule, it is only in superficially placed bones, such as the tibia, ulna, clavicle, mandible, or phalanges, that tuberculous disease in the marrow gives rise to signs sufficiently definite to allow of its clinical recognition. In the vertebræ, or in the bones of deeply seated joints, such as the hip or shoulder, the existence of tuberculous lesions in the marrow can only be inferred from indirect signs—such, for example, as rigidity and curvature in the case of the spine, or from the symptoms of grave and persistent joint-disease in the case of the hip or shoulder.

With few exceptions, tuberculous disease in the interior of a bone does not reveal its presence until by extension it reaches one or other of the surfaces of the bone. In the shaft of a long bone its eruption on the periosteal surface is usually followed by the formation of a cold abscess in the overlying soft parts. When situated in the articular ends of bones, the disease more often erupts in relation to the reflection of the synovial membrane or directly on the articular surface—in either case giving rise to disease of the joint (Fig. 156).

Diffuse Tuberculous Osteomyelitis in the shaft of a long bone is comparatively rare, and has been observed chiefly in the tibia and the ulna in children (Fig. 126). It commences at the growing extremity of the diaphysis, and spreads along the medulla to a variable extent; it is attended by the formation of vascular and porous bone on the surface, which causes thickening of the diaphysis; this is most marked at the ossifying junction and tapers off along the shaft. The infection not only spreads along the medulla, but it invades the spongy bone surrounding this, and then the cortical bone, and is only prevented from reaching the soft parts by the new bone formed by the periosteum. The bone is replaced by granulation tissue, and disappears, or part of it may become sclerosed and in time form a sequestrum. In the

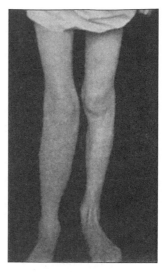

FIG. 126. Diffuse Tuberculous Osteomyelitis of Right Tibia. (Photograph lent by Sir H. J. Stiles.)

macerated specimen, the sequestrum appears small in proportion to the large cavity in which it lies. All these changes are revealed in a good skiagram, which not only confirms the diagnosis, but, in many instances, demonstrates the extent of the disease, the presence or absence of a sequestrum, and the amount of new bone on the surface. Finally the periosteum gives way, and an abscess forms in the soft parts; and if left to itself ruptures externally, leaving a sinus. The most satisfactory *treatment* is to resect sub-periosteally the diseased portion of the diaphysis.

In cancellous bones, such as those of the tarsus, there is a similar caseous infiltration in the marrow, and this may be attended with the formation of a sequestrum either in the interior of the bone or involving its outer shell, as shown in Fig. 127. The situation and extent of the disease are shown in X-ray photographs. After the tuberculous granulation tissue erupts through the cortex of the bone, it gives rise to a cold abscess or infects adjacent joints or tendon sheaths.

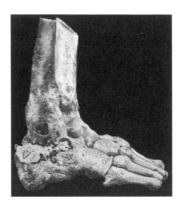

FIG. 127. Advanced Tuberculous Disease in region of Ankle. The ankle-joint is ankylosed, and there is a large sequestrum in the calcaneus. (Specimen in Anatomical Museum, University of Edinburgh.)

If an exact diagnosis is made at an early stage of the disease—and this is often possible with the aid of X-rays—the affected bone is excised subperiosteally or its interior is cleared out with the sharp spoon and gouge, the latter procedure being preferred in the case of the *calcaneus* to conserve the stability of the heel. When several bones and joints are simultaneously affected, and there are sinuses with mixed infection, amputation is usually indicated, especially in adults.

Tuberculous dactylitis is the name applied to a diffuse form of the disease as it affects the phalanges, metacarpal or metatarsal bones. The lesion presents, on a small scale, all the anatomical changes that have been described as occurring in the medulla of the tibia or ulna, and they are easily followed in skiagrams. A periosteal type of dactylitis is also met with.

The *clinical features* are those of a spindle-shaped swelling of a finger or toe, indolent, painless, and interfering but little with the function of the digit. Recovery may eventually occur without suppuration, but it is common to have the formation of a cold abscess, which bursts and forms one or more sinuses. It may be difficult to differentiate tuberculous dactylitis from the enlargement of the phalanges in inherited syphilis (syphilitic dactylitis), especially when the tuberculous lesion occurs in a child who is the subject of inherited syphilis.

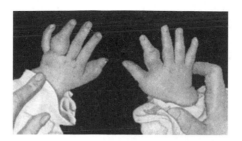

FIG. 128. Tuberculous Dactylitis.

In the syphilitic lesion, skiagrams usually show a more abundant formation of new bone, but in many cases the doubt is only cleared up by observing
the results of the tuberculin test or the effects of anti-syphilitic treatment.

Sarcoma of a phalanx or metacarpal bone may closely resemble a dactylitis both clinically and in skiagrams, but it is rare.

Treatment.—Recovery under conservative measures is not uncommon, and
the functional results are usually better than those following upon operative
treatment, although in either case the affected finger is liable to be dwarfed
(Fig. 129). The finger should be immobilised in a splint, and a Bier's bandage
applied to the upper arm. Operative interference is indicated if a cold abscess
develops, if there is a persistent sinus, or if a sequestrum has formed, a point
upon which information is obtained by examination with the X-rays. When a
toe is affected, amputation is the best treatment, but in the case of a finger it is
rarely called for. In the case of a metacarpal or metatarsal bone, sub-periosteal
resection is the procedure of choice, saving the articular ends if possible.

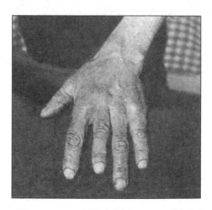

FIG. 129. Shortening of Middle Finger of Adult, the result
of Tuberculous Dactylitis in childhood.

437

SYPHILITIC DISEASE

Syphilitic affections of bone may be met with at any period of the disease, but the graver forms occur in the tertiary stage of acquired and inherited syphilis. The virus is carried by the blood-stream to all parts of the skeleton, but the local development of the disease appears to be influenced by a predisposition on the part of individual bones.

Syphilitic diseases of bone are much less common in practice than those due to pyogenic and tuberculous infectious, and they show a marked predilection for the tibia, sternum, and skull. They differ from tuberculous affections in the frequency with which they attack the shafts of bones rather than the articular ends, and in the comparative rarity of joint complications.

Evanescent periostitis is met with in acquired syphilis during the period of the early skin eruptions. The patient complains, especially at night, of pains over the frontal bone, ribs, sternum, tibiæ, or ulnæ. Localised tenderness is elicited on pressure, and there is slight swelling, which, however, rarely amounts to what may be described as a *periosteal node*.

In the later stages of acquired syphilis, *gummatous periostitis and osteomyelitis* occur, and are characterised by the formation in the periosteum and marrow of circumscribed gummata or of a diffuse gummatous infiltration. The framework of the bone is rarefied in the area immediately involved, and sclerosed in the parts beyond. If the gummatous tissue degenerates and breaks down, and especially if the overlying skin is perforated and septic infection is superadded, the bone disintegrates and exhibits the condition known as *syphilitic caries*; sometimes a portion of bone has its blood supply so far interfered with that it dies—*syphilitic necrosis*. Syphilitic sequestra are heavier and denser than normal bone, because sclerosis usually precedes death of the bone. The bones especially affected by gummatous disease are: the skull, the septum of the nose, the nasal bones, palate, sternum, femur, tibia, and the bones of the forearm.

In the bones of the skull, gummata may form in the peri-cranium, diploë, or dura mater. An isolated gumma forms a firm elastic swelling, shading off into the surroundings. In the macerated bone there is a depression or an actual perforation of the calvaria; multiple gummata tend to fuse with one another at their margins, giving the appearance of a combination of circles: these sometimes surround an area of bone and cut it off from its blood supply (Fig. 130). If the overlying skin is destroyed and septic infection superadded, such an isolated area of bone is apt to die and furnish a sequestrum; the separation of the dead bone is extremely slow, partly from the want of vascularity in the sclerosed bone round about, and partly from the density of the sequestrum. In exceptional cases the necrosis involves the entire vertical plate of the frontal bone. Pus is formed between the bone and the dura (suppurative pachymeningitis), and this may be followed by cerebral abscess or by pyæmia. Gummatous disease in the wall of the orbit may cause displacement of the eye and paralysis of the ocular muscles.

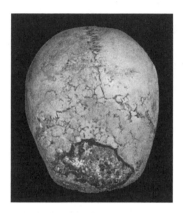

FIG. 130. Syphilitic Disease of Skull, showing a sequestrum in process of separation.

On the inner surface of the skull, the formation of gummatous tissue may cause pressure on the brain and give rise to intense pain in the head, Jacksonian epilepsy, or paralysis, the symptoms varying with the seat and extent of the disease. The cranial nerves may be pressed upon at the base, especially at their points of exit, and this gives rise to symptoms of irritation or paralysis in the area of distribution of the nerves affected.

In the septum of the nose, the nasal bones, and the hard palate, gummatous disease causes ulceration, which, beginning in the mucous membrane, spreads to the bones, and being complicated with septic infection leads to caries and necrosis. In the nose, the disease is attended with stinking discharge (ozoena), the extrusion of portions of dead bone, and subsequently with deformity characterised by loss of the bridge of the nose; in the palate, it is common to have a perforation, so that the air escapes through the nose in speaking, giving to the voice a characteristic nasal tone.

439

Syphilitic disease of the tibia may be taken as the type of the affection as it occurs *in the long bones.* Gummatous disease in the periosteum may be localised and result in the formation of a well-defined node, or the whole shaft may become the seat of an irregular nodular enlargement (Fig. 132). If the bone is macerated, it is found to be heavier and bulkier than normal; there is diffuse sclerosis with obliteration of the medullary canal, and the surface is uneven from heaping up of new bone—hyperostosis (Fig. 131). If a periosteal gumma breaks down and invades the skin, a syphilitic ulcer is formed with carious bone at the bottom. A central gumma may eat away the surrounding bone to such an extent that the shaft undergoes pathological fracture. In the rare cases in which it attacks the articular end of a long bone, gummatous disease may implicate the adjacent joint and give rise to syphilitic arthritis.

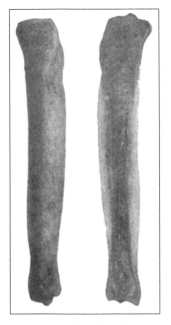

FIG. 131. Syphilitic Hyperostosis and Sclerosis of Tibia, on section and on surface view.

Clinical Features.—There is severe boring pain—as if a gimlet were being driven into the bone. It is worst at night, preventing sleep, and has been ascribed to compression of the nerves in the narrowed Haversian canals.

The *periosteal gumma* appears as a smooth, circumscribed swelling which is soft and elastic in the centre and firm at the margins, and shades off into the surrounding bone. The gumma may be completely absorbed or it may give place to a hard node. In some cases the gumma softens in the centre, the skin becomes adherent, thin, and red, and finally gives way. The opening in the skin persists as a sinus, or develops into a typical ulcer with irregular, crescentic margins; in either case a probe reveals the presence of carious bone or of a sequestrum. The health may be impaired as a result of mixed infection, and the absorption of toxins and waxy degeneration in the viscera may ultimately be induced.

A *central gumma* in a long bone may not reveal its presence until it erupts through the shell and reaches the periosteal surface or invades an adjacent joint. Sometimes the first manifestation is a fracture of the bone produced by slight violence.

In radiograms the appearance of syphilitic bones is usually characteristic. When there is hyperostosis and sclerosis, the shaft appears denser and broader than normal, and the contour is uneven or wavy. When there is a central gumma, the shadow is interrupted by a rounded clear area, like that of a chondroma or myeloma, but there is sclerosis round about.

Diagnosis.—The conditions most liable to be mistaken for syphilitic disease of bone are chronic staphylococcal osteomyelitis, tuberculosis, and sarcoma; and the diagnosis is to be made by the history and progress of the disease, the result of examination with the X-rays, and the results of specific tests and treatment.

Treatment.—The general health is to be improved by open air, by nourishing food, and by the administration of cod-liver oil, iron, and arsenic. Anti-syphilitic remedies should be given, and if they are administered before there is any destruction of tissue, the benefit derived from them is usually marked.

Radiograms show the rapid absorption of the new bone both on the surface and in the marrow, and are of value in establishing the therapeutic diagnosis.

In certain cases, and particularly when there are destructive changes in the bone complicated with pyogenic infection, specific remedies have little effect. In cases of persistent or relapsing gummatous disease with ulceration of skin, it is often necessary to remove the diseased soft parts with the sharp spoon and scissors, and to gouge or chisel away the unhealthy bone, on the same lines as in tuberculous disease. When hyperostosis and sclerosis of the bone is attended with severe pain which does not yield to blistering, the periosteum may be incised and the sclerosed bone perforated with a drill or trephine.

Lesions of Bone in Inherited Syphilis.—*Craniotabes*, in which the flat bones of the skull undergo absorption in patches, was formerly regarded as syphilitic, but it is now known to result from prolonged malnutrition from any cause. *Bossing of the skull* resulting in the formation of Parrot's nodes is also being withdrawn from the category of syphilitic affections. The lesions in infancy—epiphysitis, bossing of the skull, and craniotabes—have been referred to in the chapter on inherited syphilis.

Epiphysitis or Syphilitic Perichondritis.—The first of these terms is misleading, because the lesion involves the ossifying junction and the shaft of the bone, and the epiphysis only indirectly. The young bone is replaced by granulation tissue, so that large clear areas are seen with the X-rays. The symptoms are referred to the joint, because it is there that the muscles are inserted and drag on the perichondrium when movement occurs; swelling is most marked in the vicinity of the joint, and it may be added to by effusion into the synovial cavity. The baby, usually under six months, is noticed to be feverish and fretful and to cry when touched. The mother discovers that the pain is caused by moving a particular limb, usually the arm, as the humerus, radius, and ulna are the bones most commonly affected; the limb, moreover, hangs useless at the side as if paralysed, and the condition was formerly described as *syphilitic pseudo-paralysis*.

The lesions met with later correspond to those of the tertiary period of the acquired disease, but as they affect bones which are still actively growing, the effects are more striking. Gummatous disease may come and go over periods of many years, with the result that the external appearance and architectural arrangement of a long bone come to be profoundly altered. In the tibia, for example, the shaft is bowed forward in a gentle curve, which is compared to the curve of a sabre—"sabre-blade" deformity (Fig. 132). The diffuse thickening all round the bone obscures the sharp margins so that the bone becomes circular in section and the anterior and mesial edges are blunted, and the comparison to a cucumber is deserved. In some cases the tibia is actually increased in length as well as in girth.

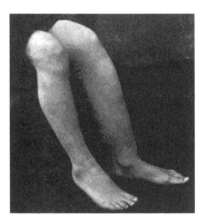

FIG. 132. Sabre-blade Deformity of Left Tibia in Inherited Syphilis. (From a photograph lent by Sir George T. Beatson.)

The contrast between the grossly enlarged and misshapen tibia and the normal or even attenuated fibula is a striking one.

Treatment is carried out on lines similar to those recommended in the acquired disease. When curving of the tibia causes disability in walking, the bone may be straightened by a cuneiform resection.

Syphilitic dactylitis is met with chiefly in children. It may affect any of the fingers or toes, but is commonest in the first phalanx of the index-finger or of the thumb. Several fingers may be attacked at the same time or in succession. The lesion consists in a gummatous infiltration of the soft parts surrounding the phalanx, or a gummatous osteomyelitis, but there is practically no tendency to break down and discharge, or to the formation of a sequestrum as is so common in tuberculous dactylitis.

The finger becomes the seat of a swelling, which is more evident on the dorsal aspect, and, according to the distribution and extent of the disease, it is acorn-shaped, fusiform, or cylindrical. It is firm and elastic, and usually painless. The movements are impaired, especially if the joints are involved. In its early stages the disease is amenable to anti-syphilitic treatment, and complete recovery is the rule.

HYDATID DISEASE

This rare disease results from the lodgment of the embryos of the tænia echinoccus, which are conveyed to the marrow by the blood-stream. The cysts are small, usually about the size of a pin-head, and they are present in enormous numbers scattered throughout the marrow. The parts of the skeleton most often affected are the articular ends of the long bones, the bodies of the vertebræ, and the pelvis.

As the cysts increase in number and in size, the framework of the bone is gradually absorbed, and there result excavations or cavities. The marrow and spongy bone first disappear, the compact tissue then becomes thin, and pathological fracture may result. The bone becomes expanded, and the cysts may escape through perforations into the surrounding cellular tissue, and when thus freed from confinement may attain considerable dimensions. Suppuration from superadded pyogenic infection may be attended with extensive necrosis, and lead to disorganisation of the adjacent joint.

Clinical Features.—The patient complains of deep-seated pains. In superficial bones, such as the tibia, there is enlargement, and it may be possible to recognise egg-shell crackling, or unequal consistence of the bone, which is hard in some parts, and doughy and elastic in others. The disease may pursue an indolent course during months or years until some complication occurs, such as suppuration or fracture. With the occurrence of suppuration the disease becomes more active, and abscesses may form in the soft parts and in the adjacent joint.

In the vertebral column, hydatids give rise to angular deformity and paraplegia. In the pelvis, there is usually great enlargement of the bones, and when suppuration occurs it is apt to infect the hip-joint and to terminate fatally.

Examination with the X-rays shows the characteristic excavations of the bone caused by the cysts. The disease is liable to be mistaken for central tumour, gumma, tuberculosis, or abscess of bone.

The *treatment* consists in thorough eradication of the parasite by operation. The bone is laid open and scraped or resected according to the extent of the disease, and the raw surfaces swabbed with 1 per cent. formalin. In advanced cases complicated with spontaneous fracture or with suppuration, amputation affords the best chance of recovery.

The lesions in the bones resulting from *actinomycosis* and from *mycetoma*, have been described with these diseases.

CONSTITUTIONAL DISEASES ATTENDED WITH LESIONS IN THE BONES

These include rickets, scurvy-rickets, osteomalacia, ostitis deformans, osteomyelitis fibrosa, fragilitas ossium, and diseases of the nervous system.

RICKETS

Rickets or rachitis is a constitutional disease associated with disturbance of nutrition, and attended with changes in the skeleton. The disease is most common and most severe among the children of the poorer classes in large cities, who are improperly fed and are brought up in unhealthy surroundings. There is evidence that the most important factors in the causation of rickets are ill-health of the mother during pregnancy, and the administration to the child after its birth of food which is defective in animal fat, proteids, and salts of lime, or which contains these in such a form that they are not readily assimilated. The occurrence of the disease is favoured, and its features are aggravated, by imperfect oxygenation of the blood as the result of a deficiency of fresh air and sunlight, want of exercise, and by other conditions which prevail in the slums of large towns.

Pathological Anatomy.—The most striking feature is the softness (malacia) of the bones, due to excessive absorption of osseous tissue, and the formation of an imperfectly calcified tissue at the sites of ossification. The affected bones lose their rigidity, so that they are bent under the weight of the body, by the traction of muscles, and by other mechanical forces.

The *periosteum* is thick and vascular, and when detached carries with it plates and spicules of soft porous bone. The new bone may be so abundant that it forms a thick crust on the surface, and in the flat bones of the skull this may be heaped up in the form of bosses or ridges resembling those ascribed to inherited syphilis.

In the epiphysial cartilages and at the ossifying junctions, all the processes concerned in ossification, excepting the deposition of lime salts, occur to an exaggerated degree. The cartilage of the epiphysial disc proliferates actively and irregularly, so that it becomes softer, thicker, and wider, and gives rise to a visible swelling, best seen at the lower end of the radius and lower end of the tibia, and at the costo-chondral junctions where the series of beaded swellings is known as the "rickety rosary."

The ossifying zone is increased in depth; the marrow is abnormally vascular; and the new bone that is formed is imperfectly calcified. The result is that the bones may never attain their normal length, and they remain stunted throughout life as in rickety dwarfs (Fig. 133), or the shafts may grow unequally and come to deviate from their normal axes as in knock-knee and bow-knee.

These changes are well brought out in skiagrams; instead of the well-defined narrow line which represents the epiphysial cartilage, there is an ill-defined, blurred zone of considerable depth.

In the shafts of the long bones, owing to the excessive absorption of bone, the cortex becomes porous, the spongy bone is rarefied, and the bones readily bend or break under mechanical influences. When the disease is arrested, a process of repair sets in which often results in the bones becoming denser and heavier than normal. In the flat bones of the skull, the absorption may result in the entire disappearance of areas of bone, leaving

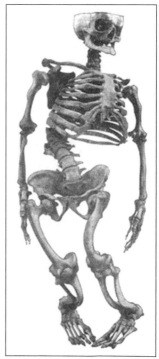

FIG. 133. Skeleton of Rickety Dwarf, known as "Bowed Joseph," leader of the Meal Riots in Edinburgh, who died in 1780. (Anatomical Museum, University of Edinburgh.)

a membrane which dimples like thin cardboard under the pressure of the finger—a condition known as *craniotabes*.

Changes in the Skeleton before the Child is able to walk.—The fontanelles remain open until the end of the second year or longer, and the frontal and parietal eminences are unduly prominent. There is sometimes hydrocephalus, and the head is characteristically enlarged. The jaws are altered so that while the upper jaw is contracted into the shape of a **V**, the lower jaw is square instead of rounded in outline, and the teeth do not oppose one another. In the *thorax*, the chief feature may be the beading at the costo-chondral junctions, principally of the fifth and sixth ribs or its walls may be contracted, particularly if respiration is interfered with as a result of bronchial catarrh or adenoids. The contraction may take the form of a vertical groove on each side, or of a horizontal groove at the level of the upper end of the xiphi-sternum; when the sternum and carti-lages form a projection in front, the deformity is known as "pigeon-breast."

The *spine* may be curved backwards—*kyphosis*—throughout its whole extent or only in one part; or it may be curved to one side—*scoliosis*.

In the *limbs*, the prominent features are the deficient growth in length of the long bones, the enlargements at the epiphysial junctions, and the bend-ing, and occasional greenstick fracture, of the shafts. The degree of enlarge-ment of the epiphysial junctions is directly proportionate to the amount of movement to which the bone is subjected (John Thomson). The curves at this stage depend on the attitude of the child while sitting or being carried—for example, the arm bones become bent in children who paddle about the floor with the aid of their arms; and in a child who lies on its back with the lower limbs everted, the weight of the limb may lead to curvature of the neck of the femur—coxa vara. The clavicle or humerus may sustain greenstick fracture from the child being lifted by the arms; the femur, by a fall. From the extreme laxity of the ligaments, the joints can be moved beyond the normal limits, and the child is often observed to twist its limbs into abnormal attitudes.

In Children who have walked.—In these children the most important defor-mities occur in the spine, pelvis, and lower extremities, and result for the most part from yielding of the softened bones under the weight of the body. Sco-liosis is the usual type of spinal curvature, and in extreme cases it may lead to a pronounced form of hump-back. The pelvis may remain small (*justo-minor pelvis*), or it may be contracted in the sagittal plane (*flat pelvis*); when the bones are unusually soft, the acetabular portions are pushed inwards by the femora bearing the weight of the body, and the pelvis assumes the shape of a trefoil, as in the malacia of women. The shaft of the femur is curved forwards and laterally; the bones of the leg laterally as in bow-leg, or forwards, or forwards and laterally just above the ankle. The deformities at the knee (genu valgum, genu varum, and genu recurvatum), and at the hip (coxa vara), will be described in the volume dealing with the Extremities.

The majority of cases seen in surgical practice suffer from the deformities resulting from rickets rather than from the active disease. The examination of a large series of children at different ages shows that the deformities become less and less frequent with each year. Those who recover may ultimately show no trace of rickets, and this is especially true of children who grow at the average rate; in those, however, in whom growth is retarded, especially from the fifth to the seventh year, the deformities are apt to be permanent. It may be noted that the scoliosis due to rickets has little tendency towards recovery.

Treatment.—The treatment of the disease consists in regulating the diet, improving the surroundings, and preventing deformity. Phosphorus in doses of 100th grain may be given dissolved in cod-liver oil, and preparations of iron and lime may be added with advantage. To avoid those postures which predispose to deformities, the child should lie as much as possible. In the well-to-do classes this is readily accomplished by the aid of a nurse and the use of a perambulator. In hospital out-patients the child is kept off its feet by the use of a light wooden splint applied to the lateral aspect of each lower extremity, and extending from the pelvis to 6 inches beyond the sole.

When deformities are already present, the treatment depends upon whether or not there is any prospect of the bone straightening naturally. Under five years of age this may, as a rule, be confidently expected; the child should be kept off its feet, and the limbs bathed and massaged. In children of five or six and upwards, the prospect of natural straightening is a diminishing one, and it is more satisfactory to correct the deformity by operation. In rickety curvature of the spine, the child should lie on a firm mattress, or, to allow of its being taken into the open air, upon a double Thomas' splint extending from the occiput to the heels; the muscles acting on the trunk should be braced up by massage and appropriate exercises.

Late Rickets or **Rachitis Adolescentium** is met with at any age from nine to seventeen, and is generally believed to be due to a recrudescence of rickets which had been present in childhood. The disease is not attended with any disturbance of the general health; the pathological changes are the same as in infantile rickets, but are for the most part confined to the ossifying junctions, especially those which are most active during adolescence, for example at the knee-joint. The patient is easily tired, complains of pain in the bones, and, unless care is taken, deformity is liable to ensue. There can be no doubt that adolescent rickets plays an important part in the production of the deformities which occur at or near puberty, especially knock-knee and bow-knee.

Scurvy-Rickets or **Infantile Scurvy.**—This disease, described by Barlow and Cheadle, is met with in infants under two years who have been brought up upon sterilised or condensed milk and other proprietary foods, and is most common in the well-to-do classes. The hæmorrhages, which are so characteristic of the disease, are usually preceded for some weeks by a cachectic condition, with listlessness and debility and disinclination for movement. Very commonly the child ceases to move one of his lower limbs—pseudo-paralysis—and screams if it is touched; a swelling is found over one of the bones, usually the femur, accompanied by exquisite tenderness; the skin is tense and shiny, and there may be some oedema. These symptoms are due to a sub-periosteal hæmorrhage, and associated with this there may be crepitus from separation of an epiphysis, rarely from fracture of the shaft of the bone. X-ray photographs show enlargement of the bone, the periosteum being raised from the shaft and new bone formed in relation to it. Hæmorrhages also occur into the skin, presenting the appearance of bruises, into the orbit and conjunctiva, and from the mucous membranes.

The *treatment* consists in correcting the errors in diet. The infant should have a wet nurse or a plentiful supply of cow's milk in its natural state. Antiscorbutics in the form of orange, lemon, or grape juice, and of potatoes bruised down in milk, may be given.

Osteomalacia.—The term osteomalacia includes a group of conditions, closely allied to rickets, in which the bones of adults become soft and yielding, so that they are unduly liable to bend or break.

One form occurs in *pregnant and puerperal women,* affecting most commonly the pelvis and lumbar vertebræ, but sometimes the entire skeleton. The lime salts are absorbed, the bones lose their rigidity and bend under the weight of the body and other mechanical influences, with the result that gross deformities are produced, particularly in the pelvis, the lumbar spine, and the hip-joints.

Neuropathic forms occur in certain chronic diseases of the brain and cord; in some cases the bones lose their lime salts and bend, in others they become brittle.

Osteomalacia associated with New Growths in the Skeleton.—When *secondary cancer* is widely distributed throughout the skeleton, it is associated with softening of the bones, as a result of which they readily bend or break, and after death are easily cut with a knife. In the disease known as *multiple myeloma*, the interior of the ribs, sternum, and bodies of the vertebræ is occupied by a reddish gelatinous pulp, the structure of which resembles sarcoma; the bones are reduced to a mere shell, and may break on the slightest pressure; the urine contains albumose, a substance resembling albumen but coagulating at a comparatively low temperature (140° F.), and the coagulum is re-dissolved on boiling, and it is readily precipitated by hydrochloric acid (Bence-Jones).

Ostitis Deformans—Paget's Disease of Bone.—This rare disease was first described by Sir James Paget in 1877. In the early stages, the marrow is transformed into a vascular connective tissue; its bone-eating functions are exaggerated, and the framework of the bone becomes rarefied, so that it bends under pressure as in osteomalacia. In course of time, however, new bone is formed in great abundance; it is at first devoid of lime salts, but later becomes calcified, so that the bones regain their rigidity. This formation of new bone is much in excess of the normal, the bones become large and bulky, their surfaces rough and uneven, their texture sclerosed in parts, and the medullary canal is frequently obliterated. These changes are well brought out in X-ray photographs. The curving of the long bones, which is such a striking feature of the disease, may be associated with actual lengthening, and the changes are sometimes remarkably symmetrical (Fig. 135). The bones forming the cranium may be enormously thickened, the sutures are obliterated, the distinction into tables and diploë is lost, and, while the general texture is finely porous, there may be areas as dense as ivory (Fig. 134).

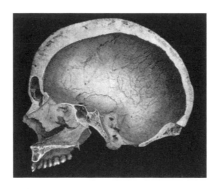

FIG. 134. Changes in the Skull resulting from Ostitis Deformans.(Anatomical Museum, University of Edinburgh.)

Clinical Features.—The disease is usually met with in persons over fifty years of age. It is insidious in its onset, and, the patient's attention may be first attracted by the occurrence of vague pains in the back or limbs; by the enlargement and bending of such bones as the tibia or femur; or by a gradual increase in the size of the head, necessitating the wearing of larger hats. When the condition is fully developed, the attitude and general appearance are eminently characteristic. The height is diminished, and, owing to the curving of the lower limbs and spine, the arms appear unnaturally long; the head and upper part of the spine are bent forwards; the legs are held apart, slightly flexed at the knees, and are rotated out as well as curved; the whole appearance suggests that of one of the large anthropoid apes. The muscles of the limbs may waste to such an extent as to leave the large, curved, misshapen bones covered only by the skin (Fig. 135). In the majority of cases the bones of the lower extremities are much earlier and more severely affected than those of the upper extremity, but the capacity of walking is usually maintained even in the presence of great deformity. In a case observed by Byrom Bramwell, the patient suffered from a succession of fractures over a period of years.

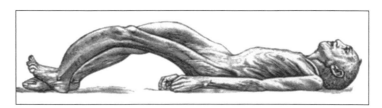

FIG. 135. Cadaver, illustrating the alterations in the Lower Limbs resulting from Ostitis Deformans.

The disease may last for an indefinite period, the general health remaining long unaffected. In a considerable number of the recorded cases one of the bones became the seat of sarcoma.

Osteomyelitis Fibrosa.—This comparatively rare disease, which was first described by Recklinghausen, presents many interesting features. Because of its causing deformities of the bones and an undue liability to fracture, and being chiefly met with in adolescents, it is regarded by some authors as a juvenile form of Paget's disease. It may be diffused throughout the skeleton—we have seen it in the skull and in the bones of the extremities—or it may be confined to a single bone, usually the femur, or, what is more remarkable, the condition may affect a portion only of the shaft of a long bone and be sharply defined from the normal bone in contact with it.

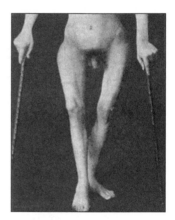

On longitudinal section of a long bone during the active stage of the disease, the marrow is seen to be replaced by a vascular young connective tissue which encroaches on the surrounding spongy bone, reducing it to the slenderest proportions; the formation of bone from the periosteum does not keep pace with the absorption and replacement going on in the interior, and the cortex may be reduced to a thin shell of imperfectly calcified bone which can be cut with a knife. The young connective tissue which replaces the marrow is not unlike that seen in osteomalacia; it is highly vascular and may show hæmorrhages of various date; there are abundant giant cells of the myeloma type,

FIG. 136. Osteomyelitis Fibrosa affecting Femora in a man æt. 19. The curving of the bones is due to multiple fractures.

and degeneration and liquefaction of tissue may result in the formation of cysts, which, when they constitute a prominent feature, are responsible for the name—*osteomyelitis fibrosa cystica*—sometimes applied to the condition.

It would appear that most of the recorded cases of *cysts of bone* owe their origin to this disease, while the abundance of giant cells with occasional islands of cartilage in the wall of such cysts is responsible for the view formerly held that they owed their origin to the liquefaction of a solid tumour, such as a myeloma, a chondroma, or even a sarcoma. Although the tissue elements in this disease resemble those of a new growth arising in the marrow, they differ in their arrangement and in their method of growth; there is no tendency to erupt through the cortex of the bone, to invade the soft parts, or to give rise to secondary growths.

Clinical Features.—The onset of the disease is insidious, and attention is usually first directed to it by the occurrence of fracture of the shaft of one of the long bones—usually the femur—from violence that would be insufficient to break a healthy bone. Apart from fracture, the great increase in the size of one of the long bones and its uneven contour are sufficiently remarkable to suggest examination with the X-rays, by means of which the condition is at once recognised. A systematic examination of the other long bones will often reveal the presence of the disease at a stage before the bone is altered externally.

Symmetrical bossing of the skull was present in the case shown in Figs. 136 and 137, and there were also scattered patches of brown pigmentation of the skin of the face, neck, and trunk, similar to those met with in generalised neuro-fibromatosis. Apart from fracture, the disease is recognised by the thickening and usually also by the curving of the shafts of the long bones. It is easy to understand the curvature of bones that have passed through a soft stage and also of those that have been broken and badly united, but it is difficult to account for the curvatures that have no such cause; for example, we have seen marked curve of the radius in a forearm of which the ulna was quite straight. The curvature probably resulted from exaggerated growth in length.

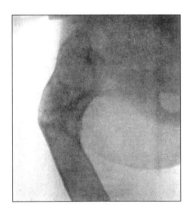

FIG. 137. Radiogram of Upper End of Femur showing appearances in Osteomyelitis Fibrosa.

The X-ray appearances vary with the stage of the malady, not estimated in time, for the condition is chronic and may become stationary, but according to whether it is progressive or undergoing repair. The shadow of the bone presents a poor contrast to the soft parts, and no trace of its original architecture; in extreme cases the shadow of the femur resembles an unevenly filled sausage (Fig. 137); there is no cortical layer, the interior shows no trabecular structure, and some of the many clear areas are probably cysts. The condition extends right up to the articular cartilage, or, in the case of adolescent bones, up to the epiphysial cartilage.

Prognosis.—The condition does not appear to affect the general health. The future is concerned with the local conditions, and, especially in the case of the femur, with its liability to fracture; so far as we know there is no time limit to this.

Treatment is confined to protecting the affected bone—usually the femur—from injury. Operative treatment may be required for lameness due to a badly united fracture.

Neuropathic Atrophy of Bone.—The conditions included under this heading occur in association with diseases of the nervous system.

Most importance attaches to the fragility of the bones met with in general paralysis of the insane, locomotor ataxia, and other chronic diseases of the brain and spinal cord. The bones are liable to be fractured by forces which would be insufficient to break a healthy bone. In *locomotor ataxia* the fractures affect especially the bones of the lower extremity, and may occur before there are any definite nerve symptoms, but they are more often met with in the ataxic stage, when the abrupt and uncontrolled movements of the limbs may play a part in their causation. They may be unattended with pain, and may fail to unite; when repair does take place, it is sometimes attended with an excessive formation of callus. Joint lesions of the nature of Charcot's disease may occur simultaneously with the alterations in the bones. In *syringomyelia* pathological fracture is not so frequent as in locomotor ataxia; it is more likely to occur in the bones of the upper extremity, and especially in the humerus. In some cases of *epilepsy* the bones break when the patient falls in a fit, and there is usually an exaggerated amount of comminution.

In these affections the bones present no histological or chemical alterations, and the X-ray shadow does not differ from the normal. It is maintained, therefore, that the disposition to fracture does not depend upon a fragility of the bone, but on the loss of the muscular sense and of common sensation in the bones, as a result of which there is an inability properly to throw the muscles into action and dispose the limbs so as to place them under the most favourable conditions to meet external violence.

Osteogenesis Imperfecta, Fragilitas Ossium, or **Congenital Osteopsath-yrosis**.—These terms are used to describe a condition in which an undue fragility of the bones dates from intra-uterine life. It may occur in several members of the same family. In severe cases, intra-uterine fractures occur, and during parturition fresh fractures are almost sure to be produced, so that at birth there is a combination of recent fractures and old fractures united and partly united, with bendings and thickenings of the bones. Large areas of the cranial vault may remain membranous.

After birth the predisposition to fracture continues, the bones are easily broken, the fractures are attended with little or no pain, the crepitus is soft, and although union may take place, it may be delayed and be attended with excess of callus. Cases have been observed in which a child has sustained over a hundred fractures.

The bones show a feeble shadow with the X-rays, and appear thin and atrophied; the medullary canal is increased at the expense of the cortex.

In young infants in whom multiple fractures occur the prognosis as to life is unfavourable, and no satisfactory treatment of the disease has been formulated. If the patient survives, the tendency to fracture gradually disappears.

Hypertrophic Pulmonary Osteo-Arthropathy.—This condition, which was described by Marie in 1890, is secondary to disease in the chest, such as chronic phthisis, empyema, bronchiectasis, or sarcoma of the lung. There is symmetrical enlargement and deformity of the hands and feet; the shafts of the bones are thickened, and the soft tissues of the terminal segments of the digits hypertrophied. The fingers come to resemble drum-sticks, and the thumb the clapper of a bell. The nails are convex, and incurved at their free ends, suggesting a resemblance to the beak of a parrot. There is also enlargement of the lower ends of the bones of the forearm and leg, and effusion into the wrist and ankle-joints. Skiagrams of the hands and feet show a deposit of new bone along the shafts of the phalanges.

TUMOURS OF BONE

New growths which originate in the skeleton are spoken of as *primary tumours*; those which invade the bones, either by metastasis from other parts of the body or by spread from adjacent tissues, as *secondary*. A tumour of bone may grow from the cellular elements of the periosteum, the marrow, or the epiphysial cartilage.

Primary tumours are of the connective-tissue type, and are usually solitary, although certain forms, such as the chondroma, may be multiple from the outset.

Periosteal tumours are at first situated on one side of the bone, but as they grow they tend to surround it completely. Innocent periosteal tumours retain the outer fibrous layer as a capsule. Malignant tumours tend to perforate the periosteal capsule and invade the soft parts.

Central or *medullary tumours* as they increase in size replace the surrounding bone, and simultaneously new bone is formed on the surface; as this is in its turn absorbed, further bone is formed beneath the periosteum, so that in time the bone is increased in girth, and is said to be "expanded" by the growth in its interior.

Primary Tumours—Osteoma.—When the tumour projects from the surface of a bone it is called an *exostosis*. When growing from bones developed in membrane, such as the flat bones of the skull, it is usually dense like ivory, and the term *ivory exostosis* is employed. When derived from hyaline cartilage—for example, at the ends of the long bones—it is known as a *cartilaginous exostosis*. This is invested with a cap of cartilage from which it continues to grow until the skeleton attains maturity.

An exostosis forms a rounded or mushroom-shaped tumour of limited size, which may be either sessile or pedunculated, and its surface is smooth or nodulated (Figs. 138 and 139). A cartilaginous exostosis in the vicinity of a joint may be invested with a synovial sac or bursa—the so-called *exostosis bursata*. The bursa may be derived from the synovial membrane of the adjacent joint with which its cavity sometimes communicates, or it may be of adventitious origin; when it is the seat of bursitis and becomes distended with fluid, it may mask the underlying exostosis, which then requires a radiogram for its demonstration.

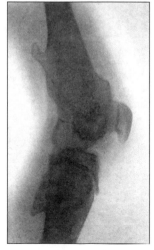

FIG. 138. Radiogram of Right Knee showing Multiple Exostoses.

Clinically, the osteoma forms a hard, indolent tumour attached to a bone. The symptoms to which it gives rise depend on its situation. In the vicinity of a joint, it may interfere with movement; on the medial side of the knee it may incapacitate the patient from riding. When growing from the dorsum of the terminal phalanx of the great toe—*subungual exostosis*—it displaces the nail, and may project through its matrix at the point of the toe, while the soft parts over it may be ulcerated from pressure (Fig. 107). It incapacitates the patient from wearing a boot. When it presses on a nerve-trunk it causes pains and cramps. In the orbit it displaces the eyeball; in the nasal fossæ and in the external auditory meatus it causes obstruction, which may be attended with ulceration and discharge. In the skull it may project from the outer table, forming a smooth rounded swelling, or it may project from the inner table and press upon the brain.

The diagnosis is to be made by the slow growth of the tumour, its hardness, and by the shadow which it presents with the X-rays (Fig. 138).

An osteoma which does not cause symptoms may be left alone, as it ceases to grow when the skeleton is mature and has no tendency to change its benign character. If causing symptoms, it is removed by dividing the neck or base of the tumour with a chisel, care being taken to remove the whole of the overlying cartilage. The dense varieties met with in the bones of the skull present greater difficulties; if it is necessary to remove them, the base or neck of the tumour is perforated in many directions with highly tempered drills rotated by some form of engine, and the division is completed with the chisel.

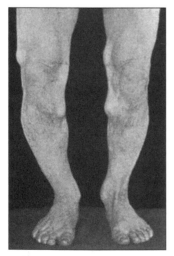

FIG. 139. Multiple Exotoses of both limbs. (Photograph lent by Sir George T. Beatson.)

Multiple Exostoses.—This disease, which, by custom, is still placed in the category of tumours, is to be regarded as a disorder of growth, dating from intra-uterine life and probably due to a disturbance in the function of the glands of internal secretion, the thyroid being the one which is most likely to be at fault (Arthur Keith). The disorder of growth is confined to those elements of the skeleton where a core of bone formed in cartilage comes to be encased in a sheath of bone formed beneath the periosteum. To indicate this abnormality the name *diaphysial aclasis* has been employed by Arthur Keith at the suggestion of Morley Roberts.

Bones formed entirely in cartilage are exempt, namely, the tarsal and carpal bones, the epiphyses of the long bones, the sternum, and the bodies of the vertebræ. Bones formed entirely in membrane, that is, those of the face and of the cranial vault, are also exempt. The disorder mainly affects the ossifying junctions of the long bones of the extremities, the vertebral border of the scapula, and the cristal border of the ilium.

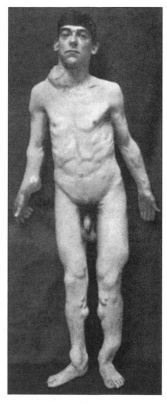

FIG. 140. Multiple Cartilaginous Exostoses in a man æt. 27. The scapular tumour projecting above the right clavicle has taken on active growth and pressed injuriously on the cords of the brachial plexus.

Clinically the disease is attended with the gradual and painless development during childhood or adolescence of a number of tumours or irregular projections of bone, at the ends of the long bones, the vertebral border of the scapula, and the cristal border of the ilium. They exhibit a rough symmetry; they rarely attain any size; and they usually cease growing when the skeleton attains maturity—the conversion of cartilage into bone being then completed. While they originate from the ossifying junctions of the long bones, they tend, as the shaft increases in length, to project from the surface of the bone at some distance from the ossifying junction and to "point" away from it. They may cause symptoms by "locking" the adjacent joint or by pressing upon nerve-trunks or blood vessels.

In a considerable proportion of cases, the disturbance of growth is further manifested by dwarfing of the long bones; these are not only deficient in length but are sometimes also curved and misshapen, which accounts for the condition being occasionally confused with the disturbances of growth resulting from rickets. In about one-third of the recorded cases there is a dislocation of the head of the radius on one or on both sides, a result of unequal growth between the bones of the forearm.

In early adult life, one of the tumours, instead of undergoing ossification, may take on active growth and exhibit the features of a chondro-sarcoma, pressing injuriously upon adjacent structures (Fig. 140) and giving rise later to metastases in the lungs.

457

The *X-ray appearances* of the bones affected are of a striking character; apart from the outgrowths of bone or "tumours" there is evident a widespread alteration in the internal architecture of the bones, which suggests analogies with other disturbances of ossification such as achondroplasia and osteomyelitis fibrosa. The condition is one that runs in families, sometimes through several generations; we have more than once seen a father and son together in the hospital waiting-room.

As regards *treatment*, there is no indication for surgical interference except when one or other tumour is a source of disability as by pressing upon a nerve-trunk or by locking a joint, in which case it is easily removed by chiselling through its neck.

Diffuse Osteoma, Leontiasis Ossea.—This rare affection was described by Virchow, and named leontiasis ossea because of the disfigurement to which it gives rise. It usually commences in adolescence as a diffuse overgrowth first of one and then of both maxillæ; these bones are enlarged in all directions and project on the face, and the nasal fossæ and the maxillary and frontal sinuses become filled up with bone, which encroaches also on the orbital cavities. In addition to the hideous deformity, the patient suffers from blocking of the nose, loss of smell, and protrusion of the eyes, sometimes followed by loss of sight. The condition is liable to spread to the zygomatic and frontal bones, the vault of the skull, and to the mandible. The base of the skull is not affected. The disease is of slow progress and may become arrested; life may be prolonged for many years, or may be terminated by brain complications or by intercurrent affections. In certain cases it is possible to remove some of the more disfiguring of the bony masses.

A less aggressive form, confined to the maxilla on one side, is sometimes met with, and, in a case of this variety under our own observation, the disfigurement, which was the only subject of complaint, was removed, after reflecting the soft parts, by paring away the excess of bone; this is easily done as the bone is spongy, and at an early stage, imperfectly calcified.

A remarkable form of *unilateral hypertrophy and diffuse osteoma of the skull*, following the distribution of the fifth nerve, has seen described by Jonathan Hutchinson and Alexis Thomson.

Chondroma.—Cartilaginous tumours, apart from those giving rise to multiple exostoses, grow from the long bones and from the scapula, ilium, ribs, or jaws. They usually project from the surface of the bone, and may attain an enormous size; sometimes they grow in the interior of a bone, the so-called *enchondroma*.

The hyaline cartilage composing the tumour frequently undergoes myxomatous degeneration, resulting in the formation of a glairy, semi-fluid jelly, and if this change takes place throughout the tumour it comes to resemble a cyst. On the other hand, the cartilage may undergo calcification or ossification. The most important transition of all is that into sarcoma, the so-called *malignant chondroma* or *chondrosarcoma*, which is associated with rapid increase

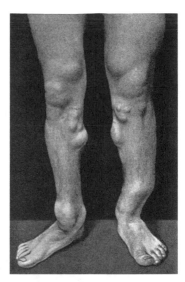

FIG. 141. Multiple Cartilaginous Exostoses in a man æt. 27, the same as in Fig. 140.

in size, and parts of the tumour may be carried off in the blood-stream and give rise to secondary growths, especially in the lungs.

Cases have been met with in which certain parts of the skeleton—only those developed in cartilage—were so uniformly permeated with cartilage that the condition has been described as a "chondromatosis" and is regarded as dating from an early period of foetal life. Unlike the condition known as multiple cartilaginous exostoses, it is a malignant disease.

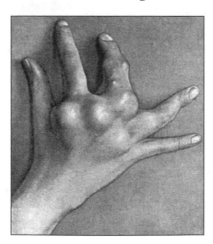

FIG. 142. Multiple Chondromas of Phalanges and Metacarpals in a boy æt. 10 (cf. Fig. 143).

The chondroma is met with as a slowly growing tumour which is specially common in the bones of the hand, often in a multiple form (Figs. 142 and 144). The surface is smooth or lobulated, and in consistence the tumour may be dense and elastic like normal cartilage, or may present areas of softening, or of bony hardness. The skin moves freely over it, except in relation to the bones of the fingers, where it may become adherent and ulcerate, simulating the appearance of a malignant tumour. Large tumours growing from the bones of the extremities may implicate the main vessels and nerves, either surrounding them or pressing on them.

Portions of a chondroma, which have undergone calcification or ossification, throw a dark shadow with the X-rays; unaltered cartilage and myxomatous tissue appear as clear areas.

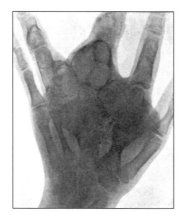

FIG. 143. Skiagram of Multiple Chondromas shown in Fig. 142.

Treatment.—It is necessary to remove the whole tumour, and in chondromas growing from the surface of the bone, especially if they are pedunculated, this is comparatively easy. When a bone, such as the scapula or mandible, is involved, it is better to excise the bone, or at least the part of it which bears the tumour. In the case of central tumours the shell of bone is removed over an area sufficient to allow of the enucleation of the tumour, or the affected portion of bone is resected. Should there be evidence of malignancy, such as increased rate of growth, a tube of radium should be inserted, and in advanced cases with destruction of tissue, amputation may be called for.

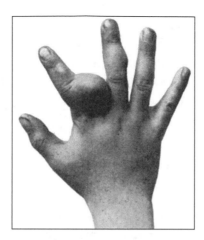

FIG. 144. Multiple Chondromas in Hand of boy æt. 8

In multiple chondromas of the hand in young subjects, it was formerly the custom to amputate the limb; an attempt should be made to avoid this by shelling out the larger tumours individually, and persevering with the application of the X-rays or of radium to inhibit the growth of the smaller ones.

Chondromas springing from the pelvic bones usually arise in the region of the sacro-iliac joint; they project into the pelvis and press on the bladder and rectum, and on the sciatic and obturator nerves; sometimes also on the iliac veins, causing oedema of the legs. They are liable to take on malignant characters, and rarely lend themselves to complete removal by operation.

Fibroma is met with chiefly as a periosteal growth in relation to the mouth and pharynx, the *simple epulis* of the alveolar margin and the *naso-pharyngeal polypus* being the most common examples. We have met with a fibroma in the interior of the lower end of the femur of an adult, causing expansion of the bone with decided increase in girth and liability to pathological fracture; it is possible that this represents the cured stage of osteomyelitis fibrosa.

Myxoma, lipoma, and *angioma* of bone are all rare.

Myeloma.—The myeloid tumour, which is sometimes classified with the sarcomas, contains as its chief elements large giant cells, like those normally present in the marrow. On section these tumours present a brownish-red or chocolate colour, and, being highly vascular, are liable to hæmorrhages, and therefore also to pigmentation, and to the formation of blood cysts. Sometimes the arterial vessels are so dilated as to impart to the tumour an aneurysmal pulsation and bruit. The enlargement or "expansion" of the bone results in the cortex being represented by a thin shell of bone, which may crackle on pressure—parchment or egg-shell crackling.

The myeloma is most often met with between the ages of twenty-five and forty in the upper end of the tibia or lower end of the femur. It grows slowly and causes little pain, and may long escape recognition unless an examination is made with the X-rays. Although these tumours have been known to give rise to metastases, they are, as a rule, innocent and are to be treated as such. When located in the shaft of a long bone, pathological fracture is liable to occur.

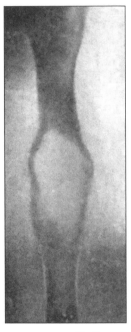

FIG. 145. Radiogram of Myeloma of Humerus. (Mr. J. W. Struthers' case.)

Diagnosis and X-ray Appearances of Myeloma.—The early diagnosis of myeloma is made with the aid of the X-rays: the typical appearance is that of a rounded or oval clear area bounded by a shell of bone of diminishing thickness (Fig. 145). The inflammatory lesions at the ends of the long bones—tubercle, syphilitic gumma, and Brodie's abscess, that resemble myeloma, are all attended with the formation of new bone in greater or lesser amount. The myeloma is also to be diagnosed from chondroma, from sarcoma, and from osteomyelitis fibrosa cystica.

Treatment.—In early cases the cortex is opened up to give free access to the tumour tissue, which is scraped out with the spoon. Bloodgood advises the use of Esmarch's tourniquet, and that the curetting be followed by painting with pure carbolic acid and then rinsing with alcohol; a rod of bone is inserted to fill the gap. In advanced cases the segment of bone is resected and a portion of the tibia or fibula from the other limb inserted into the gap; a tube of radium should also be introduced.

The coexistence of diffuse myelomatosis of the skeleton and albumosuria (Bence-Jones) is referred to on p. 474. Myeloma occurs in the jaws, taking origin in the marrow or from the periosteum of the alveolar process, and is described elsewhere.

Sarcoma and **endothelioma** are the commonest tumours of bone, and present wide variations in structure and in clinical features. Structurally, two main groups may be differentiated: (1) the soft, rapidly growing cellular tumours, and (2) those containing fully formed fibrous tissue, cartilage, or bone.

(1) The *soft cellular tumours* are composed mainly of spindle or round cells; they grow from the marrow of the spongy ends or from the periosteum of the long bones, the diploë of the skull, the pelvis, vertebræ, and jaws. As they grow they may cause little alteration in the contour of the bone, but they eat away its framework and replace it, so that the continuity of the bone is maintained only by tumour tissue, and pathological fracture is a frequent result. The small round-celled sarcomas are among the most malignant tumours of bone, growing with great rapidity, and at an early stage giving rise to secondary growths.

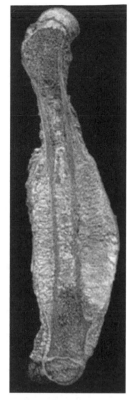

FIG. 146. Periosteal Sarcoma of Femur in a young subject

(2) The second group includes the *fibro-*, *osteo-*, and *chondro-sarcomas*, and combinations of these; in all of them fully formed tissues or attempts at fully formed tissues predominate over the cellular elements. They grow chiefly from the deeper layer of the periosteum, and at first form a projection on the surface, but later tend to surround the bone (Fig. 150), and to invade its interior, filling up the marrow spaces with a white, bone-like substance; in the flat bones of the skull they may traverse the diploë and erupt on the inner table. The tumour tissue next the shaft consists of a dense, white, homogeneous material, from which there radiate into the softer parts of the tumour, spicules, needles, and plates, often exhibiting a fan-like arrangement (Fig. 151). The peripheral portion consists of soft sarcomatous tissue, which invades the overlying soft parts. The articular cartilage long resists destruction. The ossifying sarcoma is met with most often in the femur and tibia, less frequently in the humerus, skull, pelvis, and jaws. In the long bones it may grow from the shaft, while the chondro-sarcoma more often originates at the extremities.

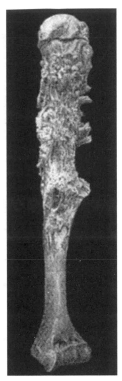

FIG. 147. Periosteal Sarcoma of Humerus, after maceration. (Anatomical Museum, University of Edinburgh.)

Sometimes they are multiple, several tumours appearing simultaneously or one after another. Secondary growths are met with chiefly in the lungs, metastasis taking place by way of the veins.

Clinical Features.—Sarcoma is usually met with before the age of thirty, and is comparatively common in children. Males suffer oftener than females, in the proportion of two to one.

In *periosteal sarcoma* the presence of a swelling is usually the first symptom; the tumour is fusiform, firm, and regular in outline, and when it occurs near the end of a long bone the limb frequently assumes a characteristic "leg of mutton" shape (Fig. 146). The surface may be uniform or bossed, the consistence varies at different parts, and the swelling gradually tapers off along the shaft. On firm pressure, fine crepitation may be felt from crushing of the delicate framework of new bone.

In *central sarcoma* pain is the first symptom, and it is usually constant, dull, and aching; is not obviously increased by use of the limb, but is often worse at night. Swelling occurs late, and is due to expansion of the bone; it is fusiform or globular, and is at first densely hard, but in time there may be parchment-like or egg-shell crackling from yielding of the thin shell. The swelling may pulsate, and a bruit may be heard over it. In advanced cases it may be impossible to differentiate between a periosteal and a central tumour, either clinically or after the specimen has been laid open.

Pathological fracture is more common in central tumours, and sometimes is the first sign that calls attention to the condition. Consolidation rarely takes place, although there is often an attempt at union by the formation of cartilaginous callus.

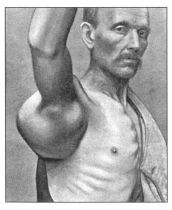

FIG. 148. Chondro-Sarcoma of Scapula in a man æt. 63; removal of the scapula was followed two years later by metastases and death.

The soft parts over the tumour for a long time preserve their normal appearance; or they become oedematous, and the subcutaneous venous network is evident through the skin. Elevation of the temperature over the tumour, which may amount to two degrees or more, is a point of diagnostic significance, as it suggests an inflammatory lesion.

The adjacent joint usually remains intact, although its movements may be impaired by the bulk of the tumour or by effusion into the cavity.

Enlargement of the neighbouring lymph glands does not necessarily imply that they have become infected with sarcoma for the enlargement may disappear after removal of the primary growth; actual infection of the glands, however, does sometimes occur, and in them the histological structure of the parent tumour is reproduced.

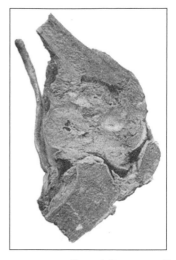

FIG. 149. Central Sarcoma of Lower End of Femur, invading the knee-joint. (Museum of Royal College of Surgeons, Edinburgh.)

To obtain a reasonable prospect of cure, the *diagnosis* must be made at an early stage. Great reliance is to be placed on information gained by examination with the X-rays.

X-ray Appearances.—In periosteal tumours that do not ossify, there is merely erosion of bone, and the shadow is not unlike that given by caries; in ossifying tumours, the arrangement of the new bone on the surface is characteristic, and when it takes the form of spicules at right angles to the shaft, it is pathognomic.

In soft central tumours, there is disappearance of bone shadow in the area of the tumour, while above and below or around this, the shadow is that of normal bone right up to the clear area. In many respects the X-ray appearances resemble those of myeloma. In tumours in which there is a considerable amount of imperfectly formed new bone, this gives a shadow which barely replaces

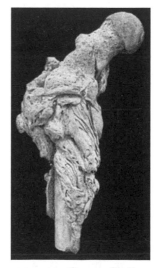

FIG. 150. Osseous Shell of Osteo-Sarcoma of Upper Third of Femur, after maceration.

that of the original bone, in parts it may even add to it—the resulting picture differing widely in different cases; but it is usually possible to differentiate it from that caused by bacterial infections of the bone and from lesions of the adjacent joint.

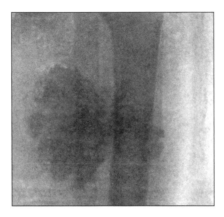

FIG. 151. Radiogram of Osteo-Sarcoma of Upper Third of Femur.

Skiagraphy is not only of assistance in differentiating new growths from other diseases of bone, but may also yield information as to the situation and nature of the tumour, which may have important bearings on its treatment by operation.

When fracture of a long bone takes place in an adolescent or young adult from comparatively slight violence, disease of the bone should be suspected and an X-ray examination made.

In difficult cases the final appeal is to exploratory incision and microscopical examination of a portion of the tumour; this should be done when the major operation has been arranged for, the surgeon waiting until the examination is completed.

The *prognosis* varies widely. In general, it may be said that periosteal tumours are less favourable than central ones, because they are more liable to give rise to metastases. Permanent cures are unfortunately the exception.

Treatment.—When one of the bones of a limb is involved, the usual practice has been to perform amputation well above the growth, and this may still be recommended as a routine procedure. There are reasons, however, which may be urged against its continuance. High amputation is unnecessary in the more benign sarcomas, and in the more malignant forms is usually unavailing to prevent a fatal issue either from local recurrence or from metastases in the lungs or elsewhere. Following the lead of Mikulicz, a considerable number of permanent cures have been obtained by resecting the portion of bone which is the seat of the tumour, and substituting for it a corresponding portion from the tibia or fibula of the other limb. In a cellular sarcoma of the humerus of a boy we resected the shaft and inserted his fibula ten years ago, and he shows no sign of recurrence. When resection is impracticable, a sub-capsular enucleation is performed, followed by the insertion of radium.

Pulsating Hæmatoma or **Aneurysm of Bone.**— A limited number of these are innocent cavernous tumours dating from a congenital angioma. The majority would appear to be the result of changes in a sarcoma, endothelioma, or myeloma. The tumour tissue largely disappears, while the vessels and vascular spaces undergo a remarkable development. The tumour may come to be represented by one large blood-containing space communicating with the arteries of the limb; the walls of the space consist of the remains of the original tumour, plus a shell of bone of varying thickness. The most common seats of the condition are the lower end of the femur, the upper end of the tibia, and the bones of the pelvis.

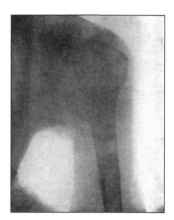

FIG. 152. Radiogram of Chondro-Sarcoma of Upper End of Humerus in a woman æt. 29.

The *clinical features* are those of a pulsating tumour of slow development, and as in true aneurysm, the pulsation and bruit disappear on compression of the main artery. The origin of the tumour from bone may be revealed by the presence of egg-shell crackling, and by examination with the X-rays.

If the condition is believed to be innocent, the treatment is the same as for aneurysm—preferably by ligation of the main artery; if malignant, it is the same as for sarcoma.

Secondary Tumours of Bone.—These embrace two groups of new growth, those which give rise to secondary growths in the marrow of bones and those which spread to bone by direct continuity.

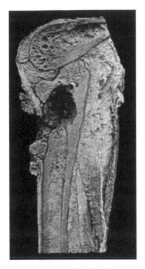

FIG. 153. Epitheliomatous Ulcer of Leg with direct extension to Tibia. (Lord Lister's specimen. Anatomical Museum, University of Edinburgh.)

Metastatic Tumours.—Excepting certain cancers which give rise to metastases by lymphatic permeation (Handley), the common metastases arising in the bone-marrow reach their destination through the blood-stream.

Secondary cancer is a comparatively common disease, and, as in metastases in other tissues, the secondary growths resemble the parent tumour. The soft forms grow rapidly, and eat away the bone, without altering its shape or form. In slowly growing forms there may be considerable formation of imperfectly formed bone, often deficient in lime salts; this condition may be widely diffused throughout the skeleton, and, as it is associated with softening and bending of the bones, it is known as *cancerous osteomalacia.* Secondary cancer of bone is attended with pain, or it suddenly attracts notice by the occurrence of pathological fracture—as, for example, in the shaft of the femur or humerus. In the vertebræ, it is attended with a painful form of paraplegia, which may involve the lower or all four extremities. On the other hand, the disease may show itself clinically as a tumour of bone, which may attain a considerable size, and may be mistaken for a sarcoma, unless the existence of the primary cancer is discovered.

The cancers most liable to give rise to metastasis in bone are those of the breast, liver, uterus, prostate, colon, and rectum; hyper-nephroma of the kidney may also give rise to metastases in bone.

Secondary tumours derived from the thyreoid gland require special mention, because they are peculiar in that neither the primary growth in the thyreoid nor the secondary growth in the bones is necessarily malignant. They are therefore amenable to operative treatment.

Secondary sarcoma, whether derived from a primary growth in the bone or in the soft parts, is much rarer than secondary cancer. Its removal by operation is usually contra-indicated, but we have known of cases terminating fatally in which the *section* revealed only one metastasis, the removal of which would have benefited the patient.

In all of these conditions, examination of the bones with the X-rays gives valuable information and often disclose unsuspected metastases.

Cancer of Bone resulting from Direct Extension from Soft Parts.—In this group there are also two clinical types. The first is met with in relation to *epithelioma of a mucous surface*—for example, the palate, tongue, gums, antrum, frontal sinus, auditory meatus, or middle ear. They will be described under these special regions.

The second type is met with in relation to *epithelioma occurring in a sinus*, the sequel of suppurative osteomyelitis, compound fracture, or tuberculous disease. The patient has usually had a discharging sinus for a great number of years: we have known it to last as many as fifty. The epithelioma originates at the skin orifice of the sinus, and spreads to the bone and into its interior, where the progress of the cancer is resisted by dense bone, which obliterates the medullary canal. Although its progress is slow, the infiltration of the bone is usually more extensive than appears externally. It is recognised clinically by the characteristic cauliflower growth at the orifice of the sinus, and by the offensive nature of the discharge. A similar epithelioma may arise in connection with a *chronic ulcer of the leg*. The cancer may infect the femoral lymph glands. The operative treatment is influenced by the extent of the disease in the soft parts overlying the bone, and consists in wide removal of the diseased tissues and resection of the bone, or in amputation.

Cysts of Bone.—With the exception of hydatid cysts, cysts in the interior of bone are the result of the liquefaction of solid tissue; this may be that of chondroma, myeloma, or sarcoma, but more commonly of the marrow in osteomyelitis fibrosa.

DISEASES OF JOINTS

Definition of Terms ◆ Ankylosis
Diseases: Errors of Development
Bacterial Diseases: Pyogenic; Gonorrhoeal;
Tuberculous; Syphilitic; Acute Rheumatism
Diseases Associated with Certain Constitutional Conditions:
Gout; Chronic Articular Rheumatism; Arthritis Deformans;
Hæmophilia ◆ Diseases Associated with Affections of the Nervous
System: Neuro-arthropathies; Charcot's Disease ◆ Hysterical or Mimetic
Affections of Joints ◆ Tumours and Cysts ◆ Loose Bodies.

Definition of Terms.—The term *synovitis* is applied to any reaction which affects the synovial membrane of a joint. It is usually associated with effusion of fluid, and this may be serous, sero-fibrinous, or purulent. As the term synovitis merely refers to the tissue involved, it should always be used with an adjective—such as gouty, gonorrhoeal, or tuberculous—which indicates its pathological nature.

The terms *hydrops, hydrarthrosis*, and *chronic serous synovitis* are synonymous, and are employed when a serous effusion into the joint is the prominent clinical feature. Hydrops may occur apart from disease—for example, in the knee-joint from repeated sprains, or when there is a loose body in the joint—but is met with chiefly in the chronic forms of synovitis which result from gonorrhoea, tuberculosis, syphilis, arthritis deformans, or arthropathies of nerve origin.

Arthritis is the term applied when not only the synovial membrane but the articular surfaces, and it may be also the ends of the bones, are involved, and it is necessary to prefix a qualifying adjective which indicates its nature. When effusion is present, it may be serous, as in arthritis deformans, or sero-fibrinous or purulent, as in certain forms of pyogenic and tuberculous arthritis. Wasting of the muscles, especially the extensors, in the vicinity of the joint is a constant accompaniment of arthritis. On account of the involvement of the articular surfaces, arthritis is apt to be followed by ankylosis.

The term *empyema* is sometimes employed to indicate that the cavity of the joint contains pus. This is observed chiefly in chronic disease of pyogenic or tuberculous origin, and is usually attended with the formation of abscesses outside the joint.

Ulceration of cartilage and *caries of the articular surfaces* are common accompaniments of the more serious and progressive forms of joint disease, especially those of bacterial origin. The destruction of cartilage may be secondary to disease of the synovial membrane or of the subjacent bone. When the disease begins as a synovitis, the synovial membrane spreads over the articular surface, fuses with the cartilage and eats into it, causing defects or holes which are spoken of as ulcers. When the disease begins in the bone, the marrow is converted into granulation tissue, which eats into the cartilage and separates it from the bone. Following on the destruction of the cartilage, the articular surface of the bone undergoes disintegration, a condition spoken of as *caries of the articular surface*. The occurrence of ulceration of cartilage and of articular caries is attended with the clinical signs of fixation of the joint from involuntary muscular contraction, wasting of muscles, and starting pains. These *starting pains* are the result of sudden involuntary movements of the joint. They occur most frequently as the patient is dropping off to sleep; the muscles becoming relaxed, the sensitive ulcerated surfaces jar on one another, which causes sudden reflex contraction of the muscles, and the resulting movement being attended with severe pain, wakens the patient with a start. Advanced articular caries is usually associated with some abnormal attitude and with shortening of the limb. It may be possible to feel the bony surfaces grate upon one another. When all its constituent elements are damaged or destroyed, a joint is said to be *disorganised*. Should recovery take place, repair is usually attended with union of the opposing articular surfaces either by fibrous tissue or by bone.

Conditions of Impaired Mobility of Joints.—There are four conditions of impaired mobility in joints: rigidity, contracture, ankylosis, and locking. *Rigidity* is the fixation of a joint by involuntary contraction of muscles, and is of value as a sign of disease in deep-seated joints, such as the hip. It disappears under anæsthesia.

Contracture is the term applied when the fixation is due to permanent shortening of the soft parts around a joint—muscles, tendons, ligaments, fasciæ, or skin. As the structures on the flexor aspect are more liable to undergo such shortening, contracture is nearly always associated with flexion. Contracture may result from disease of the joint, or from conditions outside it—for example, disease in one of the adjacent bones, or lesions of the nerves.

Ankylosis is the term applied when impaired mobility results from changes involving the articular surfaces. It is frequently combined with contracture. Three anatomical varieties of ankylosis are recognised—(a) The *fibrous*, in which there are adhesions between the opposing surfaces, which may be in the form of loose isolated bands of fibrous tissue, or may bind the bones so closely together as to obliterate the cavity of the joint. The resulting stiffness, therefore, varies from a mere restriction of the normal range of movement, up to a close union of the bones which prevents movement. Fibrous ankylosis may follow upon injury, especially dislocation or

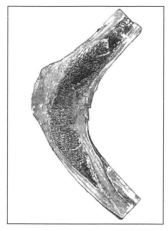

FIG. 154. Osseous Ankylosis of Femur and Tibia in position of flexion.

fracture implicating a joint, or it may result from any form of arthritis. (b) *Cartilaginous ankylosis* implies the fusion of two apposed cartilaginous surfaces. It is often found between the patella and the trochlear surface of the femur in tuberculous disease of the knee. The fusion of the cartilaginous surfaces is preceded by the spreading of a vascular connective tissue, derived from the synovial membrane, over the articular cartilage. Clinically, it is associated with absolute immobility, (c) *Bony ankylosis* or *synostosis* is an osseous union between articulating surfaces (Figs. 154 and 155). It may follow upon fibrous or cartilaginous ankylosis, or may result from the fusion of two articular surfaces which have lost their cartilage and become covered with granulations. In the majority of cases it is to be regarded as a reparative process, presenting analogies with the union of fracture.

The term *arthritis ossificans* has been applied by Joseph Griffiths to a condition in which the articular surfaces become fused without evident cause.

The occurrence of ankylosis in a joint before the skeleton has attained maturity does not appear to impair the growth in length of the bones affected; ankylosis of the temporo-maxillary joints, however, greatly impairs the growth of the mandible. When there is arrest of growth accompanying anky-losis, it usually depends on changes in the ossifying junctions caused by the original disease.

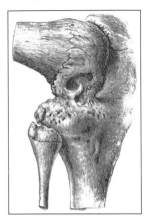

FIG. 155. Osseous Ankylosis of Knee in the flexed position following upon Tuberculous Arthritis. (Anatomical Museum, University of Edinburgh.)

To differentiate by manipulation between muscular fixation and ankylosis, it may be necessary to anæsthetise the patient. The nature and extent of ankylosis may be learned by skiagraphy; in osseous ankylosis the shadow of the two bones is a continuous one. In fibrous as contrasted with osseous ankylosis mobility may be elicited, although only to a limited extent; while in osseous ankylosis the joint is rigidly fixed, and attempts to move it are painless.

The *treatment* is influenced by the nature of the original lesion, the variety of the ankylosis, and the attitude of the joint. When there is restriction of movement due to fibrous adhesions, these may be elongated or ruptured. Elongation of the adhesions may be effected by manipulations, exercises, and the use of special forms of apparatus—such as the application of weights to the limb. It may be necessary to administer an anæsthetic before rupturing strong fibrous adhesions, and this procedure must be carried out with caution, in view of such risks as fracture of the bone—which is often rarefied—or separation of an epiphysis. There is also the risk of fat embolism, and of re-starting the original disease. The giving way of adhesions may be attended with an audible crack; and the procedure is often followed by considerable pain and effusion into the joint, which necessitate rest for some days before exercises and manipulations can be resumed.

Operative treatment may be called for in cases in which the bones are closely bound to one another by fibrous or by osseous tissue.

Arthrolysis, which consists in opening the joint and dividing the fibrous adhesions, is almost inevitably followed by their reunion.

Arthroplasty.—Murphy of Chicago devised this operation for restoring movement to an ankylosed joint. It consists in transplanting between the bones a flap of fat-bearing tissue, from which a bursal cavity lined with endothelium and containing a fluid rich in mucin is ultimately formed.

Arthroplasty is most successful in ankylosis following upon injury; when the ankylosis results from some infective condition such as tuberculosis or gonorrhoea, it is liable to result in failure either because of a fresh outbreak of the infection or because the ankylosis recurs.

When arthroplasty is impracticable, and a movable joint is desired—for example at the elbow—a considerable amount of bone, and it may be also of periosteum and capsular ligament, is resected to allow of the formation of a false joint.

When bony ankylosis has occurred with the joint in an undesirable attitude—for example flexion at the hip or knee—it can sometimes be remedied by osteotomy or by a wedge-shaped resection of the bone, with or without such additional division of the contracted soft parts as will permit of the limb being placed in the attitude desired.

Bony ankylosis of the joints of a finger, whether the result of injury or disease, is difficult to remedy by any operative procedure, for while it is possible to restore mobility, the new joint is apt to be flail-like.

Locking.—A joint is said to lock when its movements are abruptly arrested by the coming together of bony outgrowths around the joint. It is best illustrated in arthritis deformans of the hip in which new bone formed round the rim of the acetabulum mechanically arrests the excursions of the head of the femur. The new bone, which limits the movements, is readily demonstrated in skiagrams; it may be removed by operative means. Locking of joints is more often met with as a result of injuries, especially in fractures occurring in the region of the elbow. In certain injuries of the semilunar menisci of the knee, also, the joint is liable to a variety of locking, which differs, however, in many respects from that described above.

Errors of Development.—These include congenital dislocations and other deformities of intra-uterine origin, such as abnormal laxity of joints, absence, displacement, or defective growth of one or other of the essential constituents of a joint. The more important of these are described along with the surgery of the Extremities.

DISEASES OF JOINTS

Bacterial Diseases.—In most bacterial diseases the organisms are carried to the joint in the blood-stream, and they lodge either in the synovial membrane or in one of the bones, whence the disease subsequently spreads to the other structures of the joint. Organisms may also be introduced through accidental wounds. It has been shown experimentally that joints are among the most susceptible parts of the body to infection, and this would appear to be due to the viscid character of the synovial fluid, which protects organisms from bactericidal agents in the tissues and fluids.

PYOGENIC DISEASES

The commoner pyogenic diseases are the result of infection of one or other of the joint structures with *staphylococci* or *streptococci*, which may be demonstrated in the exudate in the joint and in the substance of the synovial membrane. The mode of infection is the same as in the pyogenic diseases of bone, the metastasis occurring most frequently from the mucous membrane of the pharynx (J. B. Murphy). The localisation of the infection in a particular joint is determined by injury, exposure to cold, antecedent disease of the joint, or other factors, the nature of which is not always apparent.

The effects on the joint vary in severity. In the milder forms, there is engorgement and infiltration of the synovial membrane, and an effusion into the cavity of the joint of serous fluid mixed with flakes of fibrin—*serous synovitis*. In more severe infections the exudate consists of pus mixed with fibrin, and, it may be, red blood corpuscles—*purulent* or *suppurative synovitis*; the synovial membrane and the ligaments are softened, and the surface of the membrane presents granulations resembling those on an ulcer; foci of suppuration may develop in the peri-articular cellular tissue and result in abscesses. In *acute arthritis*, all the structures of the joint are involved; the articular cartilage is invaded by granulation tissue derived from the synovial membrane, and from the marrow of the subjacent bone; it presents a worm-eaten or ulcerated appearance, or it may undergo necrosis and separate, exposing the subjacent bone and leading to disintegration of the osseous trabeculæ—*caries*. With the destruction of the ligaments, the stability of the joint is lost, and it becomes disorganised.

The *clinical features* vary with the extent of the infection. When this is confined to the synovial and peri-synovial tissues—*acute serous* and *purulent synovitis*—there is the usual general reaction, associated with pyrexia and great pain in the joint. The part is hot and swollen, the swelling assuming the shape of the distended synovial sac, fluctuation can usually be elicited, and the joint is held in the flexed position.

When the joint is infected by extension from the surrounding cellular tissue, the joint lesion may not be recognised at an early stage because of the swollen condition of the limb, and because there are already symptoms of toxæmia. We have observed a case in which both the hip and knee joints were infected from the cellular tissue.

If the infection involves all the joint structures—*acute arthritis*—the general and local phenomena are intensified, the temperature rises quickly, often with a rigor, and remains high; the patient looks ill, and is either unable to sleep or the sleep is disturbed by starting pains. The joint is held rigid in the flexed position, and the least attempt at movement causes severe pain; the slightest jar—even the shaking of the bed—may cause agony. The joint is hot, tensely distended, and there may be oedema of the peri-articular tissues or of the limb as a whole. If the pus perforates the joint capsule, there are signs of abscess or of diffuse suppuration in the cellular tissue. The final disorganisation of the joint is indicated by abnormal mobility and grating of the articular surfaces, or by spontaneous displacement of the bones, and this may amount to dislocation. In the acute arthritis of infants, the epiphysis concerned may be separated and displaced.

When the *joint is infected through an external wound*, the anatomical features are similar to those observed when the infection has reached the joint by the blood-stream, but the destructive changes tend to be more severe and are more likely to result in disorganisation.

The *terminations* vary with the gravity of the infection and with the stage at which treatment is instituted. In the milder forms recovery is the rule, with more or less complete restoration of function. In more severe forms the joint may be permanently damaged as a result of fibrous or bony ankylosis, or from displacement or dislocation. From changes in the peri-articular structures there may be contracture in an undesirable position, and in young subjects the growth of the limb may be interfered with. The persistence of sinuses is usually due to disease in one or other of the adjacent bones. In the most severe forms, and especially when several joints are involved, death may result from toxæmia.

The *treatment* is carried out on the same principles as in other pyogenic infections. The limb is immobilised in such an attitude that should stiffness occur there will be the least interference with function. Extension by weight and pulley is the most valuable means of allaying muscular spasm and relieving intra-articular tension and of counteracting the tendency to flexion; as much as 15 or 20 pounds may be required to relieve the pain.

The induction of hyperæmia is sometimes remarkably efficacious in relieving pain and in arresting the progress of the infection. If the fluid in the joint is in sufficient quantity to cause tension, if it persists, or if there is reason to suspect that it is purulent, it should be withdrawn without delay; an exploring syringe usually suffices, the skin being punctured with a tenotomy knife, and, as practised by Murphy, 5 to 15 c.c. of a 2 per cent. solution of formalin in glycerin are injected and the wound is closed. In virulent infections the injection may be repeated in twenty-four hours. Drainage by tube or otherwise is to be condemned (Murphy). A vaccine may be prepared from the fluid in the joint and injected into the subcutaneous cellular tissue.

Suppuration in the peri-articular soft parts or in one of the adjacent bones must be looked for and dealt with.

When convalescence is established, attention is directed to the restoration of the functions of the limb, and to the prevention of stiffness and deformity by movements and massage, and the use of hot-air and other baths.

At a later stage, and especially in neglected cases, operative and other measures may be required for deformity or ankylosis.

METASTATIC FORMS OF PYOGENIC INFECTION

In **pyæmia,** one or more joints may fill with pus without marked symptoms or signs, and if the pus is aspirated without delay the joint often recovers without impairment of function.

In **typhoid fever,** joint lesions result from infection with the typhoid bacillus alone or along with pyogenic organisms, and run their course with or without suppuration; there is again a remarkable absence of symptoms, and attention may only be called to the condition by the occurrence of dislocation.

Joint lesions are comparatively common in **scarlet fever,** and were formerly described as scarlatinal rheumatism. The most frequent clinical type is that of a serous synovitis, occurring within a week or ten days from the onset of the fever. Its favourite seat is in the hand and wrist, the sheaths of the extensor tendons as well as the synovial membrane of the joints being involved. It does not tend to migrate to other joints, and rarely lasts longer than a few days. It is probably due to the specific virus of scarlet fever.

At a later stage, especially in children and in cases in which the throat lesion is severe, an arthritis is sometimes observed that is believed to be a metastasis from the throat; it may be acute and suppurative, affect several joints, and exhibit a septicæmic or pyæmic character.

The joints of the lower extremity are especially apt to suffer; the child is seriously ill, is delirious at night, develops bed-sores over the sacrum and, it may happen that, not being expected to recover, the legs are allowed to assume contracture deformities with ankylosis or dislocation at the hip and flexion ankylosis at the knees; should the child survive, the degree of crippling may be pitiable in the extreme; prolonged orthopædic treatment and a series of operations—arthroplasty, osteotomies, and resections—may be required to restore even a limited capacity of locomotion.

Pneumococcal affections of joints, the result of infection with the pneumococcus of Fraenkel, are being met with in increasing numbers. The local lesion varies from a *synovitis* with infiltration of the synovial membrane and effusion of serum or pus, to an *acute arthritis* with erosion of cartilage, caries of the articular surfaces, and disorganisation of the joint. The knee is most frequently affected, but several joints may suffer at the same time. In most cases the joint affection makes its appearance a few days after the commencement of a pneumonia, but in a number of instances, especially among children, the lung is not specially involved, and the condition is an indication of a generalised pneumococcal infection, which may manifest itself by endocarditis, empyema, meningitis, or peritonitis, and frequently has a fatal termination. The differential diagnosis from other forms of pyogenic infection is established by bacteriological examination of the fluid withdrawn from the joint. The treatment is carried out on the same lines as in other pyogenic infections, considerable reliance being placed on the use of autogenous vaccines.

In **measles, diphtheria, smallpox, influenza, and dysentery**, similar joint lesions may occur.

The joint lesions which accompany **acute rheumatism** or "rheumatic fever" are believed to be due to a diplococcus. In the course of a general illness in which there is moderate pyrexia and profuse sweating, some of the larger joints, and not infrequently the smaller ones also, become swollen and extremely sensitive, so that the sufferer lies in bed helpless, dreading the slightest movement. From day to day fresh joints are attacked, while those first affected subside, often with great rapidity. Affections of the heart-valves and of the pericardium are commonly present. On recovery from the acute illness, it may be found that the joints have entirely recovered, but in a small proportion of cases certain of them remain stiff and pass into the crippled condition described under chronic rheumatism. There is no call for operative interference.

Gonococcal Affections of Joints.—These include all forms of joint lesion occurring in association with gonorrhoeal urethritis, vulvo-vaginitis, or gonorrhoeal ophthalmia. They may develop at any stage of the urethritis, but are most frequently met with from the eighteenth to the twenty-second day after the primary infection, when the organisms have reached the posterior urethra; they have been observed, however, after the discharge has ceased. There is no connection between the severity of the gonorrhoea and the incidence of joint disease. In women, the gonorrhoeal nature of the discharge must be established by bacteriological examination.

As a complication of ophthalmia, the joint lesions are met with in infants, and occur more commonly towards the end of the second or during the third week.

The gonococcus is carried to the joint in the blood-stream and is first deposited in the synovial membrane, in the tissues of which it can usually be found; it may be impossible to find it in the exudate within the joint. The joint lesions may be the only evidence of metastasis, or they may be part of a general infection involving the endocardium, pleura, and tendon sheaths.

The joints most frequently affected are the knee, elbow, ankle, wrist, and fingers. Usually two or more joints are affected.

Several clinical types are differentiated. (1) A *dry poly-arthritis* met with in the joints and tendon sheaths of the wrist and hand, formerly described as gonorrhoeal rheumatism, which in some cases is trifling and evanescent, and in others is persistent and progressive, and results in stiffness of the affected joints and permanent crippling of the hand and fingers.

(2) The commonest type is a *chronic synovitis* or *hydrops*, in which the joint— very often the knee—becomes filled with a serous or sero-fibrinous exudate. There are no reactive changes in the synovial membrane, cellular tissue, or skin, nor is there any fever or disturbance of health. The movements are free except in so far as they are restricted by the amount of fluid in the joint. It usually subsides in two or three weeks under rest, but tends to relapse.

(3) An _acute synovitis_ with peri-articular phlegmon is most often met with in the elbow, but it occurs also in the knee and ankle. There is a sudden onset of severe pain and swelling in and around the joint, with considerable fever and disturbance of health. The slightest movement causes pain, and the part is sensitive to touch. The skin is hot and tense, and in the case of the elbow may be red and fiery as in erysipelas.

The deposit of fibrin on the synovial membrane and on the articular surfaces may lead t o the formation of adhesions, sometimes in the form of isolated bands, sometimes in the form of a close fibrous union between the bones.

(4) A *suppurative arthritis*, like that caused by ordinary pus microbes, may be the result of gonococcal infection alone or of a mixed infection. Usually only one joint is affected, but the condition may be multiple. The articular cartilages are destroyed, the ends of the bones are covered with granulations, extra-articular abscesses form, and complete osseous ankylosis results.

The *diagnosis* is often missed because the possibility of gonorrhoea is not suspected.

The denial of the disease by the patient is not always to be relied upon, especially in the case of women, as they may be ignorant of its presence. The chief points in the differential diagnosis from acute articular rheumatism are, that the gonorrhoeal affection is more often confined to one or two joints, has little tendency to wander from joint to joint, and its progress is not appreciably influenced by salicylates, although these drugs may relieve pain. The conclusive point is the recognition of a gonorrhoeal discharge or of threads in the urine.

The disease may persist or may relapse, and the patient may be laid up for weeks or months, and may finally be crippled in one or in several joints.

The *treatment*—besides that of the urethral disease or of the ophthalmia—consists in rest until all pain and sensitiveness have disappeared. The pain is relieved by salicylates, but most benefit follows weight extension, the induction of hyperæmia by the rubber bandage and hot-air baths; if the joint is greatly distended, the fluid may be withdrawn by a needle and syringe. Detoxicated vaccines should be given from the first, and in afebrile cases the injection of a foreign protein, such as anti-typhoid vaccine, is beneficial (Harrison).

Murphy has found benefit from the introduction into the joint, in the early stages, of from 5 to 15 c.c. of a 2 per cent. solution of formalin in glycerin. This may be repeated within a week, the patient being kept in bed with light weight extension. In the chronic hydrops the fluid is withdrawn, and about an ounce of a 1 per cent. solution of protargol injected; the patient should be warned of the marked reaction which follows.

After all symptoms have settled down, but not till then, for fear of exciting relapse or metastasis, the joint is massaged and exercised. Stiffness from adhesions is most intractable, and may, in spite of every attention, terminate in ankylosis even in cases where there has been no suppuration. Forcible breaking down of adhesions under anæsthesia is not recommended, as it is followed by great suffering and the adhesions re-form. Operation for ankylosis—arthroplasty—should not be undertaken, as the ankylosis recurs.

TUBERCULOUS DISEASE

Tuberculous disease of joints results from bacillary infection through the arteries. The disease may commence in the synovial membrane or in the marrow of one of the adjacent bones, and the relative frequency of these two seats of infection has been the subject of considerable difference of opinion. The traditional view of König is that in the knee and most of the larger joints the disease arises in the bone and in the synovial membrane in about equal proportion, and that in the hip the number of cases beginning in the bones is about five times greater than that originating in the membrane. This estimate, so far as the actual frequency of bone lesions is concerned, has been generally accepted, but recent observers, notably John Fraser, do not accept the presence of bone lesions as necessarily proving that the disease commenced in the bones; he maintains, and we think with good grounds, that in many cases the disease having commenced in the synovial membrane, slowly spreads to the bone by way of the blood vessels and lymphatics, and gives rise to lesions in the marrow.

Morbid Anatomy.—Tuberculous disease in the articular end of a long bone may give rise to *reactive changes* in the adjacent joint, characterised by effusion and by the extension of the synovial membrane over the articular surfaces. This may result in the formation of adhesions which obliterate the cavity of the joint or divide it into compartments. These lesions are comparatively common, and are not necessarily due to actual tuberculous infection of the joint.

The *infection of the joint* by tubercle originating in the adjacent bone may take place at the periphery, the osseous focus reaching the surface of the bone at the site of reflection of the synovial membrane, and the infection which begins at this point then spreads to the rest of the membrane. Or it may take place in the central area, by the projection of tuberculous granulation tissue into the joint following upon erosion of the cartilage (Fig. 156).

Changes in the Synovial Membrane.—In the majority of cases there is a *diffuse thickening of the synovial membrane*, due to the formation of granulation tissue, or of young connective tissue, in its substance. This new tissue is arranged in two layers—the outer composed of fully formed connective or fibrous tissue, the inner of embryonic tissue, usually permeated with miliary tubercles. On opening the joint, these tubercles may be seen on the surface of the membrane, or the surface may be covered with a layer of fibrinous or caseating tissue. Where there is greater resistance on the part of the tissues, there is active formation of young connective tissue which circumscribes or encapsulates the tubercles, so that they remain embedded in the substance of the membrane, and are only seen on cutting into it.

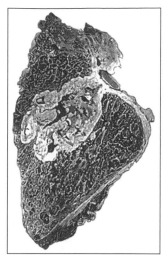

FIG. 156. Section of Upper End of Fibula, showing caseating focus in marrow, erupting on articular surface and infecting joint.

The thickened synovial membrane is projected into the cavity of the joint, filling up its pouches and recesses, and spreading over the surface of the articular cartilage "like ivy growing on a wall." Wherever the synovial tissue covers the cartilage it becomes adherent to and fused with it. The morbid process may be arrested at this stage, and fibrous adhesions form between the opposing articular surfaces, or it may progress, in which case further changes occur, resulting in destruction of the articular cartilage and exposure of the subjacent bone.

In rare instances the synovial membrane presents nodular masses or lumps, resembling the tuberculous tumours met with in the brain; they project into the cavity of the joint, are often pedunculated, and may give rise to the symptoms of loose body. The fringes of synovial membrane may also undergo a remarkable development, like that observed in arthritis deformans, and described as arborescent lipoma. Both these types are almost exclusively met with in the knee.

The Contents of Tuberculous Joints.—In a large proportion of cases of synovial tuberculosis the joint is entirely filled up by the diffuse thickening of the synovial membrane. In a small number there is an abundant serous exudate, and with this there may be a considerable formation of fibrin, covering the surface of the membrane and floating in the fluid as flakes or masses; under the influence of movement it may assume the shape of melon-seed bodies. More rarely the joint contains pus, and the surface of the synovial membrane resembles the wall of a cold abscess.

Ulceration and Necrosis of Cartilage.—The synovial tissue covering the carti-lage causes pitting and perforation of the cartilage and makes its way through it, and often spreads widely between it and the subjacent bone; the cartilage may be detached in portions of considerable size. It may be similarly ulcer-ated or detached as a result of disease in the bone.

Caries of Articular Surfaces.—Tuberculous infiltration of the marrow in the sur-face cancelli breaks up the spongy framework of the bone into minute irregular fragments, so that it disintegrates or crumbles away—caries. When there is an absence of caseation and suppuration, the condition is called *caries sicca*.

The pressure of the articular surfaces against one another favours the progress of ulceration of cartilage and of articular caries. These processes are usually more advanced in the areas most exposed to pressure—for example, in the hip-joint, on the superior aspect of the head of the femur, and on the posterior and upper segment of the acetabulum.

The occurrence of *pathological dislocation* is due to softening and stretch-ing of the ligaments which normally retain the bones in position, and to some factor causing displacement, which may be the accumulation of fluid or of granulations in the joint, the involuntary contraction of muscles, or some movement or twist of the limb. The occurrence of dislocation is also favoured by destructive changes in the bones.

Peri-articular tubercle and abscess may result from the spread of disease from the bone or joint into the surrounding tissues, either directly or by way of the lymphatics. A peri-articular abscess may spread in several directions, sometimes invading tendon sheaths or bursæ, and finally reaching the skin surface by tortuous sinuses.

Reactive changes in the vicinity of tuberculous joints are of common occurrence, and play a considerable part in the production of what is clinically known as *white swelling*. New connective tissue forms in the peri-articular fat and between muscles and tendons. It may be tough and fibrous, or soft, vascular, and oedematous, and the peri-articular fat becomes swollen and gelatinous, constituting a layer of considerable thickness. The fat disappears and is replaced by a mucoid effusion between the fibrous bundles of connective tissue. This is what was formerly known as *gelatinous degeneration* of the synovial membrane. In the case of the wrist the newly formed connective tissue may fix the tendons in their sheaths, interfering with the movements of the fingers. In relation to the bones also there may be reactive changes, resulting in the formation of spicules of new bone on the periosteal surfaces and at the attachment of the capsular and other ligaments; these are only met with where pyogenic infection has been superadded.

Terminations and Sequelæ.—A natural process of cure may occur at any stage, the tuberculous tissue being replaced by scar tissue. Recovery is apt to be attended with impairment of movement due to adhesions, ankylosis, or contracture of the peri-articular structures. Caseous foci in the interior of the bones may become encapsulated, and a cure be thus effected, or they may be the cause of a relapse of the disease at a later date. Interference with growth is comparatively common, and may involve only the epiphysial junctions in the immediate vicinity of the joint affected, or those of all the bones of the limb. This is well seen in adults who have suffered from severe disease of the hip in childhood—the entire limb, including the foot, being shorter and smaller than the corresponding parts of the opposite side.

Atrophic conditions are also met with, the bones undergoing fatty atrophy, so that in extreme cases they may be cut with a knife or be easily fractured. These atrophic conditions are most marked in bedridden patients, and are largely due to disuse of the limb; they are recovered from if it is able to resume its functions.

Clinical Features.—These vary with the different anatomical forms of the disease, and with the joint affected.

Sometimes the disease is ushered in by a febrile attack attended with pains in several joints—described by John Duncan as *tuberculous arthritic fever*. This is liable to be mistaken for rheumatic fever, from which, however, it differs in that there is no real migration from joint to joint; there is an absence of sweating and of cardiac complications; and no benefit follows the administration of salicylates.

In exceptional cases, tuberculous joint disease follows an acute course resembling that of the pyogenic arthritis of infants. This has been observed in children, especially in the knee, the lesion being in the synovial membrane, and attended with an accumulation of pus in the joint. If promptly treated by incision and drainage, recovery is rapid, and free movement of the joint, may be preserved.

The onset and early stages of tuberculous disease, however, are more often insidious, and are attended with so few symptoms that the disease may have obtained a considerable hold before it attracts notice. It is not uncommon for patients or their friends to attribute the condition to injury, as it often first attracts attention after some slight trauma or excessive use of the limb. The symptoms usually subside under rest, only to relapse again with use of the limb.

The initial local symptoms may be due to the presence of a focus in the neighbouring bone, perhaps causing neuralgic pains in the joint, or weakness, tiredness, stiffness, and inability to use the limb, these symptoms improving with rest and being aggravated by exertion.

It is rarely possible by external examination to recognise deep-seated osseous foci in the vicinity of joints; but if they are near the surface in a superficial bone—such as the head of the tibia—there may be local thickening of the periosteum, oedema, pain, and tenderness on pressure and on percussion.

X-ray Appearances of Tuberculous Joints.—Gross lesions such as caseous foci in the marrow of the adjacent bone show as clear areas with an ill-defined margin; a sclerosed focus gives a denser shadow than the surrounding bone, and a sequestrum presents a dark shadow of irregular contour, and a clear interval between it and the surrounding bone.

Caries of the articular surface imparts a woolly appearance or irregular contour in place of the well-defined outline of the articular end of the bone. In bony ankylosis the shadow of the two bones is a continuous one, the joint interval having been filled up. The minor changes are best appreciated on comparison with the normal joint of the other limb.

Wasting of muscles is a constant accompaniment of tuberculous joint disease. It is to be attributed partly to want of use, but chiefly to reflex interference with the trophic innervation of the muscles. It is specially well seen in the extensor and adductor muscles of the thigh in disease of the knee, and in the deltoid in disease of the shoulder. The muscles become soft and flaccid, they exhibit tremors on attempted movement, and their excitability to the faradic current is diminished. The muscular tissue may be largely replaced by fat.

Impairment of the normal movements is one of the most valuable diagnostic signs, particularly in deeply seated joints such as the shoulder, hip, and spine. It is due to a protective contraction of the muscles around the joint, designed to prevent movement. This muscular fixation disappears under anæsthesia.

Abnormal attitudes of the limb occur earlier, and are more pronounced in cases in which pain and other irritative symptoms of articular disease are well marked, and are best illustrated by the attitudes assumed in disease of the hip. They are due to reflex or involuntary contraction of the muscles acting on the joint, with the object of placing it in the attitude of greatest ease; they also disappear under anæsthesia. With the lapse of time they not only become exaggerated, but may become permanent from ankylosis or from contracture of the soft parts round the joint.

Startings at night are to be regarded as an indication that there is progressive disease involving the articular surfaces.

The formation of extra-articular abscess may take place early, or it may not occur till long after the disease has subsided. The abscess may develop so insidiously that it does not attract attention until it has attained considerable size, especially when associated with disease of the spine, pelvis, or hip. The position of the abscess in relation to different joints is fairly constant and is determined by the anatomical relationships of the capsule and synovial membrane to the surrounding tissues. The bursæ and tendon sheaths in the vicinity may influence the direction of spread of the abscess and the situation of resulting sinuses. When the abscess is allowed to burst, or is opened and becomes infected with pyogenic bacteria, there is not only the risk of aggravation of the disease and persistent suppuration, but there is a greater liability to general tuberculosis.

The sinuses may be so tortuous that a probe cannot be passed to the primary focus of disease, and their course and disposition can only be demonstrated by injecting the sinuses with an emulsion of bismuth and taking X-ray photographs.

Tuberculous infection of the lymph glands of the limb is exceptional, but may follow upon infection of the skin around the orifice of a sinus.

A slight rise of temperature in the evening may be induced in quiescent joint lesions by injury or by movement of the joint under anæsthesia, or by the fatigue of a railway journey. When sinuses have formed and become infected with pyogenic bacteria, there may be a diurnal variation in the temperature of the type known as hectic fever (Fig. 11).

Relative Frequency of Tuberculous Disease in Different Joints.—Hospital statistics show that joints are affected in the following order of frequency: Spine, knee, hip, ankle and tarsus, elbow, wrist, shoulder. The hip and spine are most often affected in childhood and youth, the shoulder and wrist in adults; the knee, ankle, and elbow show little age preference.

Clinical Variations of Tuberculous Joint Disease.—The above description applies to tuberculous joint disease in general; it must be modified to include special manifestations or varieties.

When the main incidence of the infection affects the synovial membrane, the clinical picture may assume the form of a *hydrops*, or of an *empyema* in which the joint is filled with pus. More common than either of these is the well-known *white swelling* or *tumor albus* (Wiseman, 1676) which is the clinical manifestation of diffuse thickening of the synovial membrane along with mucoid degeneration of the peri-synovial cellular tissue. It is well seen in joints which are superficial—such as the knee, ankle, elbow, and wrist. The swelling, which is the first and most prominent clinical feature, develops gradually and painlessly, obliterating the bony prominences by filling up the natural hollows. It appears greater to the eye than is borne out by measurement, being thrown into relief by the wasting of the muscles above and below the joint. In the early stage the swelling is elastic, doughy, and non-sensitive, and corresponds to the superficial area of the synovial membrane involved, and there is comparatively little complaint on the part of the patient, because the articular surfaces and ligaments are still intact. There may be a feeling of weight in the limb, and in the case of the knee and ankle the patient tires on walking and drags the leg with more or less of a limp. Movements of the joint are permitted, but are limited in range. The disability is increased by use and exertion, but, for a time at least, it improves under rest.

If the disease is not arrested, there follow the symptoms and signs of involvement of the articular surfaces.

Influence of Tuberculous Joint Disease on the General Health.—Experience shows that the early stages of tuberculous joint disease are compatible with the appearance of good health. As a rule, however, and especially if there is mixed infection, the health suffers, the appetite is impaired, the patient is easily tired, and there may be some loss of weight.

Treatment.—In addition to the general treatment of tuberculosis, local measures are employed. These may be described under two heads—the conservative and the operative.

Conservative treatment is almost always to be employed in the first instance, as by it a larger proportion of cures is obtained with a smaller mortality and with better functional results than by operation.

Treatment by rest implies the immobilisation of the diseased limb until pain and tenderness have disappeared. The attitude in which the limb is immobilised should be that in which, in the event of subsequent stiffness, it will be most serviceable to the patient. Immobilisation may be secured by bandages, splints, extension, or other apparatus. *Extension* with weight and pulley is of value in securing rest, especially in disease of the hip or knee; it eliminates muscular spasm, relieves pain and startings at night, and prevents abnormal attitudes of the limb. If, when the patient first comes under observation, the limb is in a deformed attitude which does not readily yield to extension, the deformity should be corrected under an anæsthetic.

The induction of hyperæmia is often helpful, the rubber bandage or the hot-air chamber being employed for an hour or so morning and evening.

Injection of Iodoform.—This is carried out on the same lines as have been described for tuberculous abscess. After the fluid contents of the joint are withdrawn, the iodoform is injected; and this may require to be repeated in a month or six weeks.

After the injection of iodoform there is usually considerable reaction, attended with fever (101° F.), headache, and malaise, and considerable pain and swelling of the joint. In some cases there is sickness, and there may be blood pigment in the urine. The severity of these phenomena diminishes with each subsequent injection.

The use of Scott's dressing and of blisters and of the actual cautery has largely gone out of fashion, but the cautery may still be employed with benefit for the relief of pain in cases in which ulceration of cartilage is a prominent feature.

The application of the X-rays has proved beneficial in synovial lesions in superficial joints such as the wrist or elbow; prolonged exposures are made at fortnightly intervals, and on account of the cicatricial contraction which attends upon recovery, the joint must be kept in good position.

Conservative treatment is only abandoned if improvement does not show itself after a thorough trial, or if the disease relapses after apparent cure.

Operative Treatment.—Other things being equal, operation is more often indicated in adults than in children, because after the age of twenty there is less prospect of recovery under conservative treatment, there is more tendency for the disease to relapse and to invade the internal organs, and there is no fear of interfering with the growth of the bones. The state of the general health may necessitate operation as the most rapid method of removing the disease. The social status of the patient must also be taken into account; the bread-winner, under existing social conditions, may be unable to give up his work for a sufficient time to give conservative measures a fair trial.

The *local conditions* which decide for or against operation are differently regarded by different surgeons, but it may be said in general terms that operative interference is indicated in cases in which the disease continues to progress in spite of a fair trial of conservative measures; in cases unsuited for conservative treatment—that is to say, where there are severe bone lesions. Operative interference is indicated also when the functional result will be better than that likely to be obtained by conservative measures, as is often the case in the knee and elbow. Cold abscesses should, if possible, be dealt with before operating on the joint.

In many cases the extent of the operation can only be decided after exploration. The aim is to remove all the disease with the least impairment of function and the minimum sacrifice of healthy tissue. The more open the method of operating the better, so that all parts of the joint may be available for inspection. The methods of Kocher, which permit of dislocating the joint, are specially to be recommended, as this procedure affords the freest possible access. Diseased synovial membrane is removed with the scissors or knife. If the cartilages are sound, and if a movable joint is aimed at, they may be left; but if ankylosis is desired, they must be removed. Localised disease of the cartilage should be removed with the spoon or gouge, and the bone beneath investigated. If the articular surface is extensively diseased, a thin slice of bone should be removed, and if foci in the marrow are then revealed, it is better to gouge them out than to remove further slices of bone, as this involves sacrifice of the cortex and periosteum.

Operative treatment of deformities resulting from tuberculous joint disease has almost entirely replaced reduction by force; the contracted soft parts are divided, and the bone is resected.

Amputation for tuberculous joint disease has become one of the rare operations of surgery, and is only justified when less radical measures have failed and the condition of the limb is affecting the general health. Amputation is more frequently called for in persons past middle life who are the subjects of pulmonary tuberculosis.

SYPHILITIC DISEASE

Syphilitic affections of joints are comparatively rare. As in tuberculosis, the disease may be first located in the synovial membrane, or it may spread to the joint from one of the bones.

In **acquired syphilis**, at an early stage and before the skin eruptions appear, one of the large joints, such as the shoulder or knee, may be the seat of pain—*arthralgia*—which is worse at night. In the secondary stage, a *synovitis* with serous effusion is not uncommon, and may affect several joints. Syphilitic *hydrops* is met with almost exclusively in the knee; it is frequently bilateral, and is insidious in its onset and progress, the patient usually being able to go about.

In the *tertiary stage* the joint lesions are persistent and destructive, and result from the formation of gummata, either in the deeper layers of the synovial membrane or in the adjacent bone or periosteum.

Peri-synovial and *peri-bursal gummata* are met with in relation to the knee-joint of middle-aged adults, especially women. They are usually multiple, develop slowly, and are rarely sensitive or painful. One or more of the gummata may break down and give rise to tertiary ulcers. The co-existence of indolent swellings, ulcers, and depressed scars in the vicinity of the knee is characteristic of tertiary syphilis.

The disease spreads throughout the capsule and synovial membrane, which becomes diffusely thickened and infiltrated with granulation tissue which eats into and replaces the articular cartilage. Clinically, the condition resembles tuberculous disease of the synovial membrane, for which it is probably frequently mistaken, but in the syphilitic affection the swelling is nodular and uneven, and the subjective symptoms are slight, mobility is little impaired, and yet the deformity is considerable.

Syphilitic osteo-arthritis results from a gumma in the periosteum or marrow of one of the adjacent bones. There is gradual enlargement of one of the bones, the patient complains of pains, which are worst at night. The disease may extend to the synovial membrane and be attended with effusion into the joint, or it may erupt on the periosteal surface and invade the skin, forming one or more sinuses. The further progress is complicated by the occurrence of pyogenic infection leading to necrosis of bone, in the knee-joint, for example, the patella or one of the condyles of the femur or tibia, may furnish a sequestrum. In such cases, anti-syphilitic treatment must be supplemented by operation for the removal of the diseased tissues. In the knee, excision is rarely necessary; but in the elbow it may be called for to obtain a movable joint.

In **inherited syphilis** the earliest joint affections are those in which there is an effusion into the joint, especially the knee or elbow; and in exceptional cases pyogenic infection may be superadded, and pus form in the joint.

In older children, a gummatous synovitis is met with of which the most striking features are: its insidious development, its chronic course, symmetrical distribution, freedom from pain, the free mobility of the joint, its tendency to relapse, and its association with other syphilitic stigmata, especially in the eyes. The knees are the joints most frequently affected, and the condition usually yields readily to anti-syphilitic treatment without impairment of function.

JOINT DISEASES ACCOMPANYING CERTAIN CONSTITUTIONAL CONDITIONS

Gout.—*Arthritis Urica.*—One of the manifestations of gout is that certain joints are liable to attacks of inflammation associated with the deposit of a chalk-like material composed of sodium biurate, chiefly in the matrix of the articular cartilage, it may be in streaks or patches towards the central area of the joint, or throughout the entire extent of the cartilage, which appears as if it had been painted over with plaster of Paris. As a result of this uratic infiltration, the cartilage loses its vitality and crumbles away, leading to the formation of what are known as gouty ulcers, and these may extend through the cartilage and invade the bone. The deposit of urates in the synovial membrane is attended with effusion into the joint and the formation of adhesions, while in the ligaments and peri-articular structures it leads to the formation of scar tissue. The metatarso-phalangeal joint of the great toe, on one or on both sides, is that most frequently affected. The disease is met with in men after middle life, and while common enough in England and Ireland, is almost unknown in hospital practice in Scotland.

The *clinical features* are characteristic. There is a sudden onset of excruciating pain, usually during the early hours of the morning, the joint becomes swollen, red, and glistening, with engorgement of the veins and some fever and disturbance of health and temper. In the course of a week or ten days there is a gradual return to the normal. Such attacks may recur only once a year or they may be more frequent; the successive attacks tend to become less acute but last longer, and the local phenomena persist, the joint remaining permanently swollen and stiff. Masses of chalk form in and around the joint, and those in the subcutaneous tissue may break through the skin, forming indolent ulcers with exposure of the chalky masses (*tophi*). The hands may become seriously crippled, especially when the tendon sheaths and bursæ also are affected; the crippling resembles that resulting from arthritis deformans but it differs in not being symmetrical.

The local *treatment* consists in employing soothing applications and a Bier's bandage for two or three hours twice daily while the symptoms are acute; later, hot-air baths, massage, and exercises are indicated. It is remarkable how completely even the most deformed joints may recover their function. Dietetic and medicinal treatment must also be employed.

Chronic Rheumatism.—This term is applied to a condition which sometimes follows upon acute articular rheumatism in persons presenting a family tendency to acute rheumatism or to inflammations of serous membranes, and manifesting other evidence of the rheumatic taint, such as chorea or rheumatic nodules.

The changes in the joints involve almost exclusively the synovial membrane and the ligaments; they consist in cellular infiltration and exudation, resulting in the formation of new connective tissue which encroaches on the cavity of the joint and gives rise to adhesions, and by contracting causes stiffness and deformity. The articular cartilages may subsequently be transformed into connective tissue, with consequent fibrous ankylosis and obliteration of the joint. The bones are affected only in so far as they undergo fatty atrophy from disuse of the limb, or alteration in their configuration as a result of partial dislocation. Osseous ankylosis may occur, especially in the small joints of the hand and foot.

The disease is generally poly-articular and may be met with in childhood and youth as well as in adult life. In some cases pain is so severe that the patient resists the least attempt at movement. In others, the joints, although stiff, can be moved but exhibit pronounced crackings. When there is much connective tissue formed in relation to the synovial membrane, the joint is swollen, and as the muscles waste above and below, the swelling is spindle-shaped. Subacute exacerbations occur from time to time, with fever and aggravation of the local symptoms and implication of other joints. After repeated recurrences, there is ankylosis with deformity, the patient becoming a helpless cripple. On account of the tendency to visceral complications, the tenure of life is uncertain.

From the nature of the disease, *treatment* is for the most part palliative. Salic-ylates are only of service during the exacerbations attended with pyrexia. The application of soda fomentations, turpentine cloths, or electric or hot-air baths may be useful. Improvement may result from the general and local therapeutics available at such places as Bath, Buxton, Harrogate, Strathpeffer, Wiesbaden, or Aix. In selected cases, a certain measure of success has followed operative inter-ference, which consists in a modified excision. The deformities resulting from chronic rheumatism are but little amenable to surgical treatment, and forcible attempts to remedy stiffness or deformity are to be avoided.

Arthritis Deformans (*Osteo-arthritis, Rheumatoid Arthritis, Rheumatic Gout, Malum Senile, Traumatic or Mechanical Arthritis*).—Under the term arthritis deformans, which was first employed by Virchow, it is convenient to include a number of joint affections which have many anatomical and clinical fea-tures in common.

The disease is widely distributed in the animal kingdom, both in domes-tic species and in wild animals in the natural state such as the larger carnivora and the gorilla; evidence of it has also been found in the bones of animals buried with prehistoric man.

The morbid changes in the joints present a remarkable combination of atrophy and degeneration on the one hand and overgrowth on the other, indicating a profound disturbance of nutrition in the joint structures. The nature of this disturbance and its etiology are imperfectly known. By many writers it is believed to depend upon some form of auto-intoxication, the toxins being absorbed from the gastro-intestinal tract, and those who suffer are supposed to possess what has been called an "arthritic diathesis."

The localisation of the disease in a particular joint may be determined by several factors, of which trauma appears to be the most important. The condition is frequently observed to follow, either directly or after an interval, upon a lesion which involves gross injury of the joint or of one of the neighbouring bones. It occurs with greater frequency after repeated minor injuries affecting the joint and its vicinity, such as sprains and contusions, and particularly those sustained in laborious occupations. This connection between trauma and arthritis deformans led Arbuthnot Lane to apply to it the term *traumatic* or *trade arthritis*.

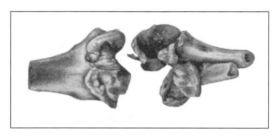

FIG. 157. Arthritis Deformans of Elbow, showing destruction of articular surfaces and masses of new bone around the articular margins. (Anatomical Museum, University of Edinburgh.)

The traumatic or strain factor in the production of the disease may be manifested in a less obvious fashion. In the lower extremity, for example, *any condition which disturbs the static equilibrium of the limb as a whole* would appear to predispose to the disease in one or other of the joints. The static equilibrium may be disturbed by such deformities as flat-foot or knock-knee, and badly united fractures of the lower extremity. In hallux valgus, the metatarso-phalangeal joint of the great toe undergoes changes characteristic of arthritis deformans.

A number of cases have been recorded in which arthritis deformans has followed upon antecedent disease of the joint, such as pyogenic or gonorrhoeal synovitis, upon repeated hæmorrhages into the knee-joint in bleeders, and in unreduced dislocations in which a new joint has been established.

Lastly, Poncet and other members of the Lyons school regard arthritis deformans as due to an attenuated form of tuberculous infection, and draw attention to the fact that a tuberculous family history is often met with in the subjects of the disease

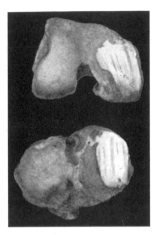

FIG. 158. Arthritis Deformans of Knee, showing eburnation and grooving of articular surfaces. (Anatomical Museum, University of Edinburgh.)

Morbid Anatomy.—The commonest type is that in which the articular surfaces undergo degenerative changes. The primary change involves the articular cartilage, which becomes softened and fibrillated and is worn away until the subjacent bone is exposed. If the bone is rarefied, the enlarged cancellous spaces are opened into and an eroded and worm-eaten appearance is brought about; with further use of the joint, the bone is worn away, so that in a ball-and-socket joint like the hip, the head of the femur and the acetabulum are markedly altered in size and shape. More commonly, the bone exposed as a result of disappearance of the cartilage is denser than normal, and under the influence of the movements of the joint, becomes smooth and polished—a change described as *eburnation* of the articular surfaces (Fig. 158). In hinge-joints such as the knee and elbow, the influence of movement is shown by a series of parallel grooves corresponding to the lines of friction (Fig. 158).

While these degenerative changes are gradually causing destruction of the articular surfaces, reparative and hypertrophic changes are taking place at the periphery. Along the line of the junction between the cartilage and synovial membrane, the proliferation of tissue leads to the formation of nodules or masses of cartilage—*ecchondroses*—which are subsequently converted into bone (Fig. 157). Gross alterations in the ends of the bone are thus brought about which can be recognised clinically and in skiagrams, and which tend to restrict the normal range of movement. The extension of the ossification into the synovial reflection and capsular ligament adds a collar or "lip" of new bone, known as "lipping" of the articular margins, and also into other ligaments, insertions of tendons and intermuscular septa giving rise to bony outgrowths or osteophytes not unlike those met with in the neuro-arthropathies.

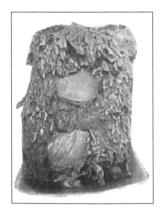

FIG. 159. Hypertrophied Fringes of Synovial Membrane in Arthritis Deformans of Knee. (Museum of Royal College of Surgeons, Edinburgh.)

Proliferative changes in the synovial membrane are attended with increased vascularity and thickening of the membrane and an enlargement of its villi and fringes. When the fatty fringes are developed to an exaggerated degree, the condition is described as an *arborescent lipoma* (Fig. 159). Individual fringes may attain the size of a hazel nut, and the fibro-fatty tissue of which they are composed may be converted into cartilage and bone; such a body may remain attached by a narrow pedicle or stalk, or this may be torn across and the body becomes loose and, unless confined in a recess of the joint, it wanders about and may become impacted between the articular surfaces. These changes in the synovial membrane are often associated with an abundant exudate or hydrops. These degenerative and hypertrophic changes, while usually attended with marked restriction of movement and sometimes by "locking" of the joint, practically never result in ankylosis.

The *ankylosing type* of chronic arthritis is fortunately much rarer than those described above, and is chiefly met with in the joints of the fingers and toes and in those of the vertebral column. The synovial membrane proliferates, grows over the cartilage, and replaces it, and when two such articular surfaces are in contact they tend to adhere, thus obliterating the joint, cavity, and resulting in fibrous or bony ankylosis. The changes progress slowly and, before they result in ankylosis, various sub-luxations and dislocations may occur with distortion and deformity which, in the case of the fingers, is extremely disabling and unsightly (Fig. 160).

Clinical Features.—It is usually observed that in patients who are still young the tendency is for the disease to advance with considerable rapidity, so that in the course of months it may cause crippling of several joints. The course of the disease as met with in persons past middle life is more chronic; it begins insidiously, and many years may pass before there is pronounced disability. The earliest symptom is stiffness, especially in the morning after rest, which passes off temporarily with use of the limb. As time goes on, the range of movement becomes restricted, and crackings occur. This stage of the disease may be prolonged indefinitely; if it progresses, stiffness becomes more pronounced, certain movements are lost, others develop in abnormal directions, and deformed attitudes add to the disablement. The disease is compatible with long life, but not with any active occupation, hence those of the hospital class who suffer from it tend to accumulate in workhouse infirmaries.

Hydrops is most marked in the knee, and may affect also the adjacent bursæ. As the joint becomes distended with fluid, the ligaments are stretched, the limb becomes weak and unstable, and the patient complains of a feeling of weight, of insecurity, and of tiredness. Pain is occasional and evanescent, and is usually the result of some extra exertion, or exposure to cold and wet. This form of the disease is extremely chronic, and may last for an indefinite number of years. It is to be diagnosed from the other forms of hydrops already considered—the purely traumatic, the pyogenic, gonorrhoeal, tuberculous, and syphilitic—and from that associated with Charcot's disease.

Hypertrophied fringes and pedunculated or loose bodies often co exist with hydrops, and give rise to characteristic clinical features, particularly in the knee. The fringes, especially when they assume the type of the arborescent lipoma, project into the cavity of the joint, filling up its recesses and distending its capsule so that the joint is swollen and slightly flexed. Pain is not a prominent feature, and the patient may walk fairly well. On grasping the joint while it is being actively flexed and extended, the fringes may be felt moving under the fingers. Symptoms from impaction of a loose body are exceptional.

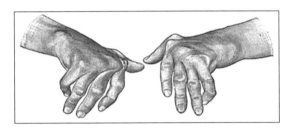

FIG. 160. Arthritis Deformans of Hands, showing symmetry of lesions, ulnar deviation of fingers, and nodular thickening at inter-phalangeal joints.

The dry form of arthritis deformans, although specially common in the knee, is met with in other joints, either as a mon-articular or poly-articular disease; and it is also met with in the joints of the spine and of the fingers as well as in the temporo-mandibular joint. In the joints of the fingers the disease is remarkably symmetrical, and tends to assume a nodular type (Heberden's nodes) (Fig. 160); in younger subjects it assumes a more painful and progressive fusiform type (Fig. 161). In the larger joints the subjective symptoms usually precede any palpable evidence of disease, the patient complaining of stiffness, crackings, and aching, aggravated by changes in the weather. The roughness due to fibrillation of the articular cartilages causes coarse friction on moving the joint, or, in the knee, on moving the patella on the condyles of the femur. It may be months or even years before the lipping and other hypertrophic changes in the ends of the bones are recognisable, and before the joint assumes the deformed features which the name of the disease suggests.

The capsular ligament, except in hydrops, is the seat of connective-tissue overgrowth, and tends to become contracted and rigid. Intra-articular ligaments, such as the ligamentum teres in the hip, are usually worn away and disappear. The surrounding muscles undergo atrophy, tendons become adherent to their sheaths and may be ossified, and the sheaths of nerves may be involved by the cicatricial changes in the surrounding tissues.

The X-ray appearances of arthritis deformans necessarily vary with the type of the disease and the joint affected; in the joints of the fingers there is a narrowing of the spaces between the articular ends of the bones as a result of absorption of the articular cartilage, and rarefaction of the cancellous tissue in the vicinity of the joints; in the larger joints there is "lipping" of the articular margins, osteophytes, and other evidence of abnormal ossification in and around the joint. Eburnation of the articular surfaces is shown by increase in the density of the shadow of the bone in the areas affected.

Treatment.—Treatment is for the most part limited to the relief of symptoms. On no account should the affected joints be kept at rest by means of splints or other apparatus. Active movements and exercises of all kinds are to be persevered with. When pain is a prominent feature, it may be relieved either by douches of iodine and hot water (tincture of iodine 1 oz. to the quart), or by the application of lint saturated with a lotion made up of chloral hydrate, gr. v, glycerin [dram]j, water [ounce]j, and covered with oil-silk. Strain and over-use of the joint and sudden changes of temperature are to be avoided. The induction of hyperæmia by means of massage, the elastic bandage, and hot-air baths is often of service. Operative interference is indicated when the disease is of a severe type, when it is mon-articular,

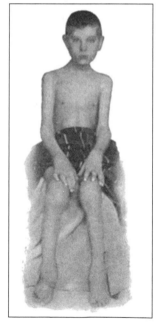

FIG. 161. Arthritis Deformans affecting several Joints, in a boy æt. 10. (Dr. Dickson's case.)

499

and when the general condition of the patient is otherwise favourable. Excision has been practised with success in the hip, knee, elbow, and temporo-mandibular joints. Limitation of movement and locking at the hip-joint when due to new bone round the edge of the acetabulum may be greatly relieved by removal of the bone—a procedure known as *cheilotomy*. Loose bodies and hypertrophied fringes if causing symptoms may also be removed by operation.

When stiffness and grating on movement are prominent features we have found the injection of from half to one ounce of sterilised white vaseline afford decided relief.

The patient should be nourished well, and there need be no restriction in the diet such as is required in gouty patients, so long as the digestion is not impaired. Benefit is also derived from the administration of cod-liver oil, and of tonics, such as strychnin, arsenic, and iron, and in some cases of iodide of potassium. Luff recommends the administration over long periods of guaiacol carbonate, in cachets beginning with doses of 5-10 grs. and increased to 15-20 grs. thrice daily. A course of treatment at one of the reputed spas—Aix, Bath, Buxton, Gastein, Harrogate, Strathpeffer, Wiesbaden, Wildbad—is often beneficial.

In some cases benefit has followed the prolonged internal administration of liquid paraffin.

On the assumption that the condition is the result of an auto-intoxication from the intestinal tract, saline purges and irrigation of the colon are indicated, and Arbuthnot Lane claims to have brought about improvement by short-circuiting or by resecting the colon.

Residence in a warm and dry climate, with an open-air life, has been known to arrest the disease when other measures have failed to give relief.

The application of radium and the ingestion of radio-active waters have also been recommended.

Hæmophilic or **Bleeder's Joint.**—This is a rare but characteristic affection met with chiefly in the knee-joint of boys who are the subjects of hæmophilia. After some trivial injury, or even without apparent cause, a hæmorrhage takes place into the joint. The joint is tensely swollen, cannot be completely extended, and is so painful that the patient is obliged to lie up. The temperature is often raised (101° to 102° F.), especially if there are also hæmorrhages elsewhere. The blood in the joint is slowly re-absorbed, and by the end of a fortnight or so, the symptoms completely disappear. As a rule these attacks are repeated; the pain attending them diminishes, but the joint becomes the seat of permanent changes: the synovial membrane is thickened, abnormally vascular, and coloured brown from the deposit of blood pigment; on its surface, and in parts of the articular cartilage, there is a deposit of rust-coloured fibrin; there may be extensive adhesions, and in some cases changes occur like those observed in arthritis deformans with erosion and ulceration of the cartilage and a form of dry caries of the articular surfaces, which may terminate in ankylosis.

As the swelling of the joint is associated with wasting of the muscles, with stiffness, and with flexion, the condition closely resembles tuberculous disease of the synovial membrane. From errors in diagnosis such joints have been operated upon, with disastrous results due to hæmorrhage.

The treatment of a recent hæmorrhage consists in securing absolute rest and applying elastic compression. The introduction of blood-serum (10-15 c.c.) into a vein may assist in arresting the hæmorrhage; anti-diphtheritic serum is that most readily obtainable.

After an interval, measures should be adopted to promote the absorption of blood and to prevent stiffness and flexion; these include massage, movements, and extension with weight and pulley.

JOINT DISEASES ASSOCIATED WITH LESIONS OF THE NERVOUS SYSTEM: NEURO-ARTHROPATHIES

In Lesions of Peripheral Nerves.—In the hand, and more rarely in the foot, when one or other of the main nerve-trunks has been divided or compressed, the joints may become swollen and painful and afterwards become stiff and deformed. Bony ankylosis has been observed.

In Affections of the Spinal Medulla.—In myelitis, progressive muscular atrophy, poliomyelitis, insular sclerosis, and in traumatic lesions, joint affections are occasionally met with.

The occurrence of joint lesions in *locomotor ataxia* (tabes dorsalis) was first described by Charcot in 1868—hence the term "Charcot's disease" applied to them. Although they usually develop in the ataxic stage, one or more years after the initial spinal symptoms, they may appear before there is any evidence of tabes. The onset is frequently determined by some injury. The joints of the lower extremity are most commonly affected, and the disease is bilateral in a considerable proportion of cases—both knees or both hips, for instance, being implicated.

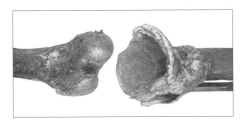

FIG. 162. Bones of Knee-joint in advanced stage of Charcot's Disease. The medial part of the head of the tibia has disappeared. (Anatomical Museum, University of Edinburgh).

Among the theories suggested in explanation of these arthropathies the most recent is that by Babinski and Barré, which traces the condition to vascular lesions of a syphilitic type in the articular arteries.

The first symptom is usually a swelling of the joint and its vicinity. There is no redness or heat and no pain on movement. The peri-articular swelling, unlike ordinary oedema, scarcely pits even on firm pressure.

In mild cases this condition of affairs may persist for months; in severe cases destructive changes ensue with remarkable rapidity. The joint becomes enormously swollen, loses its normal contour, and the ends of the bones become irregularly deformed (Fig. 162). Sometimes, and especially in the knee, the clinical features are those of an enormous hydrops with fibrinous and other loose bodies and hypertrophied fringes—and great oedema of the peri-articular tissues (Fig. 163). The joint is wobbly or flail-like from stretching and destruction of the controlling ligaments, and is devoid of sensation. In other cases, wearing down and total disappearance of the ends of the bones is the prominent feature, attended with flail-like movements and with coarse grating. Dislocation is observed chiefly at the hip, and is rather a gross displacement with unnatural mobility than a typical dislocation, and it is usually possible to move the bones freely upon one another and to reduce the displacement. A striking feature is the extensive formation of

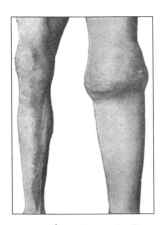

FIG. 163. Charcot's Disease of Left Knee. The joint is distended with fluid and the whole limb is oedematous.

new bone in the capsular ligament and surrounding muscles. The enormous swelling and its rapid development may suggest the growth of a malignant tumour. The most useful factor in diagnosis is the entire absence of pain, of tenderness, and of common sensibility. The freedom with which a tabetic patient will allow his disorganised joint to be handled requires to be seen to be appreciated.

The rapidity of the destructive changes in certain cases of tabes, and the entire absence of joint lesions in others, would favour the view that special parts of the spinal medulla must be implicated in the former group.

In *syringomyelia*, joint affections (gliomatous arthropathies) are more frequent than in tabes, and they usually involve the upper extremity in correspondence with the seat of the spinal lesion, which usually affects the lower cervical and upper thoracic segments. Except that the joint disease is seldom symmetrical, it closely resembles the arthropathy of tabes. The completeness of the analgesia of the articular structures and of the overlying soft parts is illustrated by the fact that in one case the patient himself was in the habit of letting out the fluid from his elbow with the aid of a pair of scissors, and that in another the joint was painlessly excised without an anæsthetic.

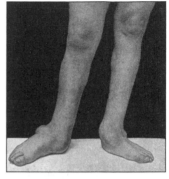

FIG. 164. Charcot's Disease of both Ankles: front view. Man, æt. 32.

The disease may become arrested or may go on to complete disorganisation; suppuration may ensue from infection through a breach of the surface, and in rare cases the joint has become the seat of tuberculosis.

Treatment, in addition to that of the nerve lesion underlying the arthropathy, consists in supporting and protecting the joint by means of bandages, splints, and other apparatus. In the lower extremity, the use of crutches is helpful in taking the strain off the affected limb. When there is much distension of the joint, considerable relief follows upon withdrawal of fluid. The best possible result being rigid ankylosis in a

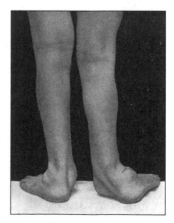

FIG. 165. Charcot's Disease of both Ankles: back view. Man, æt. 32.

good position, it may be advisable to bring this about artificially by arthrodesis or resection. Operation is indicated when only one joint is affected and when the cord lesion is such as will permit of the patient using the limb. The wounds heal well, but the victims of tabes are unfavourable subjects for operative interference, on account of their liability to intercurrent complications. When the limb is quite useless, amputation may be the best course.

In cerebral lesions attended with hemiplegia, joint affections, characterised by evanescent pain, redness, and swelling, are occasionally met with. The secondary changes in joints which are the seat of paralytic contracture are considered with the surgery of the Extremities.

In cases of *hysteria* and other *functional affections of the nervous system*, an intermittent neuropathic hydrops has been observed—especially in the knee. Without apparent cause, the joint fills with fluid and its movements become restricted, and after from two to eight days the swelling subsides and the joint returns to normal. A remarkable feature of the condition is that the effusion into the joint recurs at regular intervals, it may be over a period of years. Psychic conditions have been known to induce attacks, and sometimes to abort them or even to cause their disappearance. Hence it has been recommended that treatment by suggestion should be employed along with tonic doses of quinine and arsenic.

HYSTERICAL OR MIMETIC JOINT AFFECTIONS

Under this heading, Sir Benjamin Brodie, in 1822, described an affection of joints, characterised by the prominence of subjective symptoms and the absence of pathological changes. Although most frequently met with in young women with an impressionable nervous system, and especially among those in good social circumstances, it occurs occasionally in men. The onset may be referred to injury or exposure to cold, or may be associated with some disturbance of the emotions or of the generative organs; or the condition may be an involuntary imitation of the symptoms of organic joint disease presented by a relative or friend.

It is characteristic that the symptoms develop abruptly without satisfactory cause, that they are exaggerated and wanting in harmony with one another, and that they do not correspond with the features of any of the known forms of organic disease. In some cases the only complaint is of severe pain; more often this is associated with excessive tenderness and with impairment of the functions of the joint. On examination the joint presents a normal appearance, but the skin over it is remarkably sensitive. A light touch is more likely to excite pain than deep and firm pressure. Stiffness is a variable feature—in some cases amounting to absolute rigidity, so that no ordinary force will elicit movement. It is characteristic of this, as of other neuroses, that the symptoms come and go without sufficient cause. When the patient's attention is diverted, the pain and stiffness may disappear. There is no actual swelling of the joint, although there may be an appearance of this from wasting of the muscles above and below. If the joint is kept rigid for long periods, secondary contracture may occur—in the knee with flexion, in the hip with flexion and adduction.

The *diagnosis* is often a matter of considerable difficulty, and the condition is liable to be mistaken for such organic lesions as a tuberculous or pyogenic focus in the bone close to the joint.

The greatest difficulty is met with in the knee and hip, where the condition may closely simulate tuberculous disease. The use of the Röntgen rays, or examination of the joint under anæsthesia, is helpful.

The *local treatment* consists chiefly in improving the nutrition of the affected limb by means of massage, exercises, baths, and electricity. Splints are to be avoided. In refractory cases, benefit may follow the application of blisters or of Corrigan's button. The general condition of the patient must be treated on the same lines as in other neuroses. The Weir-Mitchell treatment may have to be employed in obstinate cases, the patient being secluded from her friends and placed in charge of a nurse. Complete recovery is the rule, but when the muscles are weak and wasted from prolonged disuse, a considerable time may elapse before the limb returns to normal.

TUMOURS AND CYSTS

New growths taking origin in the synovial membrane are rare, and are not usually diagnosed before operation. They are attended with exudation into the joint, and in the case of *sarcoma* the fluid is usually blood-stained. If the tumour projects in a polypoidal manner into the joint, it may cause symptoms of loose body. One or two cases have been recorded in which a *cartilaginous tumour* growing from the synovial membrane has erupted through the joint capsule and infiltrated the adjoining muscles. *Multiple cartilaginous tumours* forming loose bodies are described on p. 504.

Cysts of joints constitute an ill-defined group which includes ganglia formed in relation to the capsular ligament. Cystic distension of bursæ which communicate with the joint is most often met with in the region of the knee in cases of long-standing hydrops. It was suggested by Morrant Baker that cystic swellings may result from the hernial protrusion of the synovial membrane between the stretched fibres of the capsular ligament, and the name "Baker's cysts" has been applied to these.

In the majority of cases, cysts in relation to joints give rise to little inconvenience and may be left alone. If interfered with at all, they should be excised.

LOOSE BODIES

It is convenient to describe the varieties of loose bodies under two heads: those composed of fibrin, and those composed of organised connective tissue.

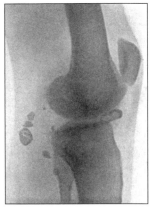

FIG. 166. Radiogram of Multiple Loose Bodies in Knee-joint and Semi-membranosus Bursa in a man æt. 38.
(Mr. J. W. Dowden's case.)

Fibrinous Loose Bodies (Corpora oryzoidea).— These are homogeneous or concentrically laminated masses of fibrin, sometimes resembling rice grains, melon seeds, or adhesive wafers, sometimes quite irregular in shape. Usually they are present in large numbers, but sometimes there is only one, and it may attain considerable dimensions. They are not peculiar to joints, for they are met with in tendon sheaths and bursæ, and their origin from synovial membrane may be accepted as proved. They occur in tuberculosis, arthritis deformans, and in Charcot's disease, and their presence is almost invariably associated with an effusion of fluid into the joint. While they may result from the coagulation of fibrin-forming elements in the exudate, their occurrence in tuberculous hydrops would appear to be the result of coagulation necrosis, or of fibrinous degeneration of the surface layer of the diseased synovial membrane. However formed, their shape is the result of mechanical influences, and especially of the movement of the joint.

Clinically, loose bodies composed of fibrin constitute an unimportant addition to the features of the disease with which they are associated. They never give rise to the classical symptoms associated with impaction of a loose body between the articular surfaces. Their presence may be recognised, especially in the knee, by the crepitating sensation imparted to the fingers of the hand grasping the joint while it is flexed and extended by the patient.

The *treatment* is directed towards the disease underlying the hydrops. If it is desired to empty the joint, this is best done by open incision.

Bodies composed of Organised Connective Tissue.—These are comparatively common in joints that are already the seat of some chronic disease, such as arthritis deformans, Charcot's arthropathy, or synovial tuberculosis. They take origin almost exclusively from an erratic overgrowth of the fringes of the synovial membrane, and may consist entirely of fat, the arborescent lipoma (Fig. 159) being the most pronounced example of this variety. Fibrous tissue or cartilage may form in one or more of the fatty fringes and give rise to hard nodular masses, which may attain a considerable size, and in course of time may undergo ossification.

Like other hypertrophies on a free surface, they tend to become pedunculated, and so acquire a limited range of movement. The pedicle may give way and the body become free. In this condition it may wander about the joint, or lie snugly in one of its recesses until disturbed by some sudden movement. A loose body free in a joint is capable of growth, deriving the necessary nutriment from the surrounding fluid. The size and number of the bodies vary widely. Single specimens have been known to attain the size of the patella. The smaller varieties may number considerably over a hundred.

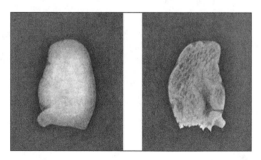

FIG. 167. Loose Body from Knee-joint of man æt. 25.
Natural size. a = Convex surface. b = Concave surface.

In arthritis deformans a rarer type of loose body is met with, a portion of the lipping of one of the articular margins being detached by injury. In

Charcot's disease, bodies composed of bone are formed in relation to the capsular and other ligaments, and may be made to grate upon one another.

The *clinical features* in this group are mainly those of the disease which has given rise to the loose bodies, and it is exceptional to meet with symptoms from impaction of the body between the articular surfaces. Treatment is to be directed towards the primary disease in the joint, as well as to the removal of the loose bodies.

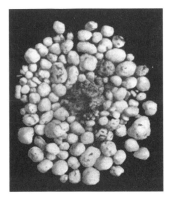

FIG. 168. Multiple partially ossified Chondromas of Synovial Membrane, from Shoulder-joint, the seat of arthritis deformans, from a man æt. 35.

Loose Bodies in Joints which are otherwise healthy.—It is in joints otherwise healthy that loose bodies causing the classical symptoms and calling for operative treatment are most frequently met with. They occur chiefly in the knee and elbow of healthy males under the age of thirty. The complaint may be of vague pains, of occasional cracking on moving the joint, or of impairment of function—usually an inability to extend or flex the joint completely. In many cases a clear account is given of the symptoms which arise when the body is impacted between the articular surfaces, namely, sudden onset of intense sickening pain, loss of power in the limb and locking of the joint, followed by effusion and other accompaniments of a severe sprain. On some particular movement, the body is disengaged, the locking disappears, and recovery takes place. Attacks of this kind may recur at irregular intervals, during a period of many years. On examining the joint, it is usually found to contain fluid, and there may be points of special tenderness corresponding to the ligaments that have been overstretched. In cases in which there has been recurrent attacks of locking, the ligaments become slack, the joint is wobbly, and the quadriceps is wasted. The patient himself, or the surgeon, may discover the loose body and feel it roll beneath his fingers, especially if it is lodged in the supra-patellar pouch in the knee, or on one or other side of the olecranon in the elbow. In most instances the patient has carefully observed his own symptoms, and is aware not only of the existence of the loose body, but of its erratic appearance at different parts of the joint. This feature serves to differentiate the lesions from a torn medial meniscus in which the pain and tenderness are always in the same spot. As the body usually contains bone, it is recognisable in a skiagram.

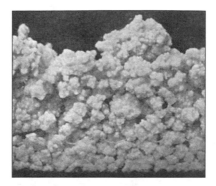

FIG. 169. Multiple Cartilaginous Loose Bodies from Knee-joint.

There are two methods of *removing the body*; the first and simpler method is applicable when the body can be palpated, usually in the supra-patellar pouch; it is preferably transfixed by a needle and can then be removed through a small incision; otherwise, the joint must be freely opened and explored, firstly to find the body and further to remove it.

The characters of this type of loose body are remarkably constant. It is usually solitary, about the size of a bean or almond, concavo-convex in shape, the convex aspect being smooth like an articular surface, the concave aspect uneven and nodulated and showing reparative changes, healing over of the raw surface, and the new formation of fibrous tissue, hyaline cartilage and bone, the necessary nutriment being derived from the synovial fluid (Fig. 167). The body is sometimes found to be lodged in a defect or excavation in one of the articular surfaces, usually the medial condyle of the femur, from which it is readily shelled out by means of an elevator. It presents on section a layer of articular cartilage on the convex aspect and a variable thickness of spongy bone beneath this.

The origin of these bodies is one of the most debated questions in surgical pathology; they obviously consist of a portion of the articular surface of one of the bones, but how this is detached still remains a mystery; some maintain that it is purely traumatic; König regards them as portions of the articular surface which have been detached by a morbid process which he calls "osteochondritis dessicans."

Multiple Chondromas and Osteomas of the Synovial Membrane.—In this rare type of loose body, the surface of the synovial membrane is studded with small sessile or pedunculated tumours composed of pure hyaline cartilage, or of bone, or of transition stages between cartilage and bone. They are pearly white in colour, pitted and nodular on the surface, rarely larger than a pea, although when compressed they may cake into masses of considerable size. With the movements of the joint many of the tumours become detached and lie in the serous exudate excited by their presence. They are found also in the diverticula of the synovial membrane, in the shoulder in the downward prolongation along the tendon of the biceps, in the hip in the bursal extension beneath the psoas.

The patient complains of increasing disability of the limb, movements of the joint becoming more and more restricted and painful. There is swelling corresponding to the distended capsule of the joint, and on palpation the bodies moving under the fingers yield a sensation as of grains of rice shifting in a bag. If the bodies are so numerous as to be tightly packed together, the impression is that of a plastic mass having the shape of the synovial sac. The stiffness and the cracking on movement may suggest arthritis deformans, but the X-ray appearances make the diagnosis an easy one. We have observed two cases of this affection in the knee-joint of adult women, one in the shoulder-joint of an adult male (Fig. 168), and Caird has observed one in the hip. The treatment consists in opening the joint by free incision and removing the bodies.

Displacement of the menisci of the knee is referred to with injuries of that joint.

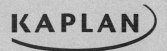
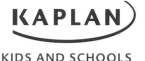
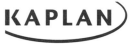
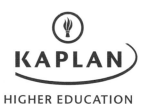
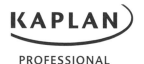